Handbook of Correctional Mental Health

Edited by

Charles L. Scott, M.D.

Joan B. Gerbasi, J.D., M.D.

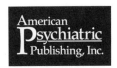
American **Psychiatric** Publishing, Inc.

Washington, DC
London, England

Copyright © 2005 American Psychiatric Publishing, Inc.
ALL RIGHTS RESERVED

Manufactured in the United States of America on acid-free paper
09   08   07   06   05   5   4   3   2   1
First Edition

Typeset in Baskerville and Caecilia.

American Psychiatric Publishing, Inc.
1000 Wilson Boulevard
Arlington, VA 22209-3901
www.appi.org

Library of Congress Cataloging-in-Publication Data
Handbook of correctional mental health / [edited by] Charles L. Scott, Joan B. Gerbasi.
     p. ; cm.
   Includes bibliographical references and index.
   ISBN 1-58562-156-0 (pbk. : alk. paper)
   1. Prisoners—Mental health services—United States—Handbooks, manuals, etc.
   [DNLM: 1. Mental Health Services. 2. Prisoners—psychology. 3. Prisons.
WA 305 H2352 2005] I. Scott, Charles L., 1960– II. Gerbasi, Joan B., 1961–
   RC451.4.P68H356 2005
   365'.66—dc22

                                                                              2005008197

British Library Cataloguing in Publication Data
A CIP record is available from the British Library.

CONTENTS

11 Management of Offenders With Mental Illnesses in Outpatient Settings 229

Erik Roskes, M.D.
The Honorable Charlotte Cooksey, Judge
Richard Feldman, LCSW-C
Sharon Lipford, LCSW-C
Jane Tambree, LCSW-C

12 Legal Issues Regarding the Provision of Mental Health Care in Correctional Settings 259

Fred Cohen, LL.B., LL.M.
Joan B. Gerbasi, J.D., M.D.

Contributors

Kenneth L. Appelbaum, M.D.
Director, Mental Health Program, UMass Correctional Health; Professor of Clinical Psychiatry, University of Massachusetts Medical School, Worcester, Massachusetts

Gary E. Beven, M.D.
Regional Medical Director, MHM Correctional Services, Columbus, Ohio

Kathryn A. Burns, M.D., M.P.H.
Assistant Clinical Professor of Psychiatry, Case Western Reserve University School of Medicine, Cleveland, Ohio

Shama B. Chaiken, Ph.D.
Chief Psychologist, California Department of Corrections, Health Care Services Division, Sacramento, California

Fred Cohen, LL.B., LL.M.
Private practice, Tucson, Arizona

The Honorable Charlotte Cooksey, Judge
District Court of Maryland for Baltimore City, Hargrove District Court, Baltimore, Maryland

Richard Feldman, LCSW-C
Senior U.S. Probation Office (Retired), Northern District of Maryland, Baltimore, Maryland

Joan B. Gerbasi, J.D., M.D.
Private practice, Davis, California

Kimberly A. Hardison, Psy.D.
Research Psychologist, Clinical Demonstration Research Unit, Napa State Hospital, Napa, California

Lindsay M. Hayes, M.S.
Project Director, National Center on Institutions and Alternatives, Mansfield, Massachusetts

Doonam Kim, M.D.
Attending Psychiatrist, Instructor of Psychiatry, Bellevue Hospital Center, New York University, New York, New York

Catherine F. Lewis, M.D.
Associate Professor of Psychiatry, Department of Psychiatry, University of Connecticut Health Center, Farmington, Connecticut

Sharon Lipford, LCSW-C
Executive Director, Harford County Mental Health Agency, Bel Air, Maryland

Avram H. Mack, M.D.
Assistant Professor of Psychiatry, Medical University of South Carolina, Charleston, South Carolina

Colin MacKenzie, M.D.
Assistant Professor of Psychiatry, University of Missouri-Kansas City, School of Medicine, Kansas City, Missouri

Kishor E. Malavade, M.D.
Attending Psychiatrist, Comprehensive Psychiatric Emergency Program, Bellevue Hospital Center, New York University, New York, New York

Barbara E. McDermott, Ph.D.
Associate Professor of Clinical Psychiatry, University of California, Davis School of Medicine, Department of Psychiatry, Division of Psychiatry and the Law, Sacramento, California; Research Director, Clinical Demonstration Unit, Napa State Hospital, Napa, California

Richard Rogers, Ph.D., ABPP
Professor of Psychology, University of North Texas, Denton, Texas

Erik Roskes, M.D.
Director, Forensic Treatment, Springfield Hospital Center, Sykesville, Maryland

Ankur U. Saraiya, M.D.
Attending Physician, Forensic Psychiatry Clinic, Bellevue Hospital Center, New York University, New York, New York

Charles L. Scott, M.D.
Chief, Division of Psychiatry and the Law; Associate Clinical Professor of Psychiatry; Director, Forensic Psychiatry Fellowship, University of California Davis Medical Center, Sacramento, California

Wendy E. Shoemaker, Psy.D.
Psychologist, California Department of Corrections, California State Prison, Sacramento, California

Jane Tambree, LCSW-C
Director, Forensic Alternative Services Team, Hargrove District Court, Baltimore, Maryland

Christopher R. Thompson, M.D.
Forensic Psychiatrist, Los Angeles, California

Michael J. Vitacco, Ph.D.
Associate Director of Research, Mendota Mental Health Institute, Madison, Wisconsin

Henry C. Weinstein, M.D.
Clinical Professor of Psychiatry, New York University School of Medicine, New York, New York

Preface

At year end 2003, more than 2.2 million individuals were incarcerated in the United States, and 1 in every 140 U.S. residents lived in a jail or prison (Harrison and Beck 2004). Correctional facilities are quickly becoming the new mental health treatment centers for individuals with mental disorders. The single largest psychiatric inpatient facility in the United States is the Los Angeles County Jail (Torrey 1999). As increasing numbers of individuals with mental disorders are living behind bars, many mental health professionals are discovering that their new workplace is located inside a jail or prison.

Despite the obvious need for mental health professionals trained to provide care to those who are incarcerated, very few general psychiatry, psychology, or social work training programs have specialized education in correctional mental health. The correctional system is a unique world with its own terminology, laws, rules, procedures, environment, and administrative management. To provide effective care to inmates, mental health care providers must understand this world.

This book was written as a practical clinical guidebook for mental health professionals who treat individuals who either are currently incarcerated or have been involved with the criminal justice system at some point in their lives. Each chapter was designed to assist the clinical practitioner in a correctional setting with understanding relevant treatment and legal issues when providing care to this population.

Chapters 1 and 2 of this book provide the reader with an introduction to the criminal justice system and to practicing psychiatry in a correctional culture. In the world of corrections, offenders are faced with numerous legal and situational challenges. Providers are faced with system challenges distinct to this treatment setting. These first two chapters provide a foundation for the reader to understand how treatment in a correctional setting differs from treatment in the outside world.

Chapter 3 provides information on the prevalence of mental illness in this population compared with individuals in the community. The authors outline types of mental health assessment and roles of various mental health providers. Special attention is given to the assessment and treatment of substance use disorders and violence risk assessments. Chapter 4 provides an important guide for assessing suicide risk and provides practical guidelines for developing suicide screening programs.

Chapters 5 and 6 focus on psychopharmacological and mental health interventions and treatment. Both chapters highlight considerations that must be taken into account when organizing a mental health treatment plan in a jail or prison. Chapter 7 assists the provider in understanding important aspects of the assessment of malingering. Pros and cons of various screening tests are highlighted to give the reader a practical guide when determining issues related to the deception of mental health symptoms.

Special populations, including female offenders and offenders with developmental disabilities, are reviewed in Chapters 8 and 9. Chapters 10 and 11 cover extremes of correctional settings, ranging from supermax prisons, where individuals may be locked down for 23 hours a day, to supervised placement in the community. The final chapter gives a practical translation of legal issues that govern why and how we must provide care to those incarcerated.

To create a meaningful, state-of-the-art text on this topic, authors recognized as national experts in their chapter topic were selected. A distinguished editorial review board was created to review and comment on each chapter prior to its submission for publication. Members of this editorial review board were Fred Cohen, LL.B., LL.M.; Joel Dvoskin, Ph.D.; Jeffrey Metzner, M.D.; and Phillip Resnick, M.D.

The chapters were carefully chosen to address common issues faced by mental heath professionals and to focus on relevant clinical and legal issues. Each chapter provides a combination of basic background information for professionals new to the world of corrections and more advanced material for seasoned correctional caregivers. Key issues are emphasized in tables throughout the chapter or in summary points at the end of the chapter. Hypothetical clinical case examples are provided that emphasize important aspects of the assessment and treatment of offenders with mental illness. An important strength of this text is the incorporation of varying viewpoints on potentially controversial treatment topics, such as the prescription of benzodiazepines to incarcerated inmates. Extensive legal and clinical references are provided that reflect current trends in correctional psychiatry.

This text is intended for a wide-ranging audience, to include psychiatrists, psychologists, social workers, nurses, correctional officers and administrators, attorneys, and judges interested in mental health issues facing inmates. The focus of this text is on synthesizing the vast literature on the treatment of offenders with mental illness into a useful practical handbook for providers. Individuals preparing for forensic psychiatry or psychology boards may also find this text helpful, as it summarizes the most important forensic clinical issues and relevant legal cases.

Charles L. Scott, M.D.

REFERENCES

Harrison PM, Beck AJ: Prisoners in 2003. Office of Justice Programs, Bureau of Justice Statistics, Washington, DC, U.S. Department of Justice, NCJ 203947, November 2004

Torrey EF: Reinventing mental health care. City Journal, Autumn 1999. Available at: http://www.city-journal.org/html/9_4_a5.html. Accessed January 24, 2005.

Acknowledgments

I wish to extend my sincere gratitude to Robert E. Hales, M.D., M.B.A, Editor-in-Chief of American Psychiatric Publishing, Inc. He possesses both the courage and the wisdom to understand the importance of a clinical textbook on correctional mental health in assisting providers who work in this environment. I am extremely grateful to each member of the Editorial Review Board, who provided valuable insight and feedback on every chapter. I wish also to thank all the wonderful chapter authors who met various deadlines and revisions with aplomb.

Finally, this project would not have been possible without the outstanding editorial assistance of David Spagnolo. Throughout his work on this project, Mr. Spagnolo demonstrated a wonderful attention to detail and amazing calm when faced with what seemed like an impossible roadblock. His professionalism and dedication are greatly appreciated.

Charles L. Scott, M.D.

CHAPTER 1

Overview of the Criminal Justice System

Charles L. Scott, M.D.

To work with offenders involved in the criminal justice system, mental health providers not only must assess them as individuals but also must understand the context in which they live. Joel Dvoskin (personal communication, January 2005) describes this unique context as follows:

> In many ways, the criminal justice system creates "communities." In some ways, these communities are similar to neighborhoods in the free world, but in other ways they are very, very different. For a person with posttraumatic stress disorder, the first day in jail can create terror that is almost beyond description. For first-time offenders, confusion about rights and expectations can dramatically increase anxiety, to pathological levels. For these reasons, it is important for mental health providers serving criminal justice clients to understand the criminal justice system itself.

The need for mental health professionals who understand the challenging world of individuals who have been arrested, charged, or sentenced for a criminal act cannot be understated. Consider that in 1955, 559,000 persons were institutionalized in state mental hospitals in the United States (out of a U.S. population of 165 million). During the next 45 years, these numbers dropped dramatically. For example, in December 2000, only 55,000 persons with mental illness were in a state hospital, though the U.S. general population had expanded to more than 275 million (Lamb et al. 2004).

In what setting do these individuals now find their treatment? The evidence increasingly suggests our nation's jails and prisons. During the period that state psychiatric inpatient beds were dramatically declining in our country, the number of jail and prison beds was on the rise. In 1985, the total number of inmates in custody was 744, 208 (Gilliard and Beck 1997). In mid-year 2003, more than 2 million persons, a significant number of whom have a mental disorder, were incarcerated in our nation's prisons and jails (Harrison and Karberg 2004). According to E. Fuller Torrey (1999), the Los Angeles County Jail houses 3,400 inmates with mental illness, making it the largest psychiatric inpatient facility in the United States.

The increased prevalence of individuals suffering from mental illness entering the criminal justice system has been referred to as the "criminalization" of the mentally ill. Reasons cited for the increasing numbers of individuals with mental illness in the criminal justice system include 1) the deinstitutionalization movement, beginning in the 1960s, that resulted in a massive discharge of psychiatric patients from state hospitals to the community; 2) more restrictive civil commitment criteria that make it more difficult to involuntarily hospitalize persons with mental illness *and* result in briefer hospital stays; 3) lack of adequate community support systems; and 4) an increased role of police officers in determining whether an arrested individual is transported to a jail or to a hospital (Lamb et al. 2004).

To provide effective mental health care in the correctional setting, the provider needs to understand this unique environment where many of their patients now live. I therefore begin this chapter by providing a definition of corrections and explaining theories of punishment. I then describe types of correctional settings, review stages of the criminal justice system, explain inmate classification schemes, and outline the process governing the return of inmates to society.

DEFINITION OF CORRECTIONS

What does the term *corrections* actually mean? Corrections includes those agencies and programs at the local, state, and federal level that interface with individuals who have been either accused of crimes (*detention*) or convicted of them (*correction*). The correctional process is integrally related to three other areas of the criminal justice system: police, prosecutors, and courts. Each of these three components plays a significant role in determining whether an individual enters the legal system at all or is subject to imposed controls from a correctional agency (Silverman 2001).

Correctional settings are wide ranging and include lockups, jails, and prisons. Other programs that may interface with the criminal justice system include mandated community alcohol and drug treatment programs and community mental health supervision and treatment. Correctional mental health involves the provision of mental health assessment and clinical treatment in a correctional setting. The term *penology* predates the concept of corrections and originates from the Latin word *poena,* which means penalty. Whereas penology represents the study of punishment, the term *corrections* encompasses a much broader area—one including both the management and the treatment of offenders—and implies an effort to "correct" the person and his or her misbehavior, presumably through some sort of rehabilitation.

The criminal justice system was created to address those actions committed by individuals that violate laws against society. These violations of laws are generally referred to as *crimes.* Each state and the federal government have a criminal code that defines specific crimes and associated sentences. In general, charges are likely to be filed in *federal* court when either 1) there is an alleged violation of federal (as opposed to state law) or 2) the alleged crime took place on federal property. The most common crimes referred to federal court include controlled substance violations, immigration law violations, mail or wire fraud, gun laws, postal offenses, child pornography, counterfeiting, and crimes that occur on federal property or in federal buildings (Federal Crime Cases 2005). Charges are filed in *state* court when an individual has violated a specific state statute and the alleged crime is not covered under federal jurisdiction.

How commonly are U.S. citizens victimized by crime? According to the 2003 National Crime Victimization Survey (NCVS), 15% of U.S. households have experienced at least one violent or property crime. This victimization rate represents a substantial drop compared with 1994, when 25% of American households reported being a victim of a violent or property crime (Klaus 2004). Proposed theories to explain this drop in victimization include changing demographics, with fewer Americans in the younger age group traditionally associated with most crime; a decline in drug trafficking; an increased police presence in the community; and longer periods of incarceration for offenders in a correctional environment.

THEORIES OF PUNISHMENT

Why punish an individual? The most common answer is because someone has done something wrong. Although this response may seem sufficient at face value, theories underlying the purposes of punishment are much more complex. In *Regina v. Dudley and Stephens* (1884), an English court grappled with the meaning and purpose of punishment in an interesting case before them. Two Englishmen, Thomas Dudley and Edwin Stephens, were indicted for the murder of a 17-year-old boy named Richard Parker. All three men were sailing on an English yacht when they encountered a severe storm on the high seas 1,600 miles from the Cape of Good Hope. As a result of the storm, they were lost and stranded. There was no supply of water and only two 1-pound tins of turnips on the boat. After 21 days of virtually no food or water, the men realized that they all would die without some type of sustenance. The 17-year-old boy was the weakest of the three and was lying at the bottom of the boat extremely malnourished by famine. Dudley and Stephens agreed that if they were not rescued by the following day, the boy would have to be killed so that they could potentially survive. On the day of the murder, the two men told the fragile boy that his time had come, put a knife to his throat, and then killed him. For 4 days the two men fed on the body and blood of the boy and on the fourth day they were rescued by a passing vessel. Both men were subsequently charged with the murder of Richard Parker, whom they had eaten. At their trial, testimony was presented that the boy would probably have died from severe famine during the 4 days prior to the rescue and therefore he would not have lived anyway. Further testimony was provided that had the two men not eaten the boy, they also would have likely died from starvation. Should these men be punished considering these circumstances? If so, what purpose would punishing them serve?

Four general principles of punishment help answer the difficult questions posed by this case: retribution, deterrence, rehabilitation, and incapacitation.

Retribution

The concept of retribution can be traced to the Latin word *retribo,* which means "I pay back." The theory of retribution involves the use of punishment in response to a law violating act simply because the offender deserves it. This philosophy can be summarized by the belief that an individual causing harm should be harmed. Historically, early legal systems almost exclusively used retribution as the guiding principle to punish. This approach was referred to as *lex talionis,* or "the law (*lex*) of retaliation." Under the law of *lex talionis,* equal and exact retribution was exacted as demonstrated in the words of the Hebrew scripture, "an eye for an eye, a tooth for a tooth, an arm for an arm, a life for a life" (Hooker 2004).

The concept known as "just deserts" is the modern equivalent of *lex talionis.* Although the individual is punished because his or her act deserves punishment, the "just deserts" approach allows consideration of punishment proportional to the severity of the crime, a factor not typically considered under strict retribution theory. It is important to note that the retribution principle is nearly entirely retrospective. Under the retribution theory, what purpose would punishing the two seamen discussed above serve?

Deterrence

Under the theory of deterrence, punishment is imposed to deter or prevent the commission of future criminal acts. The concept of deterrence involves both specific and general deterrence. The theory of specific deterrence holds that punished individuals are less likely to reoffend if there are imposed sanctions on their law-violating behavior. The theory of general deterrence proposes that by holding an individual accountable for his or her illegal actions, other members of the general public will also be less likely to offend because of their fear of legal consequences. In our example of the lost and hungry seamen, specific deterrence theorists would argue that punishment would help deter these men from eating other people in the future in the unlikely event that they were to run out of food. Under the general deterrence principle, citizens, on learning that punishment was imposed on these men, would theoretically be deterred from cannibalism, even if near starvation.

Does the theory of deterrence work in reality? An argument that specific deterrence is not achieved through punishment is supported by the high re-arrest rate of U.S. prisoners after they are released from incarceration. In a study of 300,000 prisoners released in 15 states in 1994, nearly 68% were re-arrested within 3 years (Langan and Levin 2002). At the same time, nearly a third of all offenders did not reoffend, suggesting that a significant minority seem to have been deterred from future criminal acts. Other studies indicate that in some situations, punished individuals are specifically deterred from future offenses. For example, arrested drunk drivers (Shapiro and Votey 1984), first-time offenders (Smith and Gartin 1989), and spouse abusers (Sherman and Berk 1984) who received severe punishment were less likely to violate the law on release when compared with those who received more lenient sentences. Three factors that are believed to affect the success or failure of criminal sanctions are the severity, certainty, and swiftness of punishment (Silverman 2001).

Rehabilitation

The rehabilitative theory of punishment involves a philosophy that individuals are incarcerated so that they have an opportunity to learn alternative behaviors to curb their deviant lifestyles. Corrections, therefore, is a system designed to correct those traits that result in criminal behavior. The rehabilitative model argues that the purpose of incarceration is to reform inmates through educational, training, and counseling programs. Under a rehabilitative model, would our English seamen require punishment? Considering the unusual circumstances of their having been lost at sea, would a training program be necessary to prevent them from eating others in the future? Likely not. Therefore, if rehabilitation was the sole theory of punishment applied in this case, incarceration would not be justified.

The rehabilitative approach to managing criminal offenders was prominent following World War II up until the 1960s (Silverman 2001). As recidivism of released prisoners continued, Americans became increasingly skeptical of the rehabilitative approach. A published review of rehabilitation programs for inmates by New York sociologist Robert Martinson and colleagues contributed to the belief that rehabilitation programs for offenders had minimal benefit. This research reviewed 231 studies of offender rehabilitation programs conducted between 1945 and 1967 (Lipton et al. 1975). In his famous 1974 article titled "What Works? Questions and Answers About Prison Reform," Martinson (1974) interpreted the results from the earlier research. In this article, he concluded, "with few and isolated exceptions, the rehabilitative efforts that have been reported so far have had no appreciable effect on recidivism." He emphasized that "our present strategies...cannot overcome, or even appreciably reduce, the powerful tendencies of offenders to continue in criminal behavior" (Martinson 1974, p. 49).

Martinson's article was widely read, and his published findings on rehabilitation were quickly renamed "Nothing works!" His persuasive arguments had far-reaching effects and played a significant role in the American penal system's moving away from the rehabilitative approach for offenders. Subsequent reviews of rehabilitation programs, using statistical analysis of treatment outcome not available to Martinson, did not replicate his findings. In their survey of 200 studies on rehabilitation conducted from 1981 through 1987, Gendreau and Ross (1987) concluded that successful rehabilitation of offenders was possible and that up to 80% reduction in recidivism had been noted in research studies examining effective programs. Despite these more encouraging results, the pendulum had already moved away from rehabilitation as a goal of punishment. As a result, a harsher theory of punishment, known as *incapacitation,* became increasingly popular throughout the United States.

Incapacitation

Under the incapacitation principle, individuals are prevented from committing future criminal acts against free citizens through detention in a secure environment. A sentence of life without the possibility of parole is an extreme form of incapacitation. The ultimate form of incapacitation is the imposition of the death penalty. Applying the incapacitation theory to the hungry yachtsman described earlier would result in their detention for the primary purpose of preventing them from ever repeating a criminal act. In reality, how likely are they to repeat this type of behavior? If their risk of eating another person in the future is actually very low, then lengthy incarceration under the incapacitation theory would not be justified.

With public concern increasing alongside the rising crime rate during the late 1980s and 1990s, many state legislatures passed laws that resulted in longer sentences (i.e., increased incapacitation). But not all incapacitation is the same. In general, there are three forms of incapacitation. Under a schema known as *collective incapacitation,* all offenders convicted of the same crime receive the exact same sentence. The anticipated effect of collective incapacitation is a substantial increase in the prison population, as there is no attempt to distinguish between high-risk versus low-risk offenders (Cohen 1983; Silverman 2001). In contrast, under *selective incapacitation,* only those offenders who are predicted to be at higher risk for reoffending are incarcerated. Legislative efforts to increase the length of incapacitation for higher-risk offenders have resulted in significant sentencing reform over the last three decades. These reforms include "truth in sentencing" (TIS) schemes and the passage of "three strikes and you're out" statutes. TIS laws require offenders to serve a substantial portion of their prison sentence, with restrictions on both parole eligibility and good-time credits (Ditton 1999a). Under "three strikes and you're out" statutes, felons found guilty of a third serious crime would be incarcerated for 25 years to life, even if the felonies themselves were relatively minor. In a third incapacitation approach, *criminal career incapacitation,* classes of criminals with known high rates of crime (rather than all criminals) receive longer sentences (Silverman 2001).

The increasing use of incapacitation as punishment is reflected in the growing prison population. Since 1995, the incarcerated population has grown an average of 3.7% annually (Harrison and Karberg 2004). At the end of 2003, 2,212,475 persons were incarcerated in U.S. jails and prisons. To put these numbers into perspective, 1 in every 140 U.S. residents was in prison or jail in 2003 at year's end (Harrison and Beck 2004).

TYPES OF CORRECTIONAL FACILITIES

The U.S. correctional system is complex and includes a federal system, 50 separate state systems, and thousands of local systems. Each individual state determines its own criminal justice and correctional system, with resulting differences in how crimes are defined, who is arrested, and what consequences are imposed for law violating behavior (Silverman 2001). Correctional housing facilities vary and are broadly classified into three types of facilities: lockups, jails, and prisons.

Lockups

Lockups are local temporary holding facilities that constitute the initial phase of the criminal justice system in a significant number of jurisdictions. The lockup is the most common type of correctional facility, with an average stay usually lasting less than 48 hours. Lockups are often located in the local police station, where only temporary detainment (such as for arrestees charged with drunk driving) is required. Approximately 30% of local police departments operate at least one lockup facility for adults separate from a jail. In jurisdictions with 500,000 or more residents, local lockups can detain up to 70 individuals, whereas lockups in jurisdictions with fewer than 10,000 residents typically house about 3 persons (Reaves and Goldberg 2000). Many jurisdictions do not have a local lockup. In this circumstance, individuals who arrested are usually detained in the local jail.

Jails

Jails are locally operated correctional facilities that confine persons before or after adjudication. Individuals who are convicted of a misdemeanor (i.e., minor crime) may receive a sentence of a year or less and complete their sentence in a jail, not a prison. Jails serve a variety of functions, including holding persons awaiting trial; punishing persons convicted of a misdemeanor; detaining violators of probation, parole, or bail; temporarily detaining juveniles pending transfer to juvenile authorities; holding mentally ill persons pending their movement to appropriate health facilities; serving as temporary destinations for transfer of inmates to federal, state, or other authorities; holding individuals for the military, for protective custody, for contempt, or for the courts as witnesses; and sometimes operating community-based programs as alternatives to incarceration.

In some circumstances individuals facing federal charges may be detained in a local jail. For example, the U.S. Citizenship and Immigration Services (USCIS) has the authority to detain certain categories of noncitizens. The U.S. Marshals Service assumes custody of persons arrested by all federal agencies. The Marshals Service houses more than 47,000 federal unsentenced detainees in federal, state, and local jails. In jurisdictions where detention space is limited, the Marshals Service uses Cooperative Agreement Program funds to improve local jail condition in exchange for guaranteed space for federal prisoners (U.S. Marshals Service 2005).

Of the total incarcerated population in the United States, approximately one-third are held in local jails (Harrison and Karberg 2004); in December 2003, 691,301 persons were held in local U.S. jails (Harrison and Beck 2004). Of individuals detained in jail, approximately 60% are awaiting some type of court action on their current charge, while the remainder are serving time for their conviction (Harrison and Karberg 2004). In the U.S. jail inmate population, nearly half (46%) were on probation or parole at the time of their arrest; half had been using drugs or alcohol at the time of their offense; half were held for a violent or drug offense; over half had grown up in a single-parent household; and nearly half (46%) had a family member who had been incarcerated (James 2004). Of jail inmates identified as mentally ill, over 30% were homeless in the year prior to the arrest, compared with 17.3% of jail inmates without an identified mental disorder (Ditton 1999b).

Among jail inmates, women are more likely than men to be drug offenders (29% of women vs. 24% of men). Furthermore, drug offenses by women more commonly involve drug possession, whereas drug offenses by men more commonly involve drug trafficking. Female jail inmates, compared with male jail inmates, more often report a past history of physical or sexual abuse. In 2002, among jail inmates, 55% of women reported a history of abuse, compared with 13% of men (James 2004).

Prisons

Prisons are confinement facilities that maintain custodial authority over individuals who have been convicted of felonies. A felony is considered a more serious crime than a misdemeanor. The imposed sentence for a felony is greater than 1 year at a minimum. Prisons are operated by both state and federal governments and are typically large facilities, often with more than 500 beds. Approximately two-thirds of the inmates serve their time in prison (Harrison and Beck 2004).

The Federal Bureau of Prisons (BOP) was established in 1930. The federal prison system includes a nationwide system of prisons and detention facilities for the incarceration of inmates awaiting trial or sentencing in federal court or who have been sentenced to a federal facility after conviction for a federal crime (Federal Bureau of Prisons 2004).

As of September 2004, there were 104 BOP facilities housing over 150,000 inmates throughout the country. In 2004, offenses committed by federal inmates were broken down as follows: drug offenses (54%); crimes involving weapons, explosives, or arson (12%); robbery (6.2%); homicide, aggravated assault, and kidnapping (3.3%); and sex offenses (1%). In 2004, drug offenders represented the majority of federal inmates, whereas they had represented only 16% of offenders in 1970 (Federal Bureau of Prisons 2005).

Thirty states and the federal system contract with private agencies to hold prisoners in privately operated facilities. There has been an increase in private contracting of correctional beds to alleviate overcrowding in the state and federal systems and to quickly obtain beds as the incarcerated population increases (McDonald et al. 1998). In 2003, more than 95,000 inmates were incarcerated in private facilities. Private facilities are concentrated primarily among Southern and Western states, with Texas and Oklahoma housing the largest numbers in 2003 (Harrison and Beck 2004).

Prison demographic data demonstrate inequalities based on ethnicity, age, and gender. For decades, minority males in their 20s and 30s have been overrepresented among prison inmates. In 2003, over 9% of black males aged 25–29 were in prison, compared with 2.6% of Hispanic males and 1.1% of white males in the same age group. Men continue to dominate the prison population and are nearly 15 times more likely than women to be incarcerated in a state or federal prison. However, the image of the typical prison inmate as one of a young male is slowly changing. In particular, the rate of female incarceration has been increasing faster than the rate for males. Since 1995, the total number of male prisoners has increased 29%, whereas the number of female prisoners has increased 48% (Harrison and Beck 2004).

Prison inmates are also getting older. In their recent review of prison inmates, Harrison and Beck (2004) found that inmates age 55 or older represent the age group with the largest increase in terms of percent change. Since 1995, this particular sector of the prison population has increased 85%. The increasing length of sentences under mandatory sentencing schemes has contributed to the aging of the correctional population. Because inmates have a constitutional right to medical care, states and counties will likely face substantial financial burdens as offenders age and require costly medical interventions.

Table 1–1 provides definitions of important aspects of the correctional system.

THE CRIMINAL JUSTICE PROCESS

Detainees face numerous court procedures and hearings throughout their incarceration that are stressful and can significantly impact their emotional state. An understanding of the sequence of events facing an individual journeying through the criminal justice system is important for clinicians working with this population.

Although the U.S. system of justice originates from English common law, there is no uniform criminal justice system in the United States. Often criminal actions are not discovered or reported to law enforcement agencies (Office of Justice Programs 2005). The majority of crimes are not solved. Under the Uniform Crime Report (UCR) Program, once a crime is reported to law enforcement, it is designated as "cleared" if at least one person is arrested, charged with the commission of an offense, and turned over to the court for prosecution. In 2003, law enforcement agencies cleared 46.5% of violent

---

TABLE 1–1. Important aspects of the correctional system

- **Lockup** A temporary holding facility with an average stay less than 48 hours
- **Jail** A locally operated correctional facility that confines persons before or after their adjudication
- **Prison** A confinement facility for housing individuals convicted of felonies
- **Misdemeanor** A crime for which the sentence is 1 year or less
- **Felony** A crime for which the sentence is greater than 1 year

---

crimes (murder, forcible rape, robbery, and aggravated assault), 16.4% of property crimes (burglary, larceny-theft, and motor vehicle theft), and 16.7% of arson offenses (Federal Bureau of Investigation 2004).

Despite some variation in the handling of criminal cases between various jurisdictions, the most common sequence of steps in response to known criminal behavior is as follows. An individual becomes a suspect in a crime following reports from victims or other witnesses, after discovery by a police officer, or from investigative work. For most crimes, especially minor crimes, police officers serve as gatekeepers in determining which persons will formally enter into the justice system. This discretionary arrest authority provides officers options other than taking the person into custody. For example, officers can warn offenders and release them or divert an offender to a mental health treatment program. In dealing with juveniles, the officer can bring the youth home to meet with the family (Finn and Sullivan 1988).

An arrest involves the taking of an individual into custody under the legal authority granted by the government. Law enforcement practices regarding who is arrested and why they are arrested vary according to the jurisdiction. In 2003, law enforcement made approximately 13.6 million arrests in the United States. Drug abuse violations represented the most common offense type for which individuals were arrested. Young adults are overrepresented among the arrestees. For example, over 46% of individuals arrested are under age 25, and nearly a third of arrestees are under age 21 (Federal Bureau of Investigation 2004).

Individuals who are arrested or charged with an offense are usually required to appear at the police station or local jail for booking. The booking process has many administrative steps following the arrest of a person. This process includes taking a mug shot, recording personal information, fingerprinting, assigning identifying case numbers, conducting medical and psychiatric screening, and beginning a new file for first-time arrestees. Nearly half of individuals who are arrested will leave the jail within 24–48 hours after they are booked. Inmates who are not released are thoroughly searched, their property is removed, and they are issued standard jail clothing (Silverman

2001). The booking process, particularly for first-time offenders, is often frightening for the arrestee. As discussed in Chapter 4 ("Suicide Prevention in Correctional Facilities"), the risk of suicide during the first 24–48 hours after a person is detained in a lockup or jail is exceptionally high because of the high stress level and overwhelming emotions.

Following the arrest and subsequent booking, law enforcement agencies provide information regarding the accused to the prosecutor. Prosecutors have broad discretionary authority. They play a significant role in determining whether to initiate prosecution and what specific charges will be filed with the court. If no charges are filed, the accused must be released. At this stage, there are several alternatives to a formal filing of charges. The prosecutor may request that the judge enter a *nolle prosequi*. *Nolle prosequi* is defined as a formal entry upon the record by the prosecuting officer in a criminal action, by which he or she declares that he or she "will no further prosecute" the case, either as to some of the defendants, or altogether. This is commonly referred to as "Nol Pros" (Office of Justice Programs 2005; Silverman 2001). Second, for individuals already involved in the criminal justice system, the prosecutor may decide to revoke probation or parole rather than initiate new charges. Third, the suspect may be civilly committed to a mental health treatment facility. Fourth, a decision to invoke civil sanctions, such as revocation of a person's driver's license, may substitute for processing the arrestee through the criminal justice system. Charges may also be reduced or dismissed in those situations in which the victim is unwilling to cooperate with prosecution or the suspect agrees to testify for the prosecution or act as an informer (Silverman 2001).

If a suspect is charged with a crime, he or she is taken before a judge or magistrate. At this initial appearance, the judge must inform the accused of the charges and decide whether there is probable cause to detain the individual. Probable cause exists when there is a reasonable belief that a crime has or is being committed and is the basis for all lawful searches, seizures, and arrests. For nonserious offenses, the judge or magistrate may determine guilt and assess a penalty at this stage. Defense counsel may also be assigned at this initial appearance. All suspects charged with serious crimes have a right to be represented by an attorney (Office of Justice Programs 2005; see Sixth Amendment to the U.S. Constitution). The court assigns an attorney for indigent suspects who cannot afford their own counsel (Office of Justice Programs 2005).

Following the assignment of a defense attorney, the accused has an initial appearance, where the court may decide to release the accused prior to trial. For individuals released prior to trial, the court may set bail (Office of Justice Programs 2005). *Bail* is money that a defendant must provide upfront (often through a contract with a bail bondsman) that must be forfeited if the accused fails to appear in court for trial. The amount of bail set is governed by multiple factors, including the seriousness of the charges, the risk of flight from the governing jurisdiction, the past legal history of the defendant, and the financial status of the defendant.

Depending on the locality, a preliminary hearing may follow the initial appearance of the defendant in court. The primary purpose of this hearing is for the court to determine if there is sufficient evidence of probable cause that the accused committed a crime. When the judge does not find probable cause, he or she must dismiss the case. If probable cause is found, or if the accused waives his or her right to a preliminary hearing, then the case may be forwarded to a grand jury (Office of Justice Programs 2005).

During the hearing before the grand jury, the prosecutor presents the evidence against the accused and the grand jury decides whether the evidence warrants the accused being brought to trial. If the grand jury determines there is sufficient evidence, they submit an indictment to the court. An *indictment* is a written summary of the facts of the offenses charged against the accused. In some jurisdictions, both misdemeanor and felony cases move forward after a document known as the *issuance of information* is provided. The issuance of information is a formal written accusation that the prosecutor submits to the court. The accused may choose to waive a grand jury indictment and accept the issuance of information (Office of Justice Programs 2005).

Following an indictment or filing of an issuance of information with the court, the accused is then scheduled for an arraignment. An *arraignment* is a hearing where the accused is informed of the charges, advised of his or her rights, and requested to enter a plea. In some situations, the defendant may chose to enter either a plea of guilty or a plea of *nolo contendere*. A plea of *nolo contendere* indicates that the defendant accepts his or her penalty without admitting guilt. If the judge accepts a guilty or a *nolo contendere* plea, a trial is not held and the case proceeds to the sentencing phase (Office of Justice Programs 2005).

When the defendant pleads not guilty or not guilty by reason of insanity, a trial date is scheduled. In serious crimes, the defendant is guaranteed a right to trial by jury, though he or she may choose to have a "bench trial," where the judge, rather than a jury, hears the case and determines guilt. At the trial, the defense and prosecution both present evidence and the judge decides on issues of law. At the conclusion of the trial, a finding of guilty or not guilty is made. Next, the defendant is scheduled for a sentencing hearing, where both mitigating and aggravating factors are presented.

Courts often review presentence investigations, completed by probation agencies, along with victim impact statements, in deciding the appropriate sentence for the convicted offender. Mental health professionals are frequently called on to present information regarding the defendant's psychiatric history as part of the sentencing process. Following the trial, the defendant may appeal his or her conviction or sentence. All states with a capital punishment provision provide an automatic appeal for defendants who receive the death penalty (Office of Justice Programs 2005).

The range of sentencing options include incarceration in a prison, jail, or other confinement facility, or release into the community on probationary status. Probation allows those convicted to remain in the community under specified restrictions, such as mandatory drug testing or required treatment programs. At year end 2003, 4,073,987 men and women were on probation. Of probationers serving time in the community, 25% had been convicted of a drug law violation, and 17% had been found guilty of driving while intoxicated (Glaze and Palla 2004).

The court may also require the convicted offender to pay a fine or make restitution through financial compensation to a victim. Certain jurisdictions provide other alternatives to incarceration that are more intense than regular probation requirements but that do not require actual incarceration. Such programs include boot camps, house arrest with electronic monitoring, intense supervision with mandated drug and/or psychiatric treatment, and community service. Jurisdictions vary significantly in how time periods of incarceration are determined. In general, offenders who receive a sentence of less than 1 year are sent to a jail. Convicted offenders who are sentenced to a period of more than 1 year serve their time in prison (Office of Justice Programs 2005).

INMATE CLASSIFICATION

At some point after an individual is placed into a correctional facility, a process known as *classification* occurs. Classification attempts to match inmates with the appropriate level of security, custody supervision, and services necessary to meet their needs. Appropriate classification is important for the following reasons: protecting inmates, protecting the public, maximizing efficient use of resources, controlling inmate behavior, and providing planning information for budgets, staffing, and program development (Silverman 2001).

For individuals who are serving time in jail, the classification procedure typically occurs in the jail in which they are housed. As a result of this process, the inmate may be placed in a particular housing unit within the jail based on either security, medical, or mental health needs. When the individual is sentenced to prison, the location of the classification process depends largely on the inmate's jurisdiction. In some areas, the inmate is sent to a central reception and diagnostic center after he or she is sentenced. After an evaluation of the level of security and special services required, the inmate is transferred to the most appropriate matched facility. In other jurisdictions, the inmate undergoes the classification process in a prison reception unit where he or she is kept until this process is completed. The inmate is then placed in general population or transferred to another facility if needed.

Classification involves determination of both the security and the custody level appropriate for the inmate. Facility security level has been defined as "the nature and number of physical design barriers available to prevent escape and control inmate behavior" (Henderson et al. 1997). Jurisdictions vary regarding how they define security levels for their correctional institutions. The BOP guidelines provide one example of how a security level system is determined. The BOP security classification scheme includes four recommended security levels.

1. *Level I prisons* comprise minimum-security facilities or federal prison camps. These facilities are characterized by dormitory housing without a surrounding fence and a relatively low staff-to-inmate ratio.
2. *Level II facilities* are termed low-security institutions and are typically surrounded by double-fenced perimeters. These facilities have strong work and program components with a higher staff-to-inmate ratio when compared with minimum security facilities.
3. *Level III facilities,* or medium-security institutions, have more secure perimeters, with electronic detection systems, cell-type housing, and greater staff-to-inmate ratios compared with level I and II facilities.
4. *Level IV facilities* are considered high-security institutions. Their perimeters are often significantly reinforced and may consist of walls with towers at each corner manned by armed correctional officers. Housing in a level IV facility is primarily single- or multiple-occupant cell housing, and close staff supervision and movement control are characteristic (Silverman 1991).

Whereas the security level refers to the number of environmental barriers to prevent escape or manage behavior, an inmate's custody level is determined by the degree of staff supervision necessary to provide adequate control of the inmate (National Institute of Corrections 1987). Under the BOP classification scheme, inmates noted as "out custody" have a relatively greater degree of movement of freedom compared to higher level custody inmates. For example, such inmates may be assigned to less-secure housing as they are eligible for work detail outside the secure perimeter of the institution, with decreased levels of staff supervision. Inmates classified as "in custody" are typically assigned to regular quarters, may have work assignments under normal levels of supervision, and are not allowed to participate in work programs outside the confines of the institution. A "maximum custody" classification label is the highest custody level assigned and requires intense control and supervision. This classification is generally given to those inmates who have demonstrated violence or disruptive behavior or who pose a serious escape risk (Silverman 2001).

Prison environments vary regarding the type of inmate received and the level of security and staffing. Traditionally, inmates who have received the death penalty have been segregated into separate housing areas known as "death row." Because persons who receive the death penalty have been viewed as dangerous and/or an increased escape risk, separate secure housing pods with increased supervision and correctional officer staffing are deemed necessary. At the end of 2002, more than 3,500 prisoners were under the sentence of death in the United States (Bonczar and Snell 2003). The average length of time for individuals executed in 2002 on death row prior to their execution was 10 years, 7 months (Bonczar and Snell 2003).

With the increasing financial burdens associated with longer periods on death row, some states have developed opportunities for inmates who have received the death penalty to be mainstreamed into the general population and/or to participate in work programs while on death row. Benefits for correctional administration cited by these policies have included costs savings, reduction in legal expenses regarding defense of standard of care lawsuits, and greater flexibility with the use of bed space. Advantages for inmates resulting from these emerging policies include increased access to legal resources, recreation time, commissary, visitation, medical care, and work programs (Lombardi et al. 1997; Silverman 2001).

No longer do inmates have to be convicted of a capital crime to be housed on a special security unit. During the last few decades, several jurisdictions have built or modified existing prison facilities that create highly isolated environments for inmates who are considered too dangerous to be maintained in a general prison population. These facilities are known by various names, such as "extended control facilities," "supermax" facilities, "maxi-max" facilities, or "security housing units." Often labeled a prison within a prison, these tightly managed facilities provide control of inmates who have exhibited violent or seriously disruptive behavior while incarcerated and who, as a result, cannot be maintained in a less restrictive environment. In 1963, the U.S. Penitentiary at Marion, located in southern Illinois, was opened to replace Alcatraz and was the highest maximum-security prison in the United States. Inmates in these types of facilities are often kept in their cell for up to 23 hours a day, with minimal, if any, interaction with other inmates. Chapter 10 ("Offenders With Mental Illness in Maximum and Supermaximum Security Settings") describes in greater detail this type of prison environment and relevant mental health issues.

RELEASE FROM PRISON

The exact amount of time an offender serves in prison depends on the type of sentencing scheme outlined in the reviewing jurisdiction. Each state's penal code provides sentencing guidelines, which are minimum and maximum time frames to be imposed for each offense. An *indeterminate* sentencing scheme provides a minimum time period the inmate must serve and a maximum time period after which the inmate must be released (Silverman 2001). Under an indeterminate sentencing scheme, a parole board (or other reviewing agency) considers whether it is appropriate for the individual to be released and placed into the community.

As a result of increasing public skepticism regarding the rehabilitative potential of inmates and appropriateness for early release, indeterminate schemes have lost their popularity over the last several decades. In its place, more jurisdictions are adopting determinate sentencing schemes. A *determinate* sentencing scheme outlines a specified number of years that the individual must serve based on the committing offense. Under a determinate sentencing scheme, the time sentenced cannot be increased or decreased. Although determinate sentences are fixed, an inmate may be granted an earlier release date through the accumulation of "good time." Depending on each jurisdiction's statutory provision, good time credits can be earned through either automatic or earned credits. Credits can be earned through participation in work or treatment programs (Silverman 2001).

Under both determinate and indeterminate sentencing schemes, a prisoner may be released prior to completing his or her sentence through the process known as parole. Parole represents the conditional release of the offender into the community. Under an indeterminate sentencing scheme, a parole board (or similarly designated authority) decides whether the inmate should be granted an early release. If the inmate is released, a separate process, known as *parole supervision,* begins and provides support, monitoring and supervision, and services to the newly released offender. Two important components often considered when deciding the appropriateness of parole are the severity of the offense and the inmate's risk of reoffending.

Inmates who have been sentenced under a determinate sentencing scheme are required to serve out their full sentence less any credits for participation in programs (known as "good time" credits). Convicted offenders who are released into the community under parole remain under the supervision of the parole officer. They must adhere to the specified conditions of parole for the remainder of their unexpired sentence; failure to adhere to the conditions of the parole can result in their being returned to prison to complete their sentence.

In 2003, the nation's parole population increased 3.1%, nearly double the average annual growth of 1.7% since 1995. Five states (North Dakota, Alabama, New Hampshire, Kentucky, New Mexico) have experienced more than a 20% increase in their parole population. As with the increasing rates of incarceration among women, the female parole population is also increasing. In 2003, female parolees represented 13% of all parolees, compared with 10% in 1995. Unfortunately, less than half of all parolees successfully meet the conditions of their supervision. Equally concerning is the fact that 9% of probations become lost to follow-up and escape supervision (Glaze and Palla 2004).

CONCLUSION

Correctional environments are multifaceted organizations. Societies have used various theories of punishment to justify the incarceration of offenders, some with the hopeful goal of decreasing future crime. Mental health practitioners play a variety of vitally important roles in the assessment, treatment, and management of offenders at virtually every point along their journey through this unique, complex, and sometimes frightening world. There are many reasons to provide mental health treatment in a correctional environment, including to ease the inmate's suffering, lessen the offender's disability so that he or she can participate in jail and prison programs, increase safety within the institution, and provide care for serious medical needs as constitutionally required. Understanding this special environment improves providers' ability to assist the inmate as they travel through the criminal justice system.

SUMMARY POINTS

- Reasons for punishment involve four key theories: retribution, deterrence, rehabilitation, and incapacitation.
- The criminal justice system is complex and includes multiple entry and exit points.
- Inmate classification assigns inmates to facilities that attempt to match the level of security, the custody supervision required, and the services necessary to meet inmate's needs.

REFERENCES

Bonczar TP, Snell TL: Capital punishment 2002 (NCJ 301848). Washington, DC, Office of Justice Programs, Bureau of Justice Statistics, U.S. Department of Justice, November 2003

Cohen J: Incapacitating criminals: recent research findings. National Institute of Justice Research in Brief. Washington, DC, National Institute of Justice, U.S. Department of Justice, December 1983

Federal Bureau of Investigation: Crime in the United States, 2003. Washington, DC, Federal Bureau of Investigation, U.S. Department of Justice, October 2004

Ditton PM: Truth in Sentencing in State Prisons (NCJ 170032). Washington, DC, Office of Justice Programs, Bureau of Justice Statistics, U.S. Department of Justice, January 1999a

Ditton PM: Mental health and treatment of inmates and probationers (NCJ 174463). Office of Justice Programs, Bureau of Justice Statistics, U.S. Department of Justice, July 1999b

Federal Bureau of Prisons: The Bureau in brief. Available at: http://www.bop.gov/ipapg/ipabib.html. Accessed November 13, 2004.

Federal Bureau of Prisons: Quick facts. Available at: http://www.bop.gov//about/facts.jsp#2. Accessed April 20, 2005.

Federal Crime Cases. Available at: http://www.gottrouble.com/legal/criminal/federal/federalcases.html. Accessed January 22, 2005.

Finn PE, Sullivan M: Police respond to special populations: handling the mentally ill, public inebriate, and the homeless. National Institute of Justice Reports 209:2–8, 1988

Gendreau P, Ross RR: Revivification of rehabilitation: evidence from the 1980s. Justice Quarterly 4:349–407, 1987

Gilliard DK, Beck AJ: Prison and jail inmates at midyear, 1996 (BJS Bulletin, NCJ 162843). Washington, DC, Office of Justice Programs, Bureau of Justice Statistics, U.S. Department of Justice, January 1997

Glaze L, Palla S: Probation and parole in the United States, 2003 (NCJ 205336). Washington, DC, Office of Justice Programs, Bureau of Justice Statistics, U.S. Department of Justice, July 2004

Harrison PM, Beck AJ: Prisoners in 2003 (NCJ 203947). Washington, DC, Office of Justice Programs, Bureau of Justice Statistics, U.S. Department of Justice, November 2004

Harrison PM, Karberg JC: Prison and jail inmates at midyear 2003 (BJS Bulletin, NCJ 203947). Washington, DC, Office of Justice Programs, Bureau of Justice Statistics, U.S. Department of Justice, May 2004

Henderson JD, Rauch WD, Phillips RL: Guidelines for the Development of a Security Program, 2nd Edition. Lanham, MD, American Correctional Association, 1997

Hooker R: Lex talionis, in World Cultures: General Glossary. Available at: http://www.wsu.edu:8080/~dee/GLOSSARY/LEXTAL.HTM. Accessed November 11, 2004.

James DJ: Profile of jail inmates, 2002 (NCJ 201932). Washington, DC, Office of Justice Programs, Bureau of Justice Statistics, U.S. Department of Justice, July 2004

Klaus PA: Crime and the nation's households, 2002 (BJS Bulletin, NCJ 206348). Washington, DC, Office of Justice Programs, Bureau of Justice Statistics, U.S. Department of Justice, October 2004

Lamb HR, Weinberger LE, Gross BH: Mentally ill persons in the criminal justice system: some perspectives. Psychiatr Q 75:107–126, 2004

Langan PA, Levin DJ: Recidivism of prisoners released in 1994 (NCJ 193427). Washington, DC, Office of Justice Programs, Bureau of Justice Statistics, U.S. Department of Justice, June 2002

Lipton DS, Martinson R, Wilks J: The Effectiveness of Correctional Treatment: A Survey of Treatment Validation Studies. New York, Praeger, 1975

Lombardi G, Sluder RD, Wallace D: Mainstreaming death-sentenced inmates: the Missouri experience and its legal significance. Federal Probationer 61:3–10, 1997

Martinson R: What works? Questions and answers about prison reform. The Public Interest 35:22–54, 1974

McDonald D, Fourneir E, Russell-Einhourn M, et al: Private prisons in the United States, Executive Summary. July 16, 1998. Available at: http://www.abtassoc. com/reports/ES-priv-report.pdf. Accessed January 25, 2005.

National Institute of Corrections: Guidelines for the Development of a Security Program. Washington, DC, National Institute of Corrections, U.S. Department of Justice, July 1987

Reaves BA, Goldberg AL: Local police departments 1997 (NCJ 173429). Washington, DC, Office of Justice Programs, Bureau of Justice Statistics, U.S. Department of Justice, February 2000

Regina v Dudley and Stephens, Queen's Bench Division, 14 Q.B.D. 273 (1884)

Shapiro P, Votey H: Deterrence and subjective probabilities of arrest: modeling individual decisions to drink and drive in Sweden. Law and Society Review 18:111–149, 1984

Sherman L, Berk R: The specific deterrent effects of arrest for domestic assault. American Sociological Review 49:261–272, 1984

Silverman IJ: The correctional process, in Corrections: A Comprehensive View, 2nd Edition. Edited by Silverman IJ. Belmont, CA, Wadsworth/Thomson Learning, 2001

Smith D, Gartin P: Specifying specific deterrence: the influence of arrest in future criminal activity. American Sociological Review 54:94–105, 1989

Office of Justice Programs: The justice system. Washington, DC, Office of Justice Programs, Bureau of Justice Statistics, U.S. Department of Justice. Available at: http://www.ojp.usdoj.gov/bjs/justsys.htm. Accessed January 25, 2005.

Torrey EF: Reinventing mental health care. City Journal, Autumn 1999. Available at: http://www.city-journal.org/html/9_4_a5.html. Accessed January 24, 2005.

U.S. Marshals Service: U.S. Marshals duties: major responsibilities of the U.S. Marshals Service. Available at http://www.usmarshals.gov/duties/index.html. Accessed January 25, 2005.

CHAPTER 2

Practicing Psychiatry in a Correctional Culture

Kenneth L. Appelbaum, M.D.

As described in the previous chapter, correctional facilities include lock-ups and jails for pretrial defendants, houses of correction for inmates convicted of misdemeanors, and prisons for sentenced felons. Institutions are typically segregated by gender, and the custodial levels range from prerelease centers to minimum, medium, or maximum security. The purpose of each of these types of facilities can have a significant effect on the overall environment. The pace and relatively rapid turnover of population in a jail, for example, contrasts with the stability of a prison. The atmosphere in a female facility often differs from that of a male facility. And as a general rule, higher-security facilities feel more stark, bleak, and oppressive.

Despite these differences, however, correctional institutions have many cultural similarities. Each contains a "society of captives" (Sykes 1958), subject to varying degrees of surveillance and control depending on the setting. As with any society, jails and prisons have unique rules, routines, and hardships. The inhabitants, both correctional staff and inmates, have well-defined roles and their own jargon.

Entering the correctional subculture for the first time can be daunting for the new psychiatrist. The loud, crowded, and austere environment typical of many institutions may lead to unease and apprehension. In the absence of clearly defined expectations, the newcomer can feel at a loss for how to behave. With the proper preparation and attitude, however, psychiatrists can find correctional work surprisingly stimulating and rewarding.

I begin this chapter by examining the correctional environment, including its mission, rules, routines, and deprivations. I then review the psychiatrist's role in the correctional culture from the perspectives of security staff, inmates, and the psychiatrists themselves. The emphasis throughout is on the special challenges and rewards encountered by the correctional psychiatrist. My focus in this chapter is on higher-security prisons, which tend to have the most pronounced cultural differences from noncorrectional settings.

ENVIRONMENT AND CULTURE

Containment and security are central to the mission of all correctional facilities, and the environment reflects this priority. Prisons are fortresses that carefully control who gets in and, more importantly, who gets out. Without proper clearance and identification, outsiders will not make it past the "front trap." Like the entryway of a castle, the front trap is the passage through the razor-wire-topped outer perimeter walls. A correctional officer in a separate control station regulates entrance to and exit from the trap through the security doors on either end of the passageway. At least one door is always closed, literally trapping, at least temporarily, all traffic as it transits through the trap. Another officer assigned to the trap may search visitors and staff when entering or leaving the facility. Additional inner traps control movement within the facility. Officers control all movement. The psychiatrist usually does not have a key.

Although the distance between two points in a prison may be short, transit time can vary considerably. Many factors affect the ease of movement. For example, delays can occur when visitors in the trap require more extensive searching and processing. Sometimes the control officer or the trap officer is temporarily distracted by other tasks. At other times, a freeze on all movement within the institution occurs because of a medical emergency, a fight, or another disturbance. These delays cannot be avoided, but even during normal operations, the speed of movement may be directly proportional to the quality of the relationship the psychiatrist has with the officers in charge. Good rapport with officers can go a long way toward improving a psychiatrist's efficiency, and as described later in this chapter, rapport can be critical in the efficacy of psychiatric assessments and interventions.

Regardless of the ease or speed of movement in a prison, one transits through a generally stark and drab environment. Whether old and dilapidated or modern and pristine, most prisons have an oppressive austerity. The architecture and the limited furnishings are utilitarian and institutional. Although inmates may attempt, within limits, to decorate their individual cells, the hallways and common areas typically remain unadorned and bleak. With little to soften them, sounds usually echo into a background din and cacophony. Musty odors of a densely populated community and the chemical scent from large-scale use of cleansers are often the prevailing smells. The overall impression of a harsh and impersonal setting strikes at both a conscious and a visceral level.

Some prisons, however, provide a more enriched experience. They take a broader view of their mission than mere incapacitation. All effective prisons seek to incapacitate inmates through containment, which prevents criminal activity in society at large, and through security, which prevents criminal activity in the prison itself. In a broader sense, however, prisons serve functions other than incapacitation. Several justifications for incarceration have waxed and waned in popularity (Packer 1968). These justifications include rehabilitation, which works from the assumption that incarceration can be a reforming experience. The reference to penal institutions as correctional facilities reflects the goal of rehabilitation. Thus, more enlightened institutions offer educational and vocational programming. Such programming helps to keep inmates constructively occupied; this can minimize the time and energy spent making mischief, and it also helps prepare inmates for reintegration to society.

The routines and rules of a prison mirror the institutional feel of the physical environment. Daily activities, such as meals, medication lines, and inmate counts, typically occur on an unchanging schedule. Controlled movement periods may limit the times when an inmate can go from one location to another. The predictable regularity of prison life adds to the dullness of incarceration.

Prison rules complement the security functions of the physical plant. Rules and guidelines typically address contraband, staff behavior, and interactions with inmates. Weapons, drugs, and handcuff keys cannot be brought into facilities, but prohibitions may also exist against bringing other less obvious items into facilities. Cell phones, computers with modems, and other devices that might allow inmates to communicate with people outside the institution can pose security risks. Items that can easily be fashioned into weapons, such as binder clips, and large sums of money may also qualify as contraband. Bringing personal mail, magazines, or other written materials that contain home addresses or phone numbers can compromise safety. Taking photographs of the prison or its inmates will likely require the knowledge and approval of the superintendent or warden.

Other behavioral guidelines may admonish staff to stay alert and to avoid potentially dangerous situations. Such situations can include entering areas without looking for possible setups, allowing an inmate to become positioned behind the back of a staff person, or allowing an inmate to become positioned between the staff person and the exit to the area.

Significant prohibitions generally apply to relationships with inmates, former inmates, and people outside the institution. Boundary violations can include touching or being touched by an inmate, except as part of a security or medical activity; bringing items into the facility for an inmate or transporting items, such as mail, out of the facility for an inmate; discussing a staff member's personal life with an inmate; providing an inmate with special favors or receiving such favors from an inmate; or becoming overly familiar in other ways with inmates. Prohibitions also apply to contact with former inmates, and when such contact occurs, it should be reported to supervisors. Sharing information or messages with people outside the institution or with an inmate's family or friends also can breach rules and security. For example, dangerous situations can arise if an inmate or his or her associates learn details of a pending outside medical appointment or other external trips.

The correctional culture also includes its own jargon, which the psychiatrist must learn. Some terms are simply abbreviations; others are uncommon in other settings or unique to corrections. For example, *seg* refers to a segregation unit that keeps some inmates isolated from the general population of the facility and usually locked down for 23 hours a day in single cells for disciplinary or administrative reasons. Officers *lug*, not take, inmates to segregation. *Pop* refers to a general population housing unit, as opposed to seg units or other special housing units (SHUs) or special management units (SMUs). Prisoners with mental illness are commonly referred to in a derogatory fashion as *bugs*. *Skinners*, or sex offenders, have low status within the inmate subculture and may end up in *PC*, or protective custody, units, to keep them safe from assault.

Failure to use proper terminology can cause offense and strain relationships. Correctional officers, for example, generally bristle if referred to as *guards*, a term perceived as not appreciating the challenges and professionalism of their work. Sergeants, lieutenants, and captains, who are recognizable respectively by two chevrons, a silver bar, or two gold bars on the sleeve or collar, might take umbrage if addressed in a way that does not acknowledge their superior rank. Mastery of the language specific to the institution helps convey familiarity with and sensitivity to the culture and can lessen the perception of the psychiatrist as an interloper.

New health care staff, including psychiatrists, generally receive an orientation that informs them about many of the aspects of the correctional environment and culture described above. All new employees must receive orientation for each of the prison accreditation standards of the National Commission on Correctional Health Care (2003; see Standard P-C-09) and the American Correctional Association (2003; see Standards 4–4082 and 4–4088).

Topics covered during orientation typically include security policies and procedures, contraband regulations, emergency situations, and inmate-staff relationships.

HOW OTHERS VIEW THE PSYCHIATRIST'S ROLE IN THE CORRECTIONAL CULTURE

Security Staff

As noted in the preceding section, the core mission of correctional staff involves containment and security. Correctional officers have the authority to enforce rules, regimentation, and sanctions. Unlike health care providers, who typically seek negotiated compliance from their patients, correctional officers have an authoritarian basis for their relationship with inmates. These disparate ideologies sometimes lead to conflict between officers and clinicians (Cormier 1973; Culbertson 1977; Cumming and Solway 1973; Kaufman 1973; Powelson and Bendix 1951; Roth 1986). Officers may view mental health professionals in particular as naïve or even indulgent with inmates, and mental health professionals may view officers as overly harsh and punitive.

The two professional groups, however, have many common interests despite their often disparate training, beliefs, methods, and purposes (Steadman et al. 1989). Neither can function effectively without the other. Correctional officers, for example, have extremely stressful jobs (Finn 2000). They identify the threat of violence by inmates as their most frequent source of stress (Finn 2000). Only police officers experience a higher rate of nonfatal workplace violence (Warchol 1998). Dysfunctional behavior and poor adaptation by inmates with mental disorders, described below, add to officer stress. Competent mental health treatment results in fewer behavioral disturbances and more tranquil facilities. Mental health professionals, for their part, cannot readily provide their services in an unsafe environment.

Effective security staff, of whom there are many, perform their tasks with professionalism. They are firm but fair. They support humane health care services, and they appreciate the contribution that psychiatrists and other mental health professionals make to operational efficiency (Steadman et al. 1989).

Achieving harmonious and collaborative relationships, however, takes time and effort. A new prison psychiatrist will likely face scrutiny by correctional officers, as well as by inmates (Robey 1998). Staff and inmate observers will closely note the psychiatrist's appearance, behavior, opinions, reactions, and interpersonal style. Showing professional respect for the challenges faced by security staff and for their knowledge and expertise can play a critical role in the ultimate acceptance of the psychiatrist. The newcomer's attitude toward security constraints, his or her temperament, and his or her approach to advocacy, privilege requests, medication use, consultation-liaison situations, forensic questions, and confidentiality, as described later in this chapter, will all affect the quality of relations with security staff.

Inmates

The deprivations of the prison environment can take a toll on inmates. In addition to tedium and boredom, inmates must cope with separation from family and social supports, limited privacy and autonomy, and fear of assault. Rape, which can have especially devastating physical and psychological consequences, is an understudied but endemic problem in correctional settings (Dumond 2003). Overcrowding, a common occurrence in many prisons (Harrison and Beck 2003), adds to the stress. Even in the absence of other traumatic events, the inherently dehumanizing experience of incarceration itself can have intensely negative psychological effects (Haney and Zimbaro 1998).

Inmates who have mental disorders are especially vulnerable to the hardships of incarceration (Human Rights Watch 2003). They risk rape (Dumond 2003) and victimization by higher-functioning inmates. The challenges of prison life can overwhelm their already limited coping skills and lead to exacerbation of symptoms, functional deterioration, and poor adaptation (Morgan et al. 1993; Sowers et al. 1999; Toch and Adams 1987). Some inmates with mental disorders have difficulty understanding and following rules and expectations. Those with schizophrenia (Morgan et al. 1993), mental retardation (Santamour and West 1982), or mental illness in general (Ditton 1999) commit more rule infractions, spend more time in lockup, and are less likely to obtain parole.

Despite the predominantly negative effects of incarceration, some inmates obtain tangible benefits (Human Rights Watch 2003). Although conditions can vary dramatically across states, many correctional systems offer services that may exceed those received by inmates prior to incarceration. Prisons sometimes provide better access to treatment, shelter, structure, and even safety than the opportunities available to homeless or unemployed people in the general community. Many inmates with mental disorders receive their first comprehensive treatment services during their incarcerations.

Attitudes of inmates toward their psychiatrists depend, in part, on the quality of care in the system and on the manner in which psychiatrists approach their role. Similar to the scrutiny done by correctional officers, inmates will usually try to appraise the attitude of a new psychiatrist. In some instances, they may test the psychiatrist in one of several ways. How will the new psychiatrist respond to requests for medications or special privileges?

Will the psychiatrist inappropriately bend rules or regulations with inmates and become open to exploitation? How will the psychiatrist handle questions of confidentiality? Will the psychiatrist treat inmates in an overly punitive or an overly indulgent manner? Although only some inmates will engage in schemes and testing with the newcomer, the psychiatrist's reputation will likely spread quickly. For the most part, however, inmates show appreciation and respect to competent, caring, and professional health care providers who offer appropriate services. A capable and considerate clinician provides welcomed relief in an often harsh environment.

Relationships between inmates and health care providers, however, do not always achieve such harmony. Inmate-patients can have both legitimate and frivolous grievances against their clinicians. Poor services and disrespectful or incompetent providers will likely receive a catalogue of complaints. Even appropriate care, however, may result in grievances when inmates pursue demands for unnecessary services, medications, or privileges.

Dissatisfaction with care may lead some inmates to seek legal redress. Unlike free persons in the general community, inmates cannot choose their medical caregivers or switch providers when displeased with services. A similar lack of alternatives binds the caregiver, who cannot refuse to provide services to the inmate-patient. Thus, malpractice lawsuits or complaints to state licensing boards may represent an inmate's attempt to gain leverage when seeking a denied service. Some psychiatrists with unblemished records and histories of good rapport with their patients may begin to accumulate legal complaints from working in prisons.

Correctional employment also exposes the psychiatrist to a legal course of action rarely encountered in other practice settings. Inmates, in comparison with other patients, disproportionately file allegations of constitutional violations against their medical and mental health caretakers. The basis for these allegations generally derives from the 1976 U.S. Supreme Court decision *Estelle v. Gamble* (1976). In *Estelle* the Court held that deliberate indifference by prison personnel to a prisoner's serious illness or injury constitutes cruel and unusual punishment that contravenes the Eighth Amendment to the U.S. Constitution. No other patient group in the United States has a constitutionally recognized right to health care. Although the Supreme Court did not explicitly include a right to treatment for mental disorders in the *Estelle* decision, which dealt with a nonpsychiatric problem, a federal court of appeals quickly found no reason to distinguish between a right to treatment for medical and psychiatric conditions (*Bowring v. Godwin* 1977). In the ensuing years, no court has found that the constitutional right to care does not extend to psychiatric cases (Cohen 1998). This constitutional right provides inmate litigants with access to federal courts. Because of the prevalence of such litigation, correctional psychiatrists should seek insurance that covers at least the expenses involved in defending against accusations of civil rights violations, along with standard malpractice coverage.

The neophyte correctional psychiatrist may fear assault more than litigation. Although this fear is not entirely without basis, such concerns usually exceed the real risk. Inmates have little to gain and much to lose from harming their health care providers. Security measures, including close monitoring and rapid response by officers, also help limit the risk. Correctional psychiatrists who have worked in other public sector mental health programs often feel much safer practicing in prisons than in other inpatient or outpatient settings.

THE PSYCHIATRIST'S ROLE IN THE CORRECTIONAL CULTURE

Appeal of Correctional Psychiatry

Although the challenges of working in a prison can seem daunting, the rewards more than compensate for many psychiatrists. Correctional work appeals to some individuals for a mix of altruistic, clinical, financial, and lifestyle-related reasons. Many health care providers, including psychiatrists, have a commitment to public service for historically underserved populations, such as inmates. In a system with adequate resources and reasonable caseloads, the practitioner can focus his or her time and energy on delivery of good clinical care instead of having to concentrate on processing paperwork and overcoming restrictions of managed care. The predictable income of a salaried position, absence of the expenses and demands of running a practice, and limited on-call responsibilities can add to the attractiveness.

Not all prison systems, however, have the same appeal. In addition to the typically stark environment, many correctional health care programs have insufficient funding and resources, which can limit staffing and services. The consequences of inadequate psychiatric staffing include high caseloads that allow for little more than cursory psychopharmacological management and insufficient time to treat any but the most seriously disturbed inmates. Other important psychiatric tasks, such as providing diagnostic consultations or serving as a liaison with correctional staff, cannot readily occur in understaffed facilities. Shortages among other licensed professionals that compose the multidisciplinary mental health treatment team also can significantly detract from the appeal of correctional employment. Underfunding in some systems affects not only staffing levels but the quality of services and programming. Such systems may have severely restricted formularies and limited access to hospitalization or intermediate care programs for inmates with rehabilitation needs. A paucity of educational, vocational, and other correctional programming can add to distress and dysfunction among inmates, compounding the effects of unmet treatment needs.

Temperament

Even in well-staffed and well-funded programs, however, the correctional psychiatrist must recognize that the prison is not a medical or mental health center (Start 1998). Clinicians typically have the status of guests: welcomed and appreciated when relationships are good, but rejected and resented when relationships are poor. In all settings, however, security constraints will almost always trump clinical agendas. For example, appointments commonly cannot be scheduled during inmate counts or other lockdown situations, and inmates sometimes fail to show for scheduled appointments because of freezes on movement within a facility or other security-related impediments. Some prisons can have surprisingly high rates of such no-show appointments considering the captive nature of the patient population.

Just as a prison's characteristics can influence its attractiveness as a work site, a psychiatrist's temperament can affect the success of adaptation to correctional work. Some individuals may experience the harsh environment, security constraints, and relationships with correctional staff and inmates as too overwhelming and stressful (Bell 1989). Attitudes and demeanor remain important even for those who do not feel overwhelmed by the overall climate. Expressed respect for correctional officers, a flexible style, acceptance of sometimes antiquated furnishings, and low expectations for special accommodations—all increase the likelihood of positive adjustment.

Prison psychiatrists also must feel comfortable with their career choices despite the historically poor image, often undeserved, of correctional health care professionals (Roth 1986; Yarvis 1996–1997). Although many competent and dedicated professionals have always chosen to work in penal settings, some correctional systems have further enhanced the desirability and prestige of employment by partnering with medical schools (Appelbaum et al. 2002).

A psychiatrist's temperament will also affect the quality of relationships with inmate-patients. Like any other patients, inmates usually respond positively when treated with respect by a competent and caring professional, but maintaining harmonious relationships poses challenges at times. Some inmates have committed heinous crimes that engender feelings of disgust. Even the most compassionate professional will have difficulty overcoming such feelings in some circumstances. Successful adaptation to prison work, however, usually involves an ability to sustain a caring and professional attitude despite an inmate's reprehensible past. At the very least, the psychiatrist needs to resist any inclination to withhold appropriate professional care because of negative feelings.

Preserving professional perspective can become even more difficult when an inmate tries to exploit the treatment relationship to obtain a desired, but often unstated, goal. With limited access to the goods, services, and privileges that free persons typically take for granted, it should come as no surprise that some inmates will use any available opportunity to gain sought after commodities. Such inmates may get branded as manipulative, but this label rarely serves a useful purpose. Instead, it conveys a pejorative and adversarial attitude toward the inmate. At best, using the term *manipulative* represents a shorthand communication that the described behavior has its roots in external incentives instead of an underlying mental disorder. Thus, treatment interventions that might be appropriate for behavior associated with a serious mental disorder become inappropriate, and even contraindicated, when the behavior denotes a calculated deception. This economy of communication, however, comes with a price. The relationship between the inmate and the psychiatrist may become a contest with an inevitable winner and loser. Because few of us enjoy losing, the psychiatrist's focus may shift away from understanding the reasons for the inmate's disruptive behaviors and toward resisting exploitation.

A more clinically useful approach begins by acknowledging that all people, including inmates, have needs. In an effort to meet those needs, people often try to manage, or manipulate, the impressions they make within a relationship. Inmates, who have few luxuries and little autonomy, may have even greater motivation than most people have to seize whatever advantages possible. By interpreting an inmate's behavior as an attempt to meet identifiable needs, the psychiatrist can better understand those needs while depersonalizing and disengaging, as much as possible, from the struggle for power and control.

An explicit identification of the goals of the inmate provides a foundation for a behavior management approach to the situation. As described elsewhere in this chapter, for example, a thoughtful and professional approach to privilege requests or to goal-directed self-injurious behavior is more helpful than pejorative labeling and adversarial interactions.

Advocacy

An especially critical aspect of the psychiatrist's temperament involves patient advocacy. Either excessive or insufficient advocacy can cause problems. A psychiatrist who overly champions the interests of inmates may lose credibility and persuasiveness as a clinical proponent. An effective advocate uses discretion when choosing which battles to fight. In the absence of some restraint, the psychiatrist may squander the ability to have influence over more significant concerns.

Excessive reticence about advocacy can also create problems. Psychiatrists have special expertise and a unique perspective about quality of care and the mental health needs of inmates. In the absence of active involvement by psychiatrists in clinical policy and administration, both inmates and correctional systems lose the benefit of an important voice. Inmates may receive less than adequate care, and systems expose themselves to potential public health, safety, and legal problems because of substandard services. Distinguishing minor concerns from important matters that effect quality of care is not always easy.

In addition to advocating for adequate resources and systemic services, correctional psychiatrists occasionally must recommend special privileges for inmates who have mental illnesses. Inmates sometimes request adjustments in housing, work assignments, or recreational opportunities, and allotment of extra services or commodities. The psychiatrist walks a fine line between supporting appropriate requests that can help inmates deal with disabling symptoms or treatment side effects and encouraging excessive demands and accommodations that can disrupt facility operations. Recommended guidelines include exploring alternatives to granting privileges, basing privilege decisions on objective data, using privileges mostly for inmates with serious mental disorders, and involving security staff in special privilege decisions (Pinta 1998).

Medication Use

An area of advocacy that falls uniquely within the competence and responsibility of psychiatrists involves access to medications. It should be axiomatic that inmates can obtain the full range of psychotropic medications available in the broader community. Psychiatrists need to play a key role in helping ensure that correctional formularies and policies do not compromise care through unreasonable restrictions. For example, clinically acceptable standards of care allow patients to receive first-line medications without having to first fail in treatment on less expensive second-line agents. At the same time, however, financial and operational concerns also warrant careful consideration.

Formulary costs have become a major fiscal challenge not only for correctional systems but also for private insurers, public mental health systems, and other community organizations. In recent years, costs have significantly increased for medications used in the treatment of mental disorders, HIV disease, hepatitis C, and other disorders. Pharmaceutical expenses, however, represent only one of many expenses associated with such disorders. Systems that fail to provide adequate access to medications will likely incur added expenses in other areas. For example, substandard pharmacological treatment of mental disorders, infectious diseases, and other serious conditions can result in otherwise avoidable suffering, disability, hospitalizations, staff injuries, and lost productivity. Because most inmates eventually return to the community, poor treatment in prison can jeopardize the health and safety of the general public. Psychiatrists can advocate for modern formularies by providing educational information about these broader costs and considerations.

Prescribing practices also have operational effects, especially for nursing and security staff. Controlled substances, such as benzodiazepines, require special procedures for storage, monitoring, and administration. These procedures, along with additional precautions such as crushing of medications, all add to the demands on often-limited nursing time. The potential for misuse and black market sale of controlled substances also has security implications. Predatory inmates might steal controlled substances from other inmates by pressuring those inmates into hiding pills in their mouths instead of swallowing them. Some inmates also feign symptoms in attempts to get medications that they do not need. Crushing controlled substances, whenever possible, eliminates much of the potential for medication stealing and black market diversion, but it does require additional nursing time as noted.

Despite appropriate precautions, prescribing controlled substances, such as benzodiazepines and stimulants, creates vexing problems for many correctional psychiatrists. Responding to inmate demands for controlled substances and attempting to distinguish truly symptomatic inmates from malingerers often requires considerable clinical time. Security staff, nurses, and nonmedical clinicians may view even appropriate prescribing practices with skepticism, and they might pressure psychiatrists to decrease or eliminate orders for these medications. Formal or de facto prohibitions on the use of these agents, however, would deprive inmates of access to safe and effective treatments that are available and widely used for patients in the general community (Moller 1999; Posternak and Mueller 2001). In addition to their well-established efficacy in generalized anxiety disorder, panic disorder, and sleep disorders, benzodiazepines can play a role in the treatment of many other conditions, including social phobia, mood disorders, schizophrenia, seizure disorders, and muscle spasms. Withholding treatment exposes patients to unnecessary suffering, and alternative pharmacological treatments often have less efficacy and/or lower safety than the benzodiazepines. Although benzodiazepines are among the most widely prescribed medications in the United States, with about 100 million prescriptions in 1999, relatively few patients seek dosage increases or engage in drug-seeking behavior (Drug Enforcement Agency 2003; Soumerai et al. 2003). Even many former substance abusers can safely benefit from treatment with benzodiazepines (Posternak and Mueller 2001). In addition, compared with people in the general community, inmates have less opportunity to misuse benzodiazepines by obtaining multiple prescriptions from different physicians or by combining benzodiazepines with illicit substances. As with any other treatment modality, both the psychiatrist and the patient need to weigh the risks and benefits of benzodiazepines against the risks and benefits of alternative interventions. The acknowledged problems associated with the prescription of controlled substances in prisons, as well as in community settings, do not justify blanket restrictions on their availability.

Correctional psychiatrists can show sensitivity to many fiscal and operational concerns in several ways without compromising clinical care. For example, strategies that focus on dosage strength and frequency can lower medication costs and demands on nursing time. For many of the newer psychotropic agents, such as the atypical antipsychotic medications, the selective serotonin reuptake inhibitors (SSRIs), and other novel antidepressants, the cost per pill does not substantially differ based on the dosage strength. Thus, providing a medication as a once-a-day dose often costs half as much as providing the same total quantity divided into two doses. Combined dosages also diminish the time that inmates spend in medication lines and nurses spend dispensing medications. Similarly, dosages that require use of multiple tablet strengths, such as 75 mg of a medication that comes only in 25-, 50-, and 100-mg strengths, can dramatically increase expenses. Fiscal sensitivity also includes careful attention to evidence-based practices that avoid use of medications without empirical or clinical justifications or unnecessarily substitute expensive preparations for equally effective generic or alternative medications.

Although correctional systems have an obligation to provide inmates with access to the same care and services that should be available in the community, incarceration can provide an opportunity to reassess an inmate's mental health needs and discontinue unnecessary treatment. Many inmates arrive in prison after accumulating multiple medications in the community, often within the context of active substance abuse that complicates their symptom and diagnostic presentation. Controlled medication tapering and observation in the prison represents a rare opportunity to carefully reassess their clinical needs. This process can reasonably occur, however, only in systems that have adequate professional staff to ensure comprehensive evaluation and ongoing follow-up to monitor the effect of these changes.

Consultation and Liaison Roles

As noted in the previous subsection, sufficient staffing levels allow mental health professionals, including psychiatrists, to provide more comprehensive services and to play broader roles within correctional systems. In addition to prescribing and monitoring psychotropic medications and responding to psychiatric emergencies, psychiatrists can participate in policy development and assist with difficult diagnostic questions and with strategies for managing disruptive behaviors. Nonpsychiatric physicians, other mental health professionals, and correctional staff can all benefit from access to the psychiatrists training and expertise.

A particularly challenging consultative situation involves inmates who engage in disruptive behaviors (e.g., flooding cells, setting fires, or smearing body wastes and fluids) or self-injurious behaviors, including cutting, inserting, swallowing, and interfering with medical treatment. Although several psychiatric disorders can be accompanied by self-injurious behavior (Winchel and Stanley 1991), other precipitants and motivators that often occur in correctional settings include isolation, loss of a sense of control, anxiety, situational stress, and attention- or drug-seeking behavior (Fulwiler et al. 1997; Martinez 1980; Thorburn 1984). Most self-injurious behavior in prisons occurs in isolation or segregation settings (Jones 1986). Segregation, and incarceration in general, severely limit an inmate's autonomy, but it is difficult, if not impossible, to control what an inmate does to his or her own body. Self-harm can return some control to the inmate, such as obtaining a transfer to a medical unit. These behaviors also sometimes relieve tension and anxiety due to situational stresses, and they may occur in reaction to sexual intimidation or assaults. Some inmates enjoy the commotion caused by their behaviors or seek the attention or medications they receive after hurting themselves.

The most difficult cases of self-injurious behaviors in prisons involve power struggles between the inmate and the correctional administration. Inmates with ulterior motives have higher rates of recurrence of these behaviors compared with inmates who self-injure with suicidal intent (Franklin 1988; Fulwiler et al. 1997). The presence of ulterior motives, however, does not necessarily indicate an absence of suicidal intent or a low risk of lethality (Dear et al. 2000; Haycock 1989; Karp et al. 1991). Some inmates miscalculate the risks of their behaviors, and others are willing to risk death in an attempt to get what they want. Regardless of the underlying intent, however, serious episodes of self-harm generally require a freeze in movement and suspension of normal operations during the response to the incident. Staff and other inmates risk exposure to potentially infectious blood and body fluids, and the need to transfer the inmate to a health services unit, emergency room, or hospital can drain staff time and financial resources.

The challenge of dealing with self-injurious inmates or with inmates who engage in other disruptive behaviors can be a source of ongoing conflict between mental health and security staff or an opportunity for communication and collaboration. Polarized and dichotomous disputes about whether the behavior represents a mental health or security problem serve little purpose except to create splitting and divisiveness. Interventions with self-injurious inmates must involve shared responsibility among medical, mental health, and security personnel, or they will have little chance of effectiveness. The role of the psychiatrist can include diagnostic assessment to rule out underlying mental disorders as a cause of the behavior, elucidating the environmental contingencies that reinforce the behavior, and helping to develop intervention plans that reshape those contingencies.

Forensic Roles

Unlike consultations that focus on management of disruptive behaviors, dual-agency consultations create fundamental conflicts for correctional psychiatrists (Belitsky 2002; Dvoskin et al. 1995; Krelstein 2002; Metzner 2002). A psychiatrist who treats inmates cannot appropriately conduct, with the same inmates, forensic evaluations, such as parole assessments or formal determinations of competence or responsibility in disciplinary proceedings. Clinical, ethical, professional, and programmatic contraindications preclude such formal assessments or opinions. The therapeutic alliance with inmate-patients would likely weaken if treatment providers assume forensic responsibilities. Clinical care can suffer if inmates become less trusting and less willing to share information. In part because of the adverse effect that a forensic evaluation can have on the therapeutic relationship, ethical guidelines assert that treating psychiatrists should generally avoid performing evaluations of their patients for forensic purposes (American Academy of Psychiatry and the Law 1995). In addition, forensic evaluations usually require third-party interviews that are not commonly a part of a therapeutic relationship and specialized knowledge, training, skills, and experience that general psychiatrists do not necessarily possess. Examiners who lack the requisite background often reach conclusions based on an unsophisticated understanding of the forensic issues. Conducting formal forensic assessments can also foster tensions between security and mental health staff and drain programmatic resources away from the primary mission of providing treatment services.

Role boundaries do not necessarily restrict appropriate informal sharing of clinical information. For example, limited sharing of information as described in the previous section may help disciplinary hearing officers to appreciate an association between an inmate's symptoms and behavior that might otherwise result in a disciplinary sanction such as placement in segregation. Even when symptoms do not have a direct relationship to the proscribed behavior, they may impair the ability of an inmate to tolerate segregation or other sanctions. Psychiatrists have an obligation to inform correctional staff of these mitigating and dispositional factors, without undertaking formal forensic roles or offering formal forensic opinions.

These informal, but potentially valuable, consultations with disciplinary officers and correctional administrators can involve general education about mental health matters as well as information about the functioning of a specific inmate in active mental health treatment. For example, inmates may receive disciplinary sanctions for failing to comply with instructions and regulations, including providing urine samples for drug screening. Some inmates, however, may claim that for psychological reasons they cannot produce a urine specimen while observed, a frequently occurring condition known as *paruresis* (Bohn and Sternbach 1997; Labbate 1996–1997; Zgourides 1987). Difficulty with public urination is one of several common social fears and phobias (Kessler et al. 1998), and it can occur with a wide range of severity among individuals or within the same person in different circumstances and times. There is no definitive or objective test that can confirm or refute the presence of paruresis. The absence of prior treatment or the ability to void in some social situations but not in others does not rule it out. Although modalities associated with the treatment of social phobias help some individuals, there is no universally effective medication or other treatment. Coercive interventions, such as forcing fluids while observing a person with paruresis, are ineffective and can cause serious medical complications. Alternatives to observed urine specimen collection for individuals who self-report paruresis include unobserved collections in a dry room, testing of hair specimens, saliva testing, sweat testing with a patch, or blood testing ("Tests for Drugs of Abuse" 2002). These alternatives preclude the need for futile attempts to differentiate inmates with true paruresis from those who fabricate complaints. Psychiatrists provide a valuable service to the disciplinary process and to inmates when they provide information about such conditions and helpful suggestions about their management.

Confidentiality

Limitations on confidentiality exist in prisons, just as they do in other settings. In addition to universally recognized exceptions to confidentiality, such as the duty to protect, some exceptions arise uniquely in correctional facilities. For example, the psychiatrist may need to report to authorities serious inmate rule violations and plans for escapes or disturbances.

Some information is hard to keep confidential in a prison. Because of medication lines and scheduled clinic visits, correctional officers and other inmates have little difficulty determining which inmates take medications or have appointments with the psychiatrist. Inmates at maximum-security facilities may require special transport and monitoring by officers during psychiatric appointments. The medical record itself is often accessible to security staff. In Massachusetts, for example, the medical record, including the mental health notes, belongs to the Department of Correction. Medical personnel have access to the record as needed for the performance of their duties. Designated correctional administrators have unrestricted access to the record, and other security personnel can receive authorization to review the record for reasons that include preserving the health or enhancing the care of the patient, protecting the health of others, or exercising a duty to warn (Commonwealth of Massachusetts Regulations, 103 DOC 607.05).

In addition, correctional officers cannot adequately fulfill their important role in observing and intervening with inmates who have mental disorders unless mental health professionals share some clinical information with them (Appelbaum et al. 2001). Compared with clinicians, who have relatively brief contact with inmates, correctional officers typically spend many hours a day in close proximity to inmates. They may have the first opportunity to observe significant changes in an inmate's behavior or mental status. Their observations can aid in diagnostic assessments and alert clinical staff to potential crisis situations. Officers can also assist functionally impaired inmates and encourage treatment compliance if they know about inmates' mental health needs. For officers to fulfill these roles effectively, clinicians must sometimes share confidential information to apprise them of concerns about an inmate. If appropriate communication between clinical and security staff does not occur, the treatment of inmates suffers and their safety can be compromised (Geller et al. 1997). Successful collaboration requires clinical staff to exercise discretion about the type and amount of information to share, and security staff to handle the clinical information that they receive with the same degree of care and confidentiality that applies to clinicians. Under Massachusetts law, for example, Department of Correction employees must keep "strictly confidential" any information that they learn regarding an inmate's medical condition (Commonwealth of Massachusetts Regulations, 103 DOC 607.05; General Laws of Massachusetts, Chapter 111, section 70E [b]).

CONCLUSION

Psychiatrists venture into a different world when they enter a prison. Within the stark, regimented, and utilitarian environment exists a culture with its own rules, customs, jargon, roles, and relationships. Unlike the health care facilities with which psychiatrists typically have the greatest familiarity, medical services occupy a peripheral place in the overall mission and organization of a prison. Nevertheless, psychiatrists can make valuable contributions to the health and well-being of inmates and to the safety and efficiency of the institution. Although not every psychiatrist has the temperament or desire to pursue a successful career in corrections, those who possess these characteristics may find rewarding opportunities in correctional work. Openness and sensitivity to the cultural differences and constraints increase the likelihood of harmonious relationships. The topics covered in this chapter provide an overview to some of the areas that make this work both challenging and interesting.

SUMMARY POINTS

An effective correctional psychiatrist

- Understands the correctional culture.
- Complies with institutional rules and regulations.
- Maintains appropriate boundaries.
- Uses correctional jargon appropriately.
- Treats inmates, security staff, and other health care professionals with respect.
- Collaborates with security staff.
- Approaches patients in a professional, nonadversarial way.
- Adapts with flexibility to the prison environment.
- Advocates selectively.
- Practices with sensitivity to fiscal and operational concerns.
- Provides consultation and liaison services.
- Balances confidentiality with sharing of necessary information.

REFERENCES

American Academy of Psychiatry and the Law: Ethics Guidelines for the Practice of Forensic Psychiatry. Bloomfield, CT, American Academy of Psychiatry and the Law, 1995

American Correctional Association: Standards for Adult Correctional Institutions, 4th Edition. Lanham, MD, American Correctional Association, 2003

Appelbaum KL, Hickey JM, Packer I: The role of correctional officers in multidisciplinary mental health care in prisons. Psychiatr Serv 52:1343–1347, 2001

Appelbaum KL, Manning TD, Noonan JD: A university-state-corporation partnership for providing correctional mental health services. Psychiatr Serv 53:185–189, 2002

Belitsky R: Commentary: mental health in the inmate disciplinary process. J Am Acad Psychiatry Law 30:500–501, 2002

Bell MH: Stress as a factor for mental health professionals in correctional facilities, in Correctional Psychiatry. Edited by Rosner R, Harmon RB. New York, Plenum, 1989, pp 145–154

Bohn P, Sternbach H: Current knowledge and research directions in the treatment of paruresis. Depress Anxiety 5:41–42, 1997

Bowring v Godwin, 551 F.2d 44 (4th Cir. 1977)

Cohen F: The Mentally Disordered Inmate and the Law. Kingston, NJ, Civic Research Institute, 1998, Chapter 4, Section 4.1

Cormier B: The practice of psychiatry in the prison society. Bull Am Acad Psychiatry Law 1:156–183, 1973

Culbertson R: Personnel conflicts in jail management. American Journal of Corrections 39:28–39, 1977

Cumming R, Solway H: The incarcerated psychiatrist. Hosp Community Psychiatry 24:631–632, 1973

Dear GE, Thomson DM, Hills AM: Self-harm in prison: manipulators can also be suicide attempters. Criminal Justice Behavior 27:160–175, 2000

Ditton PM: Mental health and treatment of inmates and probationers (BJS Special Report, NCJ 174463). Washington, DC, Office of Justice Programs, Bureau of Justice Statistics, U.S. Department of Justice, July 1999

Drug Enforcement Agency: DEA Briefs and Background, Drugs and Drug Abuse, Drug Descriptions: Benzodiazepines. Available at: http://www.usdoj.gov/dea/concern/benzodiazepines.html. Accessed December 18, 2003.

Dumond RW: Confronting America's most ignored crime problem: the Prison Rape Elimination Act of 2003. J Am Acad Psychiatry Law 31:354–360, 2003

Dvoskin JA, Petrila J, Stark-Riemer S: Case note: Powell v Coughlin and the application of the professional judgment rule to prison mental health. Ment Phys Disabil Law Rep 19:108–114, 1995

Estelle v Gamble, 429 U.S. 97 (1976)

Finn P: Addressing correctional officer stress: programs and strategies (NJC 183474). Washington, DC, National Institute of Justice, December 2000. Available at: http://www.ncjrs.org/pdffiles1/nij/183474.pdf. Accessed November 8, 2004.

Franklin RK: Deliberate self-harm: self-injurious behavior within a correctional mental health population. Criminal Justice Behavior 15:210–218, 1988

Fulwiler C, Forbes C, Santangelo SL, et al: Self-mutilation and suicide attempt: distinguishing features in prisoners. J Am Acad Psychiatry Law 25:69–77, 1997

Geller J, Appelbaum K, Dvoskin J, et al: Report on the psychiatric management of John Salvi in Massachusetts Department of Correction facilities 1995–1996. Submitted to the Massachusetts Department of Correction by the University of Massachusetts Medical Center, January 31, 1997.

Haney C, Zimbaro P: The past and future of U.S. prison policy: twenty-five years after the Stanford Prison Experiment. Am Psychol 53:709–727, 1998

Harrison PM, Beck AJ: Prisoners in 2002 (NCJ 200248). Washington, DC, Office of Justice Programs, Bureau of Justice Statistics, U.S. Department of Justice, July 2003, p 7

Haycock J: Manipulation and suicide attempts in jails and prisons. Psychiatr Q 60:85–98, 1989

Human Rights Watch: Ill-Equipped: U.S. Prisons and Offenders With Mental Illness. New York, Human Rights Watch, 2003. Available at: http://www.hrw.org. Accessed November 8, 2004.

Jones A: Self-mutilation in prison: a comparison of mutilators and nonmutilators. Criminal Justice Behavior 13:286–296, 1986

Karp JG, Whitman L, Convit A: Intentional ingestion of foreign objects by male prison inmates. Hosp Community Psychiatry 42:533–535, 1991

Kaufman E: Can comprehensive mental health care be provided in an overcrowded prison system? J Psychiatry Law 1:243–262, 1973

Kessler RC, Stein MB, Berglund P: Social phobia subtypes in the National Comorbidity Survey. Am J Psychiatry 155:613–619, 1998

Krelstein MS: The role of mental health in the inmate disciplinary process: a national survey. J Am Acad Psychiatry Law 30:488–496, 2002

Labbate LA: Paruresis and urine drug testing. Depress Anxiety 4:249–252, 1996–1997

Martinez ME: Manipulative self-injurious behavior in correctional settings: an environmental treatment approach. Journal of Offender Counseling, Services and Rehabilitation 4:275–283, 1980

Metzner JL: Commentary: the role of mental health in the inmate disciplinary process. J Am Acad Psychiatry Law 30:497–499, 2002

Moller H-J: Effectiveness and safety of benzodiazepines. J Clin Psychopharmacol 19(6, suppl 2):2S–11S, 1999

Morgan DW, Edwards AC, Faulkner LR: The adaptation to prison by individuals with schizophrenia. Bull Am Acad Psychiatry Law 21:427–433, 1993

National Commission on Correctional Health Care: Standards for Health Services in Prisons. Chicago, IL, National Commission on Correctional Health Care, 2003

Packer HL: Justifications for criminal punishment, in The Limits of the Criminal Sanction. Stanford, CA, Stanford University Press, 1968, pp 35–61

Pinta ER: Evaluating privilege requests from mentally ill prisoners. J Am Acad Psychiatry Law 26:259–265, 1998

Posternak MA, Mueller TI: Assessing the risks and benefits of benzodiazepines for anxiety disorders in patients with a history of substance abuse or dependence. Am J Addict 10:48–68, 2001

Powelson H, Bendix R: Psychiatry in prison. Psychiatry 14:73–86, 1951

Robey A: Stone walls do not a prison psychiatrist make. J Am Acad Psychiatry Law 26:101–105, 1998

Roth L: Correctional psychiatry, in Forensic Psychiatry and Psychology: Perspectives and Standards for Interdisciplinary Practice. Edited by Curran WJ, McGarry AL, Shah SA. Philadelphia, FA Davis, 1986, pp 429–468

Santamour MB, West B: The mentally retarded offender: presentation of the facts and a discussion of issues, in The Retarded Offender. Edited by Santamour MB, Watson PS. New York, Praeger, 1982

Soumerai SB, Simoni-Wastila L, Singer C, et al: Lack or relationship between long-term use of benzodiazepines and escalation to high dosages. Psychiatr Serv 54:1006–1011, 2003

Sowers W, Thompson K, Mullins S: Mental Health in Corrections: An Overview for Correctional Staff. Lanham, MD, American Correctional Association, 1999

Start A: Interaction between correctional staff and health care providers in the delivery of medical care, in Clinical Practice in Correctional Medicine. Edited by Puisis M. St Louis, Mosby, 1998, pp 26–31

Steadman HJ, McCarty DW, Morrissey JP: Scope and frequency of conflict between mental health and correctional staffs, in The Mentally Ill in Jail: Planning for Essential Services. New York, Guilford, 1989, pp 90–104

Sykes GM: The Society of Captive: A Study of a Maximum Security Prison. Princeton, NJ, Princeton University Press, 1958

Tests for drugs of abuse. The Medical Letter on Drugs and Therapeutics, 44:W1137A, August 19, 2002

Thorburn KM: Self-mutilation and self-induced illness in prison. J Prison Jail Health 4:40–51, 1984

Toch H, Adams K: The prisoner as dumping ground: mainlining disturbed offenders. J Psychiatry Law 15:539–553, 1987

Warchol G: Workplace violence, 1992–96 (BJS Special Report, NCJ 168634). Washington, DC, Office of Justice Programs, Bureau of Justice Statistics Special Report, U.S. Department of Justice, 1998

Winchel RM, Stanley M: Self-injurious behavior: a review of the behavior and biology of self-mutilation. Am J Psychiatry 148:306–316, 1991

Yarvis RM: Correctional psychiatry, in Psychiatry, Vol 3. Edited by Michels R, Cooper AM, et al. Philadelphia, Lippincott-Raven, 1996–1997, pp 1–16

Zgourides GD: Paruresis: overview and implications for treatment. Psychol Rep 60:1171–1176, 1987

CHAPTER 3

Prevalence and Assessment of Mental Disorders in Correctional Settings

Henry C. Weinstein, M.D.

Doonam Kim, M.D.

Avram H. Mack, M.D.

Kishor E. Malavade, M.D.

Ankur U. Saraiya, M.D.

The provision of mental health care in a correctional setting can be a daunting endeavor; however, significant numbers of offenders with mental illness that live behind the walls that confine them need mental health care. In this chapter, we provide an overview that compares the prevalence of mental disorders among individuals in correctional settings with rates of mental disorders in the community. We review key components of mental health service delivery in correctional environments and discuss substance abuse disorders (SUDs) and violence risk assessments among inmates. We also describe the roles and responsibilities of various correctional providers responsible for mental health care delivery.

PREVALENCE OF PSYCHIATRIC DISORDERS

Overall Prevalence Estimates

Prevalence estimates of mental illness in correctional settings range from 6% to 20% for severe mental disorders (i.e., schizophrenia and major affective disorders) with even higher lifetime prevalence rates when all mental disorders are considered (Teplin 1994; Teplin et al. 1996; Veysey and Bichler-Robertson 2002). Three important points emerge in reviewing the prevalence of mental illness in correctional settings: 1) the prevalence of severe mental illness in correctional facilities is significantly higher than the prevalence in the community; 2) females have higher rates of mental illness than males in both adult and youth correctional settings; and 3) comorbidity of substance use with mental illness is prominent.

Prevalence of Mental Illness in Jails

Because jails and lockups have frequent transition of inmates, they are difficult places to gather prevalence data. Teplin (1990, 1994) performed the first rigorous epidemiological study of mental illness prevalence on a random sample of 728 male urban jail detainees. Using the Diagnostic Interview Schedule (DIS), Teplin compared prevalence rates of severe mental disorders (defined as schizophrenia, schizophreniform disorder, and major affective disorders) in the Cook County jail with Epidemiologic Catchment Area (ECA) data (Teplin 1990, 1994). Teplin found that 6% of male jail detainees in the Cook County jail had a current (within 2 weeks of arrest) severe mental disorder, and 9% had had a severe mental disorder at some point during their lifetime (Teplin 1994). After differences in demographics were controlled for, the jail prevalence rates were two to three times higher than those in the community (Teplin 1990, 1994).

Steadman and colleagues (1995) found, as did Teplin in her 1994 study, that over 6% of jail detainees have a severe mental disorder. The National Commission on Correctional Health Care (NCCHC) estimated that on any given day, approximately 1% of individuals admitted to U.S. jails had schizophrenia or a psychotic disorder; 2%–3% had experienced a manic episode; and 8%–15% had experienced a major depressive episode within the 6 months prior to being booked (Kessler et al. 1994; Veysey and Bichler-Robertson 2002). Prevalence rates for female jail detainees are significantly higher than rates for women in the general population and male jail detainees (see Teplin et al. 1996). An excellent review of prevalence rates of mental illness in female detainees is provided in Chapter 8 ("Female Offenders in Correctional Settings").

Prevalence of Mental Illness in Prisons

Census-based prevalence studies are easier to conduct in prisons than in jails because prisons contain more stable populations. Steadman and colleagues (1991) surveyed a random sample of 3,684 inmates in the New York State prison system to determine the prevalence of psychiatric and functional disability. They estimated that 5% of inmates had a severe psychiatric or functional disability and 10% had a significant psychiatric disability.

The NCCHC found that on any given day, between 2% and 4% of inmates in state prisons were estimated to have schizophrenia or a psychotic disorder and between 2% and 4% were estimated to have a manic episode. Between 13% and 18% of prisoners were estimated to have experienced a major depressive episode during their lifetime (Veysey and Bichler-Robertson 2002). Both state and federal prison rates of mental illness were higher than the rates reported in a nationally representative population used in the National Comorbidity Survey (NCS) (Kessler et al. 1994; Veysey and Bichler-Robertson 2002). In the largest epidemiological survey of prevalence rates of female inmates in a U.S. prison, researchers found rates of lifetime major depressive episode, dysthymia, and alcohol abuse or dependence (Jordan et al. 1996) that were nearly equal to the rates found among incarcerated women in jail (Teplin et al. 1996).

MENTAL HEALTH SERVICES IN CORRECTIONAL SETTINGS

The essential mental health services that should be provided in correctional facilities are set out in the guidelines for psychiatric services in jails and prisons of the American Psychiatric Association (2000). These guidelines are based on the NCCHC standards (National Commission on Correctional Health Care 2003a, 2003b), which divide mental health services in correctional settings into three components: identification, treatment, and discharge planning.

Identification

Identification of mental illness involves the recognition of offenders with signs or symptoms of mental illness. The various opportunities for this recognition in a correctional setting are described below.

Screening and Referral

At every stage of the criminal justice process, from the time of apprehension and arrest through discharge into the community, sufficient mechanisms to identify an individual's mental health care needs must be in place. These mechanisms are commonly referred to as *screening*. Considering the legal requirements, as well as the litigation risks presented in the corrections context, screening is arguably the most important aspect of mental health care (Dvoskin et al. 2003). The American Psychiatric Association's *Guidelines on Psychiatric Services in Jails and Prisons* specify two types of screening: 1) receiving mental health screening and 2) intake mental health screening (American Psychiatric Association 2000).

Receiving mental health screening.   Receiving mental health screening occurs immediately upon arrival at the lockup or jail (during booking) or on entry into prison. This screening includes both inmate observation and a structured inquiry into the inmate's mental health history. This initial screening usually includes questions regarding suicide potential, prior psychiatric hospitalizations and treatment, and current and past medications. This screening has several purposes, including the following:

- Determining whether the inmate, as a result of mental illness, may be dangerous to himself/herself or others
- Evaluating if the inmate is so mentally ill that he or she requires immediate referral for evaluation by a mental health professional
- Assessing if the inmate requires nonemergent mental health assessment
- Providing recommendations for specific required treatment during the criminal justice process

Depending on the type of receiving facility, an acutely mentally ill or suicidal inmate may require transfer to an outside mental health treatment facility, admission to the jail psychiatric unit, assignment to a special evaluation and housing unit, or placement on special observation within the jail.

Various professional staff (such as the booking officer, custodial personnel, medical intake nurse, or mental health provider) may be involved in the receiving screening process. Specific training in mental health screening and referral is required for individuals responsible for conducting the receiving screening. The correctional psychiatrist usually has a limited role in the receiving screening process. Nevertheless, important roles of the correctional psychiatrist in the screening process may include 1) developing appropriate screening forms and procedures, 2) training officers and health care personnel to use the screening forms and to make appropriate referrals, and 3) working with facility officials to write referral procedures for high-risk inmates identified during the screening.

Intake mental health screening.   The second general type of screening, termed *intake mental health screening,* is a more comprehensive examination performed on each newly booked inmate, usually within 14 days after arrival. This form of screening includes a review of the medical and mental health screening, behavioral observation, inquiry into any mental health history, and an assessment of suicide potential. In contrast to receiving screening, the intake mental health screening should be conducted by a mental health care professional. The procedure and the questions asked should be standardized. Observations and staff interventions should also be documented and made a part of the permanent health record. If no referral is deemed necessary after the intake mental health screening, the inmate should be provided information regarding how to access mental health services in their particular facility.

Postclassification referral.   Inmates, who do not receive a mental health referral during one of the screening processes, may subsequently demonstrate a need for mental health services. *Postclassification referral* is the process by which an inmate is brought to the attention of mental health staff for either a brief mental health assessment or a comprehensive mental health evaluation. Specific written procedures for postclassification referral should be part of the facility's mental health services plan. Custodial administration must be alert to the potential for emotional crises during important events in an inmate's life. Significant stressors include court dates, probation or parole hearings, adverse news from legal counsel, and the learning of distressing personal/family news. Mental health emergency services should be accessible on a 24-hour basis. Training health care and custody staff should be done on an ongoing basis, with information provided on both how and when to make a referral to mental health services.

Brief Mental Health Assessment

The brief mental health assessment is a mental health examination that serves as a new triage for individuals who have previously received a mental health screening or evaluation. This assessment occurs when an inmate reports mental health concerns to custody or writes to the mental health team with specific concerns, or when custody becomes concerned regarding an inmate's behavior or mental status. This assessment should be conducted by an appropriately trained mental health professional within 72 hours of any positive mental health screening or postclassification referral (American Psychiatric

Association 2000; National Commission on Correctional Health Care 2003a, 2003b). The findings should be recorded on a standard form that is part of the confidential mental health record. The correctional psychiatrist may have one or all of the following roles in relationship to the brief mental health assessment: 1) developing the procedure for the brief mental health assessment, 2) conducting the assessment if the sole available mental health practitioner, 3) supervising mental health staff conducting the assessment, and 4) consulting with other medical, administrative, and custody personnel in the facility as appropriate.

Comprehensive Mental Health Evaluation

The comprehensive mental health evaluation includes a face-to-face interview of the inmate, a review of all available health care records and collateral information, a diagnostic formulation, and an initial treatment plan. A comprehensive mental health evaluation may be indicated if treatment for a serious mental disorder is being contemplated and a brief mental health assessment is not deemed adequate. A comprehensive mental health evaluation should be conducted by a psychiatrist or other appropriately credentialed mental health professional within a time frame appropriate to the level of urgency. The findings should be recorded in a standardized format that becomes part of the confidential mental health record.

A correctional psychiatrist may perform all or part of the comprehensive mental health assessment when necessary (e.g., when an inmate is already taking psychotropic medications). In addition, a psychiatrist may undertake responsibility for supervision of the mental health staff, for administration of the mental health services, and for liaison with other medical and administrative personnel in the facility. A comprehensive mental health evaluation should include access to psychological and neuropsychological services when indicated, as well as access to clinical laboratory and neuroimaging procedures.

Mental Health Treatment

Timely and effective access to mental health treatment is the hallmark of adequate mental health care (American Psychiatric Association 2000). The American Psychiatric Association's (2000) *Guidelines for Psychiatric Services in Jails and Prisons* states that "the fundamental policy goal for correctional mental health treatment is to provide the same level of mental health services to each patient in the criminal justice process that should be available in the community" (p. 6). The purposes of mental health treatment in jails and prisons include 1) enabling patients to avail themselves of the rights of due process; (i.e., those ju-

TABLE 3–1.   Essential services in a jail or prison

- Psychiatric inpatient resources
- Seven-day-a-week mental health coverage (including coverage with a board-certified or board-eligible psychiatrist)
- Written treatment plan for each inmate receiving mental health services
- Full range of psychotropic medications, including involuntary medication, with the capacity to administer them in an emergency
- Procedures developed and monitored by a psychiatrist to ensure that psychotropic medications are distributed by qualified medical personnel
- Psychiatrist to prescribe and monitor psychotropic medications
- Seven-day-a-week, 24-hour nursing coverage in any area in which people with acute or emergent psychiatric problems are housed
- Special observation, seclusion, or restraint capability
- Supportive and informative verbal interventions in an individual or group context as clinically appropriate
- Programs that provide productive out-of-cell activity that teach necessary psychosocial and living skills
- Training of all custodial staff in the recognition of mental disorders

dicial proceedings or other governmental activities designed to safeguard their legal rights); 2) making the correctional facility safer for everyone who lives, works, or visits there; 3) relieving unnecessary extremes of human suffering; and 4) permitting inmates the opportunity to make use of offered programs.

In the correctional setting, the goal of treatment is the alleviation of mental health symptoms that significantly interfere with an inmate's ability to function. Because of the short-term nature of most jail confinements, treatment typically emphasizes crisis intervention, treatment with psychotropic medication, brief or supportive therapies, and patient education. Table 3–1 summarizes the essential treatment services that should be provided in a jail or prison.

Discharge Planning

Timely and effective discharge planning is essential to continuity of care and an important component of mental health treatment (American Psychiatric Association 2000). Discharge planning is required both in preparation for the transfer of the inmate to another correctional facility and in preparation for their reentry into the community (Osher et al. 2002). Important discharge planning factors to consider for inmates with mental illness who are being released into the community include 1) arranging appointments with mental health agencies or assisting the inmate in arranging the appointment, 2) providing prescriptions or opportunity for renewal of medication evaluation, 3) sharing mental health record information with community providers as appropriate for purposes of care, 4) evaluating for appropriateness of a community referral, and 5) providing linkages to community-based services or agencies capable of providing ongoing treatment.

SUBSTANCE USE DISORDERS

Prevalence

Substance use and SUDs are epidemic in this population. In a study of newly admitted inmates, researchers found that 66% of males and 60% of females had consumed alcohol in the 3 months prior to admission, with 33% of those using alcohol reporting daily intake (Conklin et al. 2000). This same study found that over 66% of newly admitted inmates reported they had used drugs (other than nicotine or alcohol) at some point in their life. Of those who reported other substance use, 80% had used in the 3 months prior to incarceration (Conklin et al. 2000).

The National Institute of Justice drug testing program, ADAM (Arrestee Drug Abuse Monitoring), provides specific information regarding what types of illicit drugs are commonly used by arrestees. According to the 2000 ADAM survey, in half of the ADAM surveyed jail sites, over 60% of adult male arrestees had recently used at least one of five drugs: cocaine, marijuana, opiates, methamphetamine, or PCP (phencyclidine). (National Institute of Justice 2003).

The negative ramifications of substance use are heightened because of the common co-occurrence of substance use diagnoses with other mental health and medical disorders in inmates. Abram and Teplin (1991) found that more than half of the inmates who had a current severe mental disorder had a co-occurring SUD or had used a substance at the time of their arrest.

Screening

Screening is vital at each intervention, and clinicians working in the correctional setting should be aware of when, whom, and how to screen for SUDs. The most fundamental SUD screening component, regardless of the setting, is the clinician's ability to distinguish between active substance-induced disorders (e.g., intoxication, withdrawal or other psychiatric syndromes secondary to substance use), which may require emergency intervention, and substance use disorders (abuse and dependence) that do not require immediate attention.

Receiving

Because arriving inmates often use a last hit of alcohol or other substance prior to their arrest, symptoms of both intoxication and/or overdose may be present at booking. Arresting officers can provide valuable information to evaluators regarding the inmate's appearance and behavior upon arrest and during transport. The initial intake is a critical time when the staff must carefully examine for signs of active intoxication or withdrawal from any substance (especially alcohol, benzodiazepines, stimulants, or other sedatives).

At booking, a nurse (or another trained staff person) typically takes the inmate's vital signs and reviews whether recent substances have been used by the inmate. Substance use screening may also involve ordering urine toxicology tests and blood alcohol levels with ongoing observation for signs of intoxication or withdrawal. Immediate medical and/or psychiatric intervention is generally required for those inmates who experience an agitated intoxication or withdrawal syndrome. In many jail facilities, nonpsychiatric medical personnel are responsible for recognizing and initiating detoxification procedures. The correctional psychiatrist plays an important role in providing input into the development of appropriate written detoxification procedures and in ensuring medical clearance prior to the inmate being referred to psychiatry for an acute psychiatric admission. Medical providers, mental health staff, and custody must have ongoing working communication in the assessment and management of inmates with acute intoxication or withdrawal syndromes. Facilities that do not have adequate medical support for management of acute substance use disorders should transfer the arrestee to a facility where specialized care is available.

Both mental health intake screening and postclassification screening provide an opportunity to obtain a comprehensive review of lifetime substance use. Important reasons for identifying a history of substance use disorders during these screening processes include the following:

1. Recognition of prolonged detoxification syndromes (primarily jail setting) that may be misdiagnosed as psychiatric in etiology
2. Consideration of malingered psychiatric symptoms in an attempt to obtain prescribed substances from the treating provider to maintain substance use
3. Evaluation of sleep disturbance that may be secondary to chronic substance use
4. Identification of primary psychiatric disorders that the inmate has attempted to treat with substances to alleviate symptoms
5. Monitoring for any ongoing illicit substance use during period of incarceration

6. Referral for appropriate medical consultation to evaluate for high-risk co-morbid medical disorders (e.g., HIV, hepatitis)
7. Referral to correctional substance abuse treatment programs and groups
8. Coordination with discharge planning regarding substance use treatment when released into the community

Despite their incarceration, some inmates continue their alcohol or substance misuse within the jail or prison. Many inmates learn to make their own alcohol from supplies obtained from the commissary and/or meals provided to them. This alcoholic brew has different names depending on geographical location. In California, inmates refer to the homemade alcohol as "pruno," whereas inmates in the southeastern United States often refer to this drink as "julep." This strong alcohol concoction is typically made in a plastic bag from a combination of oranges or fruit, a can of fruit cocktail, sugar cubes, and ketchup. After the ingredients are heated under hot water, the mixture ferments, resulting in a pungent alcoholic beverage. Changes in mental status or aggressive behavior may result following the ingestion of this substance.

Inmates also obtain illicit substances that are smuggled into the correctional facility or through the misuse and alteration of prescribed medications. Because of concerns regarding ongoing illicit substance abuse within the jail setting, nearly 70% of jail jurisdictions reported in 1998 that they had a policy that permitted drug testing of jail inmates. Of these facilities, 10% of drug tests of inmates conducted in June 1998 were positive for one or more drugs (Wilson 2000). Finding inmates with substance misuse is important to ensure that dangerous paraphernalia is not available and that the substances cannot be used for harm; to identify cases for treatment; to decrease the risk of violence inside the facility; and to assist the inmate to eventual return to the community (Hiller et al. 1999).

Screening Instruments for Detecting Substance Use

Numerous screening instruments useful in detecting alcohol and substance use have been developed. One diagnostic instrument that can easily be used in screening for alcohol disorders in a correctional environment is the CAGE questionnaire. CAGE is an acronym for the four questions that appear on this instrument. The questions involve asking the inmate if they have had an attempt to Cut back on drinking; have experienced Annoyance at others' criticism of one's drinking; have felt Guilt about drinking; and have needed an Eye opener (a drink first thing in the morning) to steady the nerves. In a study of hospital admissions (noncorrectional), three or more positive responses to the four CAGE questions carried a .99 predictive value for alcohol abuse or dependence (Bush et al. 1987). In a 1997 study of state and federal prisoners that examined inmate's alcohol history with the CAGE questionnaire, over 24% of state prisoners and 16% of federal prisoners gave three or more positive answers. Nearly 80% of state prisoners who answered three of the CAGE questions positively also reported a past history of binge drinking, defined as an equivalent of 20 drinks in one day (Mumola 1999).

Other instruments that have been used to screen for alcohol and substance use include the Alcohol Dependence Scale (ADS; Ross et al. 1990; Skinner and Horn 1984), the Addiction Severity Index (ASI; McLellan et al. 1980, 1985), the Drug Abuse Screening Test (DAST; Staley and El Guebaly 1990); and the Michigan Alcoholism Screening Test (MAST) and short version of the MAST (SMAST) (McHugo et al. 1993; Storgaard et al. 1994; Willenbring et al. 1987). In a survey of community corrections programs for parolees and probationers, the National Institute of Corrections found that the ASI was the most commonly used instrument to assess substance use (Clem 2003).

Two less familiar instruments include the Simple Screening Instrument (SSI; Center for Substance Abuse Treatment 1994), a 16-item screening instrument that examines symptoms of alcohol and drug dependency, and the Texas Christian University Drug Screen (TCUDS; Broome at al. 1996; Simpson 1995; Simpson et al. 1997). The TCUDS includes 19 items, derived from a substance abuse diagnostic instrument, developed by the Texas Christian University Institute of Behavioral Research, that examines diagnostic symptoms of drug use.

In a study conducted in a Texas prison, 400 male inmates were administered eight different substance abuse screening instruments. On the basis of the positive predictive value, sensitivity, and overall accuracy, the TCUDS, the SSI, and a combined instrument (Alcohol Dependence Scale/Addiction Severity Index–Drug Use Section) were found to be the most effective in identifying substance abuse and dependence disorders (Peters et al. 2000). Because of the high prevalence of substance use disorders, the use of screening instruments would likely identify the vast majority of inmates as needing some type of substance use treatment.

Treatment

Treatment for substance use disorders is increasingly recommended for offenders during the early phase of the judicial process. Numerous jurisdictions have developed drug courts (a special court docket within the criminal division) that provide alternatives to incarceration through the provision of mandated alcohol and drug treatment programs. In general, cases assigned to the drug court docket are those in which the defendant is charged with a nonviolent crime (e.g., drug possession) that is considered part of his or her drug use or addiction pattern. Of the 800 drug court programs in the United States, over 90% are postplea, postconviction, and/or for probation violators. Drug courts report that recidivism is substantially reduced for participants who complete the mandated treatment program (Cooper 2003).

The majority of inmates not referred to a substance use treatment program in lieu of incarceration nevertheless have a substance use disorder. However, there is no constitutional right for inmates to receive rehabilitative treatment for substance abuse or dependence. In *Marshall v. United States* (1974), the U.S. Supreme Court held that there was no fundamental right to rehabilitation from drug addiction at public expense after an individual has been convicted of a crime. Five years later, a New Jersey District Court was asked to determine whether failure to provide treatment for prisoners with alcoholism violated the Eighth Amendment's ban on cruel and unusual punishment. In *Pace v. Fauver* (1979), the court held that failure or refusal of a prison to provide rehabilitative treatment for alcoholism did not represent cruel and unusual punishment. Rulings that govern the right to rehabilitation should be distinguished from the constitutional obligation of providers to treat serious medical needs that may result from substance use, intoxication, or withdrawal.

Although the Supreme Court has not ruled that there is a constitutional obligation to provide rehabilitation for substance use disorders, many correctional facilities have recognized the importance of treatment in this area and have established drug and alcohol treatment programming. How common is it for jails to provide drug or alcohol treatment? The answer depends on which study is cited. For example, Peters and May (1992) found that only 28% of jails offered treatment for substance use disorders. In contrast, a Department of Justice (DOJ) study noted that over 70% of 800 jails surveyed provided some type of substance abuse treatment. In the DOJ study, the definition of treatment included detoxification, professional counseling, a residential stay, and/or maintenance drug programs. Other treatment programs cited in the DOJ survey included programs such as Alcoholics Anonymous (AA), Narcotics Anonymous (NA), and other groups that emphasize either self-help or drug or alcohol education and awareness (Wilson 2000).

During the past decade, more intensive jail-based substance user treatment programs were developed. In an analysis of five such programs, researchers found several factors that predicated those inmates who were more likely to remain in treatment for substance abuse while in jail. Factors predicting successful completion of treatment included being age 26 or older, not having used methadone, and having already received a sentence. The two programs described in this study with the highest efficacy of substance treatment retention were the DEUCE (Deciding, Educating, Understanding, Counseling, and Evaluation) jail program in Contra Costa County, California, and the

SAID (Substance Abuse Intervention Division) jail program in New York (Krebs et al. 2003).

Jail substance-based treatment programs have demonstrated efficacy in decreasing criminal recidivism on release into the community. In a longitudinal study of a jail treatment drug and alcohol program in Monroe County, New York, researchers found that three different cohorts of nonviolent, short-term inmates were substantially less likely to be criminal recidivists during a 1-year follow-up period when compared with an inmate control group (Turley et al. 2004).

Prison-based substance abuse services have also demonstrated significant treatment efficacy. The use of therapeutic community within a prison for inmates with substance use disorders is associated with significant advantages for management of the institution. These benefits include lower rates of infractions, reduced absenteeism among correctional staff, markedly low illicit drug use among inmates (Prendergast et al. 2001), decreased grievances, and improved inmate perceptions of their living environment (Dietz et al. 2003). Research has also shown that focused rehabilitation-oriented treatment for substance use can lead to favorable outcomes following incarceration (Gendreau 1996; Knight et al. 1999), especially if aftercare is provided (Griffith et al. 1999). In a study conducted by the Federal Bureau of Prisons, 3% of prisoners who had received drug treatment were rearrested in the 6 months after release, compared with 12% of inmates who had not received treatment (Curley 1999).

RISK ASSESSMENT OF INMATE VIOLENCE

Correctional settings house a large number of violent offenders in confined quarters under stressful circumstances over lengthy periods of time. The resulting environment can lead to significant aggression by inmates toward other inmates, treatment providers, and custodial staff. Assessment of an inmate's risk of future violence is an ongoing process that occurs from the moment the individual is arrested until he or she is released from the criminal justice system. Disciplines responsible for assessing an inmate's risk of future violence include the arresting police officer, sentencing judge, custodial staff, correctional officers, medical and mental health staff, disciplinary boards, review boards, and parole/probation officers. These disciplines conduct their own violence risk assessments that are used for purposes unique to that discipline. Correctional administrators and officers are responsible for assigning inmates to a particular jail floor, cell, or prison facility on the basis of their understanding of the inmate's risk of violence. Failure to make an appropriate risk assessment could result in two individuals at risk for serious conflicts with each other being housed in the same cell, with serious physical violence resulting. Mental health clinicians may be asked to clinically assess an inmate's risk of future dangerousness. Although violence is not always an indicator of a psychiatric problem, psychiatrists can play an important role in assessing violence risk and may be requested to assist in decisions regarding placement, housing, work programs, disciplinary proceedings, and reentry of the inmate into general population or the community.

Types of Violence Risk Assessments

What tools and techniques are used to accomplish these risk assessments under such a variety of circumstances? Three general approaches to violence risk assessment are unaided clinical assessments, actuarial risk assessments, and structured professional judgment risk assessments.

Unaided Clinical Assessments

Unaided clinical assessments are violence risk assessments based on clinical interview or intuition but unaided by an actuarial risk assessment instrument. The arresting officer performs an unaided clinical assessment at the crime scene by observing risk factors exhibited by the individual and the surrounding environment. Likewise, correctional mental health clinicians typically use unaided clinical assessments when asked to conduct a violence risk assessment. Clinical professional judgment assessing future risk of violence involves an examination of both static and dynamic factors associated with violence risk. Static factors include those areas in a person's history that are not easily subject to change, such as past history of violence, age at time of arrest, gender, and intelligence. Dynamic factors represent areas that are subject to change and therefore subject to intervention to decrease violence risk. Dynamic factors include areas such as active drug and alcohol use, current psychotic symptoms, access to weapons, and negative peer associations (see Leong et al. 2003).

In conducting a clinical violence risk assessment, the examiner should carefully consider the inmate's past history of violence. Research repeatedly demonstrates that the best predictor of future behavior is a past history of behavior (Klassen and O'Connor 1988). Important areas to consider when reviewing the inmate's prior violence history include an evaluation of prior treatment responses, the inmate's understanding of triggers and motivations for violent behavior, any discrepancies between the inmate's account of violence and other sources of information, discussion of the inmate's behaviors before and after an aggressive act, and future situations with the inmate that may likely precipitate future violent behavior (Litwack and Schlesinger 1999).

The clinical violence risk assessment also includes a careful assessment regarding the role of mental health symptoms in violent behavior. The evaluator should pay close attention to the individual's affect, as individuals who are angry and lack empathy are at increased risk for violent behavior (Borum et al. 1996; Menzies et al. 1985). The evaluator should also screen for symptoms of fear and paranoia. In paranoid psychotic patients, violence is usually well planned and in line with their false beliefs (Krakowski et al. 1986). In two studies, the presence of "threat control override" delusions were noted to increase the risk of violence (Link et al. 1993; Wessely et al. 1993). Threat control override delusions involve the following beliefs: that the person's mind is dominated by forces beyond the person's control, that the person is being followed, that people are wishing the person harm, and that thoughts are being put into the person's head (Link et al. 1993). Although the MacArthur Study of Mental Disorder and Violence did not find that threat control override delusions increased risk of violence in their study of more than 900 released civil committees, the study did report that nondelusional suspiciousness, such as misperceiving others' behavior as indicating hostile intent, appeared linked to subsequent violence (MacArthur Foundation 2001).

In a review of seven controlled studies examining the relationship between command hallucinations and violence, no study demonstrated a positive relationship between command hallucinations and violence, and one found an inverse relationship (Rudnick 1999). A positive relationship between violence in the presence of command hallucinations was found when the voice was familiar to the person and when the act commanded was less serious. Junginger (1990) reported that command hallucinations are also more likely to be followed in the presence of a delusion whose content is related to the hallucination. In the MacArthur Foundation Violence Risk Assessment Study (MacArthur Foundation 2001), there was no relationship between the presence of general hallucinations or nonviolent command hallucinations and violence. However, there was a relationship between command hallucinations to commit violence and actual violence (MacArthur Foundation 2001; Monahan et al. 2001).

Other important clinical factors to consider are a person's ability to tolerate attacks on his or her self-esteem and the person's capacity for empathy. A review of the research literature identified four fundamental personality dimensions that increase the risk for violence: low impulse control, low affect regulation, a paranoid cognitive personality style, and susceptibility for narcissistic injury (Nestor 2002). Gathering collateral information from correctional officers who have observed the inmate can provide extremely valuable information regarding the inmate's behavior, level of functioning, and change in mental status. While the clinical model has been described as informal, subjective, and impressionistic, it is more sensitive to violence risk factors unique for a particular individual (Borum 1996; Douglas et al. 2003). In addition, clinical assessment allows the clinician to consider active psychiatric symptoms that are not typically included in the actuarial instruments described in the next subsection.

Actuarial Risk Assessments

Actuarial risk assessments involve gathering information about a specified number of factors correlated with an increased violence risk as demonstrated by longitudinal research studies. These risk factors are then converted into a scoring system that assigns a degree of risk to the inmate based on this score. The actuarial model has been described as more formal, reliable, and statistically accurate than the clinical judgment model (Borum 1996; Douglas et al. 2003).

Correctional systems routinely use some type of actuarial instrument to screen inmates for potentially dangerous behaviors. Internal management systems used by correctional facilities incorporate actuarial instruments to determine what housing is most appropriate for the inmate on the basis of their degree of risk to the safe operation of the facility. Two such actuarial instruments are the Adult Internal Management System (AIMS) and the Prisoner Management Classification System (PMC) (Austin and McGinnis 2004). The AIMS attempts to identify inmates who may be incompatible in terms of housing and who may pose a threat to the security of the facility. The PMC utilizes a semistructured interview and 11 historical factors to provide guidelines for safe management of the inmate in their housing unit and recommendations to assist in planning the inmate's reentry into the community.

Other actuarial instruments include those instruments designed to assess criminal behavior, likelihood of recidivism, and potential for rehabilitation. According to the 2003 National Institute of Corrections (NIC) survey, 43% of community corrections programs have developed in-house actuarial instruments to assess violence risk in general population offenders (Clem 2003). Many of these in-house instruments use known risk factors correlated with prison misbehavior. Table 3–2 summarizes several factors noted by the National Institute of Corrections that are considered predictive and not predictive of prisoner violent behavior (Austin 2003).

Two actuarial assessments that are not unique to any one institution include the so-called Wisconsin-model instruments and the Level of Service Inventory–Revised (LSI-R; Andrews and Bonta 1995). The term *Wisconsin model* refers to an assessment and classification system developed by the Wisconsin Department of Corrections in the 1970s. This instrument was designed to measure the relative risk of offenders and their level of service need. (Clem 2003, pp. 5–6) The LSI-R is a combined risk and needs assessment tool

TABLE 3–2. National Institute of Corrections factors found predictive or not predictive of prisoner violent behavior

Factors found *predictive* of violent behavior in prison

• Younger age

• Male

• Recent history of violence

• Mental illness history

• Gang membership

• Lack of prison program involvement or program completion

• Recent disciplinary action (past 12 months)

Factors found *not predictive* of violent behavior in prison

• Detainer

• Drug and alcohol use

• History of escape

• Sentence length

• Severity of offense

• Time left to serve

Source.   Austin 2003.

developed in Canada whose measurements have been validated in North America. The LSI-R consists of 54 items and is composed of 10 subscales. The LSI-R score suggests the likelihood of recidivism and provides interventions based on the score.

Numerous actuarial schemes have been developed for mental health clinicians to use when asked to assess future violence. Examples of these actuarial tools include the Hare Psychopathy Checklist–Revised (PCL-R; Hare 1991) and the Violence Risk Appraisal Guide (VRAG; Rice and Harris 1995), which includes the PCL-R score. Although these instruments are increasingly used in forensic hospital settings and for forensic assessments of dangerousness outside of corrections, the 2003 NIC survey of community corrections noted that only 2 of 73 responding agencies cited the use of one of these standard actuarial instruments to assess a general offender's violence risk (Clem 2003).

Actuarial models, when used exclusively, have inherent limitations. Specific criticisms of actuarial instruments include the following: 1) they provide only approximations of risk, 2) their use is not applicable beyond the studied populations on which they are based, 3) they are rigid and lacking sensitivity to change, and 4) they fail to inform violence prevention and risk management (Douglas et al. 2003; Leong et al. 2003). Although actuarial models attempt to standardize the practice of dangerousness assessment, they are not designed to be the sole standard for violence assessment. Actuarial tools are useful in assisting clinicians in reaching reasonable conclusions based on research findings (Borum 1996).

Structured Professional Judgment Risk Assessments

Structured risk assessments use tools that blend both actuarial assessments and clinical judgment. In structured professional judgments, the evaluator reviews all relevant clinical data to determine the presence of risk factors found to be specifically associated with violence. The decision-making process is structured by using empirically supported and operationalized risk factors and fixed scoring guidelines. In addition, these tools provide guidance for making final decisions (Douglas et al. 2003). Examples of such tools are the Historical Clinical Risk Management–20 (HCR-20; Webster et al. 1997) and the Violence Prediction Scheme (Webster et al. 1994), a combination of the VRAG and the clinical scheme called the ASSESS-LIST.

PROFESSIONAL ROLES AND RESPONSIBILITIES

Correctional mental health care is not a homogenous profession, but rather a diverse collection of services that varies from setting to setting. Each facility is unique, and mental health treatment teams comprise different combinations of mental health professionals (American Psychiatric Association 2000). The differences among services are dictated by availability of various professionals, funding, and geographic licensing and certification requirements. As such, the roles played by members of the different disciplines in the correctional settings may vary and overlap at the same time. The roles and responsibilities of psychiatrists who work in a correctional setting are described in detail in various chapters throughout this book. Other important providers in this setting include psychologists, nursing staff, social workers, correctional officers, and other counselors.

Psychologists

Psychologists are the most frequently employed mental health professional in the correctional setting and may perform tasks usually undertaken by other mental health professionals in other settings (Fagan and Ax 2003). While the inmate population has continued to increase during the last decade, the psychologist-to-inmate ratio is approximately half of what it was during the 1980s (Boothby and Clements 2000). Psychologists often run the treatment team and may be responsible for overseeing quality assurance programs and the evaluation of service delivery. They may also perform initial brief evaluations as well as more comprehensive evaluations. Psychologists provide a large proportion of the treatment that typically includes both individual and group therapy (e.g., anger management). Despite limited resources, a survey of correctional psychologists found that one-to-one therapy was the preferred treatment modality (Boothby and Clements 2000).

An area of expertise specific to psychologists is psychological testing, which can assist the mental health team in evaluating personality characteristics, cognitive functioning, degree of psychosis, and level of impairment from mental health symptoms. Psychologists may also assist in the assessment of malingering through the use of testing such as the Structured Interview of Reported Symptoms (SIRS; Rogers et al. 1992). In Chapter 7 ("Assessment of Malingering in Correctional Settings"). Vitacco and Rogers provide an excellent overview of the use of psychological testing in the assessment of malingering in a correctional setting.

Nursing Staff

In inpatient settings, nurses are the professionals most often on the front-line in terms of the regularity of contact with inmates and the amount of time they spend observing and working with inmates. Nursing staff who work on inpatient psychiatric units inside the jail or prison play a crucial role in making suicide assessments, carrying out suicide prevention, identifying the signs and symptoms of mental illness, assessing treatment efficacy, and consulting with other team members and custody to ensure continuity of psychiatric treatment (Johnson 2003). Correctional nurses also assist in the assessment of malingering, as they have the opportunity to observe the inmate and assist in the differentiation between genuine psychiatric symptoms and symptoms or behaviors that are reported for other reasons. Nurses' daily contact with correctional staff provides support, education, and guidance in managing mentally ill prisoners and is invaluable to day-to-day operations (Johnson 2003).

Nurses also administer medications to inmates either on an inpatient unit or during pill call, which is generally conducted in the inmate's pod or housing unit. This activity is extremely important as it provides an additional opportunity for the nurse to interact with the inmate and observe for any clinical signs of improvement or deterioration. In addition, because there is a risk that some inmates may "cheek" their medications to use for nontreatment purposes, the nurse plays an important role in ensuring and verifying that the inmate takes his or her medication as prescribed. When inmates refuse medications, the correctional nurse typically documents this medication refusal on a standardized form. The correctional psychiatrist and nurse should work together to ensure that treatment refusals are communicated to the mental health team so that follow-up evaluations of the inmate may be conducted.

Social Workers

In addition to providing mental health counseling, social workers mobilize social services for the inmate. Inmates often distrust social service agencies, and this distrust may prevent them from accessing available services both inside and outside the correctional environment. Assisting an inmate in the utilization of available services may play a vital role in improving the ultimate quality of life for the inmate. As in most settings, the roles of social workers in the correctional setting are quite diverse. Social workers can serve as deliverers of clinical care in both individual and group therapy. An important component of social work intervention is the assessment of family functioning and in finding avenues to access and improve community support systems. Social workers may also serve as intermediaries between inmates and the legal system as well as between inmates and their support systems.

Correctional Officers

Correctional officers not only maintain the secure environment but also draw on their unique relationship with the inmates as a useful tool in the assessment and management of mental health issues. In jails and prisons, correctional officers are the staff members who spend the largest amount of time with the inmates.

Basic mental health training for correctional officers is extremely important, as they are more likely than any other staff member to face an inmate situation requiring deescalation (Dvoskin and Spiers 2004). Correctional officers need not be "amateur psychotherapists" (Anthony and Carkhuff 1977), but they can provide supportive interventions and basic coping skills to the inmate (Anthony and Carkhuff 1977; Dvoskin and Spiers 2004). In administrative segregation units, correctional officers play an even more crucial role in using their training and experience to help achieve a positive outcome for very difficult inmates. In some segregation units, behavioral contingency plans (designed to award or remove privileges for inmates) rely heavily on input from officers. Officers' input into behavioral intervention plans includes the identification of reinforcers, development of behavioral management schedules, and assessment of improvement (Dvoskin and Spiers 2004).

The Federal Bureau of Prisons has adopted an approach known as unit team management in which the correctional officer is routinely considered part of the treatment team. The advantages of having an officer part of the treatment team include cross-disciplinary consultation, assistance in making security decisions, and improvement in officer morale, as they have the opportunity to observe positive progress in the inmates they supervise (Dvoskin and Spiers 2004; Holt 2001).

Clearly officers' first priority is safety. It is important to realize, however, that the proper identification and treatment of psychiatric symptoms serves the interests of safety. As a consequence, line staff should feel comfortable making referrals to mental health services when they have a concern regarding the emotional status of an inmate. To facilitate referrals from correctional officers, mental health professionals must find ways to establish trust with the line staff. Important steps in developing trust with the line staff include establishing open bidirectional communication while demonstrating respect, seeking out the impressions and opinions regarding the inmate's functioning, giving assistance and feedback on interventions that may be potentially useful, and providing training on basic mental health assessment and interventions (Dvoskin and Spiers 2004).

A potential source of conflict between security and health care staff comprises issues surrounding possible malingered symptoms and suicidal gestures. All reports of suicide should be taken seriously. If trust between the line staff and mental health team has been established and communication channels are open, both professions can work together to properly evaluate potential malingered symptoms and to identify actual suicide attempts versus suicidal gestures.

Other Mental Health Professionals

As previously described, SUDs are extremely common in the incarcerated population. Because SUDs are the most common diagnosis in this population, *substance use counselors* can play a vital role in mental health service delivery. Substance use counselors can serve as individual therapists, run organized substance use groups, and serve as liaisons to various treatment services in the community.

Activity therapists have also been used in a correctional environment. There are limited data on how commonly various activity therapists are employed in the correctional setting. As correctional health care becomes more sophisticated and more and more emphasis is placed on rehabilitation and reintegration into society to avoid re-incarceration, the importance of this discipline is being recognized. Potential roles of activity therapists (e.g., recreational therapy) include conducting basic life skills group on an inpatient psychiatric unit, assisting in the development of activities programs for offenders with mental illness, and running interactive groups in general population.

CONCLUSION

Correctional mental health care providers have important roles and responsibilities that vary depending on the stage of the criminal justice process and

the type of correctional housing facility. These responsibilities are wide ranging and may include program development, establishment of policies and
procedures, consultation and education, and the provision of clinical care.

The prevalence of mental illness in an incarcerated population is strik-
ingly high. In addition, increased rates of co-occurring medical disorders and
substance use disorders are found in this same population. The overwhelming prevalence of substance use disorders emphasizes the significance of detecting and treating such co-occurring disorders.

The threat of inmate violence is ever present, as many inmates have per-
petrated violent crimes. Screening techniques for potentially violent behavior
are critical to the safety of the facility and important when mental health services are being provided. Although different professional staff members work
in the same environment, the ultimate goal is safety for inmates and staff combined with effective treatment. This goal can be accomplished. The key is cooperation, mutual respect, and the understanding that all staff can and should
work together to make one another's jobs more effective.

SUMMARY POINTS

- The prevalence of severe mental illness in correctional settings is
  higher for men and women than in the community.
- Mental health services in correctional settings include identification, treatment, and discharge planning.
- Substance use disorders are extremely common.
- Various types of violence risk assessments are used to classify and
  assess inmates.
- Correctional mental health is multidisciplinary and includes valuable input from correctional officers.

REFERENCES

Abram KM, Teplin LA: Co-occurring disorders among mentally ill jail detainees: im-
 plications for public policy. Am Psychol 46:1036–1045, 1991
American Psychiatric Association: Psychiatric Services in Jails and Prisons: A Task
 Force Report of the American Psychiatric Association, 2nd Edition. Washington,
 DC, American Psychiatric Association, 2000
Andrews D, Bonta J: LSI-R: The Level of Service Inventory–Revised Users' Manual.
 Toronto, ON, Multi-Health Systems, 1995
Anthony WA, Carkhuff RR: The functional professional therapeutic agent, in Effective
 Psychotherapy. Edited by Gurman AS, Razin AM. Oxford, England, Pergamon,
 1977
Austin J: Findings in Prison Classification and Risk Assessment. Washington, DC,
 National Institute of Corrections, U.S. Department of Justice, June 2003

Austin J, McGinnis K: Classification of high-risk and special management prisoners: a national assessment of current practices (NIC 019468). Washington, DC, National Institute of Corrections, U.S. Department of Justice, June 2004

Boothby JL, Clements CB: A national survey of correctional psychologists. Criminal Justice Behavior 27:716–732, 2000

Borum R: Improving the clinical practice of violence risk assessment. Am Psychol 51:945–956, 1996

Borum R, Swartz M, Swanson J: Assessing and managing violence risk in clinical practice. Journal of Practical Psychiatry and Behavioral Health 4:205–215, 1996

Broome KM, Knight K, Joe G, et al: Evaluating the drug-abusing probationer: clinical interview versus self-administered assessment. Criminal Justice Behavior 23:593–606, 1996

Bush B, Shaw S, Cleary P, et al: Screening for alcohol abuse using the CAGE questionnaire. Am J Med 82:231–235, 1987

Center for Substance Abuse Treatment: Simple Screening Instruments for Outreach for Alcohol and Other Drug Abuse Infectious Diseases (Treatment Improvement Protocol Series, No 11). Rockville, MD, U.S. Department of Health and Human Services, 1994

Clem C: Topics in Community Corrections: Annual Issue 2003: Offender Assessment. Washington, DC, National Institute of Corrections, U.S. Department of Justice, 2003. Available at: http://www.nicic.org. Accessed January 8, 2005.

Conklin TJ, Lincoln T, Tuthill RW: Self-reported health and prior health behaviors of newly admitted correction inmates. Am J Public Health 90:1939–1941, 2000

Cooper CS: Drug courts: current issues and future perspectives. Subst Use Misuse 38:1671–1711, 2003

Curley R: Treatments' last frontier? The criminal justice system is trying to build a culture of compassion. Will it promote recovery? Behav Healthc Tomorrow 8:10–15, 1999

Dietz EF, O'Connell DJ, Scarpitti FR: Therapeutic communities and prison management: an examination of the effects of operating an in-prison therapeutic community on levels of institutional disorder. International Journal of Offender Therapy and Comparative Criminology 47:210–223, 2003

Douglas KS, Ogloff JRP, Hart SD: Evaluation of a model of violence risk assessment among forensic psychiatric patients. Psychiatr Serv 54:1372–1379, 2003

Dvoskin JE, Spiers EM: On the role of correctional officers in prison mental health. Psychiatr Q 75:41–59, 2004

Dvoskin JE, Spiers EM, Metzner JL, et al: The structure of correctional mental health services, in Principles and Practice of Forensic Psychiatry, 2nd Edition. Edited by Rosner R. New York, Oxford University Press, 2003, pp 489–504

Fagan TJ, Ax RK: Correctional Mental Health Handbook. Thousand Oaks, CA, Sage, 2003

Gendreau P: Offender rehabilitation: what we know and what needs to be done. Criminal Justice and Behavior 23:144–161, 1996

Griffith JD, Hiller M, Knight K, et al: A cost-effectiveness analysis of in-prison therapeutic community treatment and risk classification. The Prison Journal 79:352–368, 1999

Hare RD: The Hare Psychopathy Checklist–Revised. Toronto, ON, Multi-Health Systems, 1991

Hiller ML, Knight K, Simpson DD: Prison-based substance abuse treatment, residential aftercare and recidivism. Addiction 94:833–842, 1999

Holt C: The correctional officer's role in mental health treatment of youthful offenders. Issues in Mental Health Nursing 22:173–180, 2001

Johnson J: Psychiatric nursing in the correctional setting, 2003. Available at: http://nsweb.nursingspectrum.com/ce/m30C-1.htm. Accessed January 2, 2004.

Jordan BK, Schlenger WE, Fairbank JA, et al: Prevalence of psychiatric disorders among incarcerated women, II: convicted women felons entering prison. Arch Gen Psychiatry 53:513–519, 1996

Junginger J: Predicting compliance with command hallucinations. Am J Psychiatry 147:245–247, 1990

Kessler RC, McGonagle KA, Zhao S, et al: Lifetime and 12-month prevalence of DSM-III-R psychiatric disorders in the United States: results from the National Comorbidity Survey. Arch Gen Psychiatry 51:8–19, 1994

Klassen D, O'Connor W: A prospective study of predictors of violence in adult male mental health admissions. Law and Human Behavior 12:143–158, 1988

Knight K, Simpson DD, Hiller ML: Three year reincarceration outcomes for in-prison therapeutic community treatment in Texas. The Prison Journal 79:337–351, 1999

Krakowski M, Volavka J, Brizer D: Psychopathology and violence: a review of literature. Compr Psychiatry 27:131–148, 1986

Krebs CP, Brady T, Laird G: Jail-based substance user treatment: an analysis of retention. Subst Use Misuse 38:1227–1258, 2003

Leong GB, Silva JA, Weinstock R: Dangerousness, in Principles and Practice of Forensic Psychiatry, 2nd Edition. Edited by Rosner R. New York, Oxford University Press, 2003, pp 564–571

Litwack TR, Schlesinger LB: Dangerousness risk assessments: research, legal, and clinical considerations, in The Handbook of Forensic Psychology. Edited by Hess AK, Weiner IB. Hoboken, NJ, Wiley, 1999, pp 195–209

Link BG, Andrews H, Cullen FT: The violent and illegal behavior of mental patients reconsidered. American Sociological Review 57:275–292, 1993

MacArthur Foundation: The MacArthur Violence Risk Assessment Study: Executive Summary, 2001. Available at: http://macarthur.virginia.edu/risk.html. Accessed February 5, 2002.

Marshall v United States, 414 U.S. 417 (1974)

McHugo GW, Paskus TS, Drake RE: Detection of alcoholism and schizophrenia using the MAST. Alcoholism: Clinical and Experimental Research 17:187–191, 1993

McLellan AT, Luborsky L, Woody GE, et al: An improved diagnostic evaluation instrument for substance abuse patients. J Nerv Ment Dis 168:26–33, 1980

McLellan AT, Luborsky L, Cacciola J, et al: New data from the Addiction Severity Index: reliability and validity in three centers. J Nerv Ment Dis 173:412–423, 1985

Menzies RJ, Webster CD, Sepejak DS: The dimensions of dangerousness: evaluating the accuracy of psychometric predictions of violence among forensic patients. Law and Human Behavior 9:49–70, 1985

Monahan J, Steadman HJ, Silver E, et al (eds): Rethinking Risk Assessment: The MacArthur Study of Mental Disorder and Violence. New York, Oxford University Press, 2001

Mumola CJ: Substance abuse and treatment of state and federal prisoners, 1997 (BJS Special Report, NCJ 172871). Washington, DC, Office of Justice Programs, Bureau of Justice Statistics, U.S. Department of Justice, January 1999

National Commission on Correctional Health Care: Standards for Health Services in Jails. Chicago, IL, National Commission on Correctional Health Care, 2003a

National Commission on Correctional Health Care: Standards for Health Services in Prisons. Chicago, IL, National Commission on Correctional Health Care, 2003b

National Institute of Justice: Annual Report 2000: Arrestee Drug Abuse Monitoring (NCJ 193013). Washington, DC, Office of Justice Programs, National Institute of Justice, U.S. Department of Justice, April 2003

Nestor PG: Mental disorder and violence: personality dimensions and clinical features. Am J Psychiatry 159:1973–1978, 2002

Osher F, Steadman HJ, Barr HA: Best Practice Approach to Community Re-entry From Jails for Inmates With Co-occurring Disorders: The APIC Model. Delmar, NY, The National GAINS Center, 2002

Pace v Fauver, 470 F.Supp. 456 (D.N.J. 1979)

Peters RH, May RL: Drug treatment services in jails, in Drug Abuse Treatment in Prisons and Jails (NIDA Publ No ADC 92–1884). Edited by Leukefeld C, Tims F. Rockville, MD, National Institute on Drug Abuse, U.S. Department of Health and Human Services, 1992, pp 38–50

Peters RH, Greenbaum PE, Steinberg ML, et al: Effectiveness of screening instruments in detecting substance use disorders among prisoners. J Subst Abuse Treat 18:349–358, 2000

Prendergast ML, Farabee D, Cartier J: The impact of in-prison therapeutic community programs on prison management. Journal of Offender Rehabilitation 32:63–78, 2001

Rice ME, Harris GT: Violent recidivism: assessing predictive validity. J Consult Clin Psychol 63:737–748, 1995

Rogers R, Bagby RM, Dickens SE: Structured Interview of Reported Symptoms (SIRS) Professional Manual. Odessa, FL, Psychological Assessment Resources, 1992

Ross HE, Gavin DR, Skinner HA: Diagnostic validity of the MAST and the Alcohol Dependence Scale in the assessment of DSM-III alcohol disorders. J Stud Alcohol 51:506–513, 1990

Rudnick A: Relations between command hallucinations and dangerous behavior. J Am Acad Psychiatry Law 27:253–257 1999

Simpson DD: TCU Forms Manual: Improving Drug Abuse Treatment, Assessment, and Research. Fort Worth, Texas Christian University, Institute of Behavioral Research, 1995

Simpson DD, Knight K, Broome KM: TCU/CJ Forms Manual: Drug Dependence Screen and Initial Assessment. Forth Worth, Texas Christian University, Institute of Behavioral Research, 1997

Skinner HA, Horn JL: Alcohol Dependence Scale: Users' Guide. Toronto, ON, Addictions Research Foundation, 1984

Staley D, El Guebaly N: Psychometric properties of the Drug Abuse Screening Test in a psychiatric patient population. Addict Behav 15:257–264, 1990

Steadman HJ, Holohean EJ, Dvoskin J: Estimating mental health needs and service utilization among prison inmates. Bull Am Acad Psychiatry Law 19:297–307, 1991

Steadman HJ, Morris SM, Dennis, DL: The diversion of mentally ill persons from jails to community-based services: a profile of programs. Am J Public Health 85:1630–1635, 1995

Storgaard H, Nielsen SD, Gluud C: The validity of the Michigan Alcoholism Screening Test. Alcohol 29:493–502, 1994

Teplin LA: The prevalence of severe mental disorders among male urban jail detainees: comparison with the Epidemiologic Catchment Area Program. Am J Public Health 80:663–669, 1990

Teplin LA: Psychiatric and substance abuse disorders among male urban jail detainees. Am J Public Health 84:290–293, 1994

Teplin LA, Abram KM, McClelland GM: Prevalence of psychiatric disorders among incarcerated women, I: pretrial jail detainees. Arch Gen Psychiatry 53:505–512, 1996

Turley A, Thornton T, Johnston C, et al: Jail drug and alcohol treatment program reduces recidivism in nonviolent offenders: a longitudinal study of Monroe County, New York's jail treatment drug and alcohol program. International Journal of Offender Therapy and Comparative Criminology 48:721–728, 2004

Veysey BM, Bichler-Robertson G: Prevalence estimates of psychiatric disorders in correctional settings, in The Health Status of Soon-to-Be-Released Inmates: A Report to Congress, Vol 2. Chicago, IL, National Commission on Correctional Health Care, 2002. Available at: http://www.ncchc.org/pubs/pubs_stbr.vol2.html. Accessed November 15, 2003.

Webster CD, Harris GT, Rice M, et al: The Violence Prediction Scheme: assessing dangerousness in high risk men. Toronto, ON, University of Toronto, Centre of Criminology, 1994

Webster CD, Douglas KS, Eaves D, et al: HCR-20: Assessing the Risk for Violence (Version 2). Vancouver, BC, Mental Health Law and Policy Institute, Simon Fraser University, 1997

Wessely S, Buchanan A, Reed A, et al: Acting on delusions, I: prevalence. Br J Psychiatry 163:69–76, 1993

Willenbring ML, Christensen KJ, Spring WD, et al: Alcoholism screening in the elderly. J Am Geriatr Soc 35:864–869, 1987

Wilson DJ: Drug use, testing, and treatment in jails (NCJ 179999). Washington, DC, Office of Justice Programs, Bureau of Justice Statistics, U.S. Department of Justice, May 2000

Suicide Prevention in Correctional Facilities

Lindsay M. Hayes, M.S.

According to available records, during the late evening of March 18, the Nathan County Sheriff's Department received information regarding a disturbance at the residence of 43-year-old James Cooper. (To ensure complete confidentiality, names of the victim, staff, and jail facility have been changed. No other modifications have been made.) When Nathan County Sheriff Jack Buck and other personnel arrived at the scene, Mr. Cooper was observed wielding a gun and pointing it at himself and others. The weapon was eventually confiscated without injury and Mr. Cooper was transported to the Nathan County Detention Facility (NCDF), arriving at approximately 9:00 P.M. Although not criminally charged, Mr. Cooper was known to suffer from mental illness and, according to NCDF documents (including the jail docket), was being held for "mental." Approximately 30 minutes later, at 9:30 P.M., Mr. Cooper was observed to be attempting suicide by hanging in a holding cell. He had tied one end of his shirt to the bunk bed and the other end around his neck. Mr. Cooper was rescued by jail staff and placed in a straitjacket. He continued his self-destructive behavior by repeatedly banging his head against the cell wall. Mr. Cooper was eventually transported to a local hospital for medical treatment and returned to the facility at approximately 11:00 P.M. He was rehoused in the holding cell in a straitjacket and without his clothes. He was ob-

69

served to be crying and again engaging in self-destructive behavior by banging his head against the wall. Mr. Cooper then was able to remove his straitjacket and began banging it against the cell door. Jail staff entered the cell and briefly chained Mr. Cooper to his bunk by waist chains and leg irons. The inmate eventually calmed down, was permitted to smoke a cigarette, and fell asleep. According to jail logs, Mr. Cooper was given a blanket at approximately 2:30 A.M. (on March 19), his clothing was returned at 12:00 P.M., and he was observed at 20-minute intervals between 2:00 A.M. to 5:15 A.M. (although these observations were not documented). Despite continuous suicidal behavior, he was never placed on suicide precautions by jail staff.

Later in the morning of March 19, Mr. Cooper was transported by sheriff's deputies to the county mental health center (CMHC) for evaluation of his need for civil commitment to a state hospital. The preevaluation screening form completed by the examining psychologist noted Mr. Cooper's prior outpatient treatment at the CMHC, history of or present danger to self ("high-risk behavior" and "self-mutilation"), depressive-like behaviors ("sadness," "crying," and "weight loss or gain"), and "beating head against wall in admitted tantrum," recently fighting with his father, and substance abuse. The examining psychologist was unaware of Mr. Cooper's suicide attempt in the county jail the previous day. Following the assessment, a certificate of examining physician/psychologist was completed, although the recommendation from the psychologist appeared unclear. A prescription for daily doses of paroxetine was also written. Mr. Cooper was then returned to the county jail and, apparently because of the unclear recommendation on the certificate of examining physician/psychologist, was released from custody the following day (March 20).

On March 25, the Nathan County Chancery Court received a resubmitted certificate of examining physician/psychologist regarding Mr. Cooper from the CMHC that clearly recommended civil commitment. The resubmitted form included boxes checked off in the areas of "grossly disturbed behavior/faulty perceptive," "substantial likelihood of physical harm as manifested by recent threat or attempt to physically harm him/herself or others," and "failure to provide necessary care for him/herself." According to a clinical note written by the CMHC examining psychologist on March 25: "Apparently the public officials misunderstood our possibly ambiguously stated intentions for him to be held until a comprehensive evaluation could be accomplished in a hospital setting. I further learned that the report that we sent was possibly incomplete. I immediately contacted Sheriff Buck and the Chancery Clerk by telephone to review our recommendations. I also faxed them a copy of the completed physician and psychologist recommendations."

During the late evening of March 29, the Nathan County Sheriff's Department again received information regarding a disturbance involving Mr.

Cooper in the community. Sheriff Buck and other personnel again responded to the scene and observed Mr. Cooper wielding a knife. The weapon was eventually confiscated without injury, and Mr. Cooper was transported to the county jail by Sheriff Buck, arriving at approximately 11:35 P.M. He was not criminally charged and, according to jail documents, was again being held for "mental." Mr. Cooper was again placed in a holding cell and observed periodically, although not placed on suicide precautions by jail staff.

At approximately 3:20 P.M. on March 31, Mr. Cooper was rehoused from the holding cell to the general population section of the jail. He was allowed to take a shower and was given all his clothing and a box of personal items. According to jail staff, who did not consult with any mental health staff prior to rehousing Mr. Cooper, the rationale for the transfer was that his "state of mind was good" and they needed to utilize the holding cell for observation of another mentally ill detainee. When commenting later about Mr. Cooper's transfer to general population, the chief jailer stated, "We treated him like any other inmate when we moved him to the back of the jail."

On April 1, Mr. Cooper attended the Nathan County Chancery Court proceeding for his civil commitment to a state hospital for mental health examination and treatment. The commitment order was signed by Mr. Cooper, his attorney, and the court, stating, in part, that Mr. Cooper was a "danger to himself and others." According to his attorney, "James Cooper agreed to and signed the commitment order, and the order was entered by the chancellor at approximately 11:00 A.M. Sheriff Buck was aware that Mr. Cooper had agreed to be committed and was present when the chancellor signed the order. James Cooper was to be kept in custody at the Nathan County Detention Facility until an opening became available at the state mental hospital. The inmate was subsequently returned to his cell.

Several hours later, at approximately 8:16 P.M. on April 1, Mr. Cooper was again observed banging his head against the wall of his cell. He appeared agitated to jail staff, observed to be crying, and requested his psychotropic medication and a cigarette. Although the officer believed that Mr. Cooper's head banging was an attempt to commit suicide, no effort was made to ensure his safety from further self-destructive behavior. Instead, at approximately 8:30 P.M., Mr. Cooper was given his medication and a cigarette (a.k.a. "smoke therapy"), and the lights in his cell were turned off. According to jail records, Mr. Cooper was not seen again for approximately 2½ hours, when he was found at approximately 11:00 P.M. hanging by a laundry bag cord that was tied to the upper bunk in his cell. The officer eventually entered the cell and cut the cord away from the victim's neck but did not initiate cardiopulmonary resuscitation. A medical emergency was called, and paramedics arrived approximately 10 minutes later. Mr. Cooper was subsequently pronounced dead.

SCOPE OF THE PROBLEM

Suicide continues to be a leading cause of death in jails across the country, where more than 400 inmates take their lives each year (Hayes 1989). The rate of suicide in county jails is estimated to be approximately five times greater than that of the general population (Stephan 2001). Overall, most jail suicide victims are young white males arrested for nonviolent offenses and intoxicated upon arrest. Many are placed in isolation and are found dead within 24 hours of incarceration (Davis and Muscat 1993; Hayes 1989). The overwhelming majority of victims are found hanging by either bedding or clothing. Most victims are not adequately screened for potentially suicidal behavior on entrance into the jail (Hayes 1989).

Research specific to suicide in urban jail facilities provides certain disparate findings. Most victims of suicide in large urban facilities are arrested for violent offenses and are dead within 1–4 months of incarceration (DuRand et al. 1995; Marcus and Alcabes 1993). Because of the extended length of confinement prior to suicide, intoxication is not always the salient factor in urban jails as it is in other types of jail facilities. Suicide victim characteristics such as age, race, gender, method, and instrument remain generally consistent in both urban and non-urban jails.

The precipitating factors of suicidal behavior in jail are well established (Bonner 1992, 2000; Winkler 1992). It has been theorized that there are two primary causes for jail suicide: 1) jail environments are conducive to suicidal behavior, and 2) the inmate is facing a crisis situation. From the inmate's perspective, certain features of the jail environment enhance suicidal behavior: fear of the unknown, distrust of authoritarian environment, lack of apparent control over the future, isolation from family and significant others, shame of incarceration, and the dehumanizing aspects of incarceration. In addition, certain factors are prevalent among inmates facing a crisis situation that could predispose them to suicide: recent excessive drinking and/or use of drugs, recent loss of stabilizing resources, severe guilt or shame over the alleged offense, current mental illness, prior history of suicidal behavior, and approaching court date. Some inmates simply are (or become) ill-equipped to handle the common stresses of confinement. As the inmate reaches an emotional breaking point, the result can be suicidal ideation, attempt, or completion. During initial confinement in a jail, this stress can be limited to fear of the unknown and isolation from family, but over time (including stays in prison) the stress may become exacerbated and include loss of outside relationships, conflicts within the institution, victimization, further legal frustration, physical and emotional breakdown, and problems of coping within the institutional environment (Bonner 1992).

While suicide is well recognized as a critical problem within jails, the issue of prison suicide has not received comparable attention, primarily because the number of jail suicides far exceeds the number of prison suicides. Suicide ranks third, behind natural causes and AIDS, as the leading cause of death in prisons (Bureau of Justice Statistics 2000). Although the rate of suicide in prison is considerably lower than in jail, it still remains greater than in the general population (Hayes 1995). Most research on prison suicide has found that the vast majority of victims are convicted of personal crimes, are housed in single cells (often some type of administrative confinement), and have histories of prior suicide attempts and/or mental illness (He et al. 2003; Salive et al. 1989; White and Schimmel 1995). Although normally serving long sentences, most victims commit suicide in the early stages of their prison confinement (New York State Department of Correctional Services 2002). Precipitating factors in prison suicide may include new legal problems, marital or relationship difficulties, and inmate-related conflicts (White and Schimmel 1995).

Finally, an inmate suicide is emotionally devastating to the victim's family and can be financially devastating to the correctional facility (and its personnel) sustaining the death. Many inmate suicides result in litigation brought against a state or local jurisdiction alleging that the death was caused by the negligence and/or deliberate indifference of facility personnel. Although the plaintiff's burden to demonstrate liability in these cases remains high (Hanser 2002), several recent federal court jury awards have well exceeded $1 million (Sanville v. Scaburdine 2002; Woodward v. Myres 2003).

COMPREHENSIVE SUICIDE PREVENTION PROGRAMMING

The literature is replete with numerous examples of how jail and prison systems have developed effective suicide prevention programs (Cox and Morschauser 1997; Goss et al. 2002; Hayes 1995, 1998; White and Schimmel 1995). New York experienced a significant drop in the number of jail suicides after implementing a statewide comprehensive prevention program (Cox and Morschauser 1997). Texas saw a 50% decrease in the number of county jail suicides, as well as almost a sixfold decrease in the rate of these suicides from 1986 through 1996, much of it attributable to increased staff training and a state requirement for jails to maintain suicide prevention policies (Hayes 1996). One researcher reported no suicides during a 7-year time period in a large county jail after the development of suicide prevention policies based on the following principles: screening; psychological support; close observation; removal of dangerous items; clear and consistent procedures; and diagnosis, treatment, and transfer of suicidal inmates to the hospital as necessary (Felthous 1994).

Comprehensive suicide prevention programming has also been advocated nationally by such organizations as the American Correctional Association (ACA), American Psychiatric Association (APA), and National Commission on Correctional Health Care (NCCHC). These groups have promulgated national correctional standards that are adaptable to individual jail, prison, and juvenile facilities. Although the ACA standards are the most widely recognized throughout the country, they provide severely limited guidance regarding suicide prevention, simply stating that institutions should have a written prevention policy that is reviewed by medical or mental health staff. ACA's broad focus on the operation and administration of correctional facilities precludes these standards from containing needed specificity (American Correctional Association 1991).

Both the APA and NCCHC standards, however, are much more instructive and offer the recommended ingredients for a suicide prevention program: identification, training, assessment, monitoring, housing, referral, communication, intervention, notification, reporting, review, and critical incident debriefing (American Psychiatric Association 2000; National Commission on Correctional Health Care 1999, 2003). Consistent with national correctional standards, the eight components discussed below (and outlined in Table 4–1) encompass a comprehensive suicide prevention policy.

Staff Training

The essential component of any suicide prevention program is properly trained correctional staff, who form the backbone of any jail or prison facility. Very few suicides are actually prevented by mental health, medical, or other professional staff, because suicides are usually attempted in inmate housing units, often during late evening hours or on weekends when inmates are generally outside the purview of program staff. These incidents, therefore, must be thwarted by correctional staff who have been trained in suicide prevention and have developed an intuitive sense about the inmates under their care. Correctional officers are often the only staff available 24 hours a day; thus, they form the front line of defense in preventing suicides. However, as is true with medical and mental health personnel, correctional staff cannot detect, assess, or prevent a suicide without training. Bluntly stated, lives will be lost and jurisdictions will incur unnecessary liability from these deaths if administrators do not create and maintain effective training programs.

All staff (including correctional, medical, and mental health personnel) should receive 8 hours of initial suicide prevention training, followed by 2 hours

TABLE 4–1. Components of a comprehensive suicide prevention policy

- Staff training
- Intake screening and assessment
- Communication
- Housing
- Levels of observation
- Intervention
- Reporting
- Follow-up and mortality review

of refresher training each year. At a minimum, initial suicide prevention training should include, but not be limited to, the following:

- Reasons why correctional environments are conducive to suicidal behavior
- Staff attitudes about suicide
- Potential predisposing factors to suicide
- High-risk suicide periods
- Warning signs and symptoms
- Identification of suicide risk despite the denial of risk
- Liability issues
- Critical incident stress debriefing
- Recent suicides and/or serious suicide attempts within the facility/agency
- Components of the facility/agency's suicide prevention policy

In addition, all staff who have routine contact with inmates should receive standard first aid and cardiopulmonary resuscitation (CPR) training. All staff should also be trained in the use of various emergency equipment located in each housing unit. In an effort to ensure an efficient emergency response to suicide attempts, "mock drills" should be incorporated into both initial and refresher training for all staff. Table 4–2 highlights the important components of staff training for suicide prevention.

Intake Screening and Assessment

Screening and assessment of inmates when they enter a facility is also critical to a correctional facility's suicide prevention efforts. Although there is no single set of risk factors that mental health and medical communities agree can be used to predict suicide, there is little disagreement about the value of screen-

---

TABLE 4–2.   Staff suicide prevention training

- Suicide risk factors
- Suicide risk factors inherent in the correctional environment
- Analysis of staff attitudes about suicide
- Identification of high-risk suicide periods
- Identification of suicide warning signs and symptoms
- Identification of suicidality despite verbal denial of risk
- Liability issues
- Critical incident stress debriefing
- Discussion about completed suicides and attempts in the facility
- Discussion about sound suicide prevention practices and the facility's written suicide prevention policy

---

ing and assessment in preventing suicide (Cox and Morschauser 1997; Hughes 1995). Intake screening for all inmates and ongoing assessment of inmates at risk are critical because research consistently reports that two-thirds or more of all suicide victims communicate their intent some time before death and that any individual with a history of one or more suicide attempts is at a much greater risk for suicide than those who have never made an attempt (Clark and Horton-Deutsch 1992; Maris 1992). Although ideation, prior attempt(s), and/or other forms of suicidal behavior are indicative of current risk, other factors such as recent significant loss, limited prior incarceration, lack of social support system, and various "stressors of confinement" can also be strongly related to suicide (Bonner 1992).

Intake screening may be contained within the medical screening form or as a separate form and should include inquiry regarding past suicidal ideation and/or attempts; current ideation, threat, and plan; prior mental health treatment/hospitalization; recent significant loss (job, relationship, death of family member/close friend, etc.); history of suicidal behavior by family member/ close friend; suicide risk during prior confinement; and arresting/transporting officer(s) belief that inmate is currently at risk. The process should also include referral procedures to mental health and/or medical personnel for assessment.

Following the intake process, if any staff hear an inmate verbalize a desire or intent to commit suicide, observe an inmate engaging any self-harm, or otherwise believe an inmate is at risk for suicide, a procedure must be in place to allow the staff member to take immediate steps to ensure that the inmate is continuously observed until appropriate assistance is obtained. Important aspects of a suicide screening form are outlined in Table 4–3.

TABLE 4–3. Suicide screening form

- Past suicidal ideation and/or attempts
- Current suicidal ideation
- Current suicide threat
- Current suicide plan
- Current suicide intent
- Prior mental health treatment/hospitalization
- Recent significant loss (job, relationship, death of family member/close friend, etc.)
- Suicide risk during prior confinement
- Arresting/transporting officer(s) view of inmate's current risk

Communication

Certain behavioral signs exhibited by the inmate may be indicative of suicidal behavior, and detection of these signs and communication of their presence to others may prevent a suicide. There are essentially three stages of communication in preventing inmate suicides: 1) communication between the arresting/transporting officer and correctional staff; 2) communication among facility staff (including correctional, medical, and mental health personnel); and 3) communication between facility staff and the suicidal inmate.

In large measure, suicide prevention begins at the point of arrest. During initial contact, what an individual says and how he or she behaves during arrest, transportation to the jail, and booking are crucial in detecting suicidal behavior. The scene of arrest is often the most volatile and emotional time for the arrestee. Arresting officers should pay close attention to the arrestee during this time because suicidal behavior, anxiety, and/or hopelessness of the situation might be manifested. Prior behavior can also be confirmed by onlookers such as family and friends. Any pertinent information regarding the arrestee's well-being must be communicated by the arresting or transporting officer to facility staff. As noted in the previous subsection, the intake screening form should document whether the arresting/transporting officer believes that the inmate is currently at risk for suicide. It is also critically important for facility staff not to create barriers of communication between themselves and the inmate's inner circle of family and friends, because this group often has pertinent information regarding the current and prior mental health status of the inmate.

Because an inmate can become suicidal at any point during incarceration, correctional officers must maintain awareness, share information, and make appropriate referrals to mental health and medical staff. At a minimum, facility officials should ensure that appropriate staff are properly informed of the status of each inmate placed on suicide precautions. Multidisciplinary team meetings (to include correctional, medical, and mental health personnel) should occur on a regular basis for the various team members to discuss the status of an inmate on suicide precautions. In addition, the authorization of suicide precautions for an inmate, any changes to those precautions, and observation of an inmate placed on suicide precautions should be documented on designated forms and distributed to appropriate staff.

Facility staff must also use various communication skills with the suicidal inmate, including active listening, staying with the inmate if they suspect immediate danger, and maintaining contact through conversation, eye contact, and body language.

Most importantly, correctional staff should trust their own judgment and observation of risk behavior, and avoid being misled by others (including mental health staff) into ignoring signs of suicidal behavior. Because correctional staff have the unique opportunity to observe inmate behavior over an extended period of time (e.g., an 8-hour shift, several days), they are generally in the best position to identify signs and symptoms of suicidal behavior. Mental health staff generally spend a brief amount of time assessing an inmate's risk for suicide, and an inmate may deny and/or mask his or her symptoms. For example, it is not uncommon for correctional staff to place an inmate on suicide precautions after observing suicidal behavior. The inmate is then referred to mental health staff for assessment. The inmate then denies any suicidal ideation, and the clinician does not observe any self-harm behavior; the inmate is released from suicide precautions and returned to his or her housing unit. The inmate again begins to engage in suicidal behavior that is observed by an officer. Should the officer discount these observations, on the basis of the recent assessment by mental health staff that concluded the inmate was not suicidal? The appropriate response would be for the officer to again place the inmate on suicide precautions, document his or her observations of the suicidal behavior, refer the inmate to mental health staff for further assessment, and share his or her observations with the clinician.

Finally, the communication breakdown between correctional, medical, and mental health personnel is a common factor found in the reviews of many inmate suicides (Anno 1985; Appelbaum et al. 1997; Hayes 1995).

Housing

While considerable energy is often devoted to the areas of staff training, identification, assessment, and observation, less thought is given to the physical plant environment. Inmates placed on suicide precautions are frequently housed in unsafe cells containing protrusions (i.e., anchoring devices) conducive to suicide by hanging. It is well established that hanging is the method of choice in the overwhelming majority of inmate suicides (Hayes 1989). Research has now begun to identify specific common anchoring devices in these deaths. One study, for example, indicated that air vent grates were used in over 50% of prison suicides by hanging (He et al. 2003). Recently, the first national study on juvenile suicides found that door knobs/hinges (21%), air vent grates (20%), bunk frames/holes (20%), and window frames (15%) were the anchoring devices used in most youth deaths (Hayes 2005). Finally, telephones with cords of varying length located inside holding cells have been shown to be dangerous in facilitating hanging attempts (Hayes 2003a; Quinton and Dolinak 2003).

Although impossible to create a "suicide-proof" cell environment within any correctional facility, it is certainly reasonable to ensure that any cell used to house a potentially suicidal inmate is free of all obvious protrusions (Atlas 1989; Hayes 2003b). Decisions regarding the location of cells designated to house suicidal inmates should be based on the ability to maximize staff interaction with those inmates. To every extent possible, suicidal inmates should be housed in the general population, mental health unit, or medical infirmary, if available, but should always be located close to staff. As a federal appeals court once stated, "It is true that prison officials are not required to build a suicide-proof jail. By the same token, however, they cannot equip each cell with a noose" (Tittle v. Jefferson County Commission 1992).

Levels of Observation

With regard to suicide attempts in correctional facilities, the promptness of the emergency response is often driven by the level of observation afforded the inmate. Medical experts warn that brain damage from strangulation caused by a suicide attempt can occur within 4 minutes, and death often takes place within 5–6 minutes (American Heart Association 1992). Standard correctional practice requires that "special management inmates," including those housed in administrative segregation, disciplinary detention, and protective custody, be observed at intervals not exceeding every 30 minutes, with mentally ill inmates observed more frequently (American Correctional Association 1991). Inmates held in medical restraints and "therapeutic seclusion" should be observed at intervals that do not exceed every 15 minutes (National Commission on Correctional Health Care 2003).

Consistent with national correctional standards and practices, two levels of supervision are generally recommended for suicidal inmates: close observation and constant observation. *Close observation* is reserved for the inmate who is not actively suicidal but expresses suicidal ideation (e.g., expressing a wish to die without a specific threat or plan) and/or an inmate who denies suicidal ideation but demonstrates other concerning behavior (through actions, current circumstances, or recent history). Staff should observe such an inmate at staggered intervals not to exceed every 15 minutes (e.g., 5, 10, 7 minutes). *Constant observation* is reserved for the inmate who is actively suicidal, either threatening or engaging in suicidal behavior. Staff should observe such an inmate on a continuous, uninterrupted basis.

In some jurisdictions, an intermediate level of observation is used with monitoring at staggered intervals that do not exceed every 5 minutes. Of course, there should never be a situation in which a suicidal inmate is placed on a 30-minute observation level, because such a time frame provides little protection for the individual. Other aids (e.g., closed-circuit television, inmate companions or watchers) can be used as a supplement to, but never as a substitute for, these observation levels. Finally, mental health staff should assess and interact with (not just observe) suicidal inmates on a daily basis.

Intervention

Many correctional officials cling to the misguided belief that suicide prevention begins when the inmate is initially screened for suicide risk during the intake process and ends when they are discharged from a level of observation by mental health personnel. Yet suicide prevention is a multidimensional issue and includes effective intervention following incidents of self-injury. More importantly, following a suicide attempt, the degree and promptness of the staff's intervention often foretell whether the victim will survive. National correctional standards and practices generally acknowledge that a facility's policy regarding intervention should be threefold (National Commission on Correctional Health Care 1999): 1) all staff who come into contact with inmates should be trained in standard first aid and CPR procedures; 2) any staff member who discovers an inmate engaging in self-harm should immediately survey the scene to assess the severity of the emergency, alert other staff to call for medical personnel, and begin standard first aid and/or CPR as necessary; and 3) staff should never presume that the inmate is dead, but rather should initiate and continue appropriate life-saving measures until relieved by arriving medial personnel. Finally, medical personnel should ensure that all equipment utilized in responding to an emergency within the facility is in working order on a daily basis.

Reporting

In the event of a completed suicide or attempt, all appropriate correctional officials should be notified through the chain of command. Following the incident, the victim's family should be notified immediately, as well as appropriate outside authorities. All staff that came into contact with the victim prior to the incident should be required to submit a statement including their full knowledge of the inmate and incident.

Follow-up and Mortality Review

An inmate suicide can be extremely stressful for staff. They may also feel ostracized by fellow personnel and administration officials. After a death, reasonable guilt is sometimes displayed by the officer, who wonders: "What if I had made my cell check earlier?" When crises occur and staff are affected by the traumatic event, they should receive appropriate assistance. One form of assistance is *critical incident stress debriefing* (CISD). A CISD team, consisting of professionals trained in crisis intervention and traumatic stress awareness (e.g., police officers, paramedics, fire fighters, clergy, and mental health personnel), provides affected staff members an opportunity to process their feelings about the incident, develop an understanding of critical stress symptoms, and develop ways of dealing with those symptoms (Meehan 1997; Mitchell and Everly 1996). For maximum effectiveness, the CISD process or other appropriate support services should occur within 24–72 hours of the critical incident.

Every completed suicide, as well as suicide attempt of high lethality (i.e., requiring hospitalization), should be examined through a mortality review process. If resources permit, clinical review through a psychological autopsy is also recommended (Aufderheide 2000; Sanchez 1999). Ideally, the mortality review should be coordinated by an outside agency to ensure impartiality. The review, separate and apart from other formal investigations that may be required to determine the cause of death, should include a critical inquiry of 1) the circumstances surrounding the incident, 2) jail procedures relevant to the incident, 3) all relevant training received by involved staff, 4) pertinent medical and mental health services/reports involving the victim, 5) possible precipitating factors leading to the suicide, and 6) recommendations, if any, for changes in policy, training, physical plant, medical or mental health services, and operational procedures.

Finally, it should be noted that quality assurance documents (i.e., mortality reviews) generated as a result of an inmate death or injury are *not* always protected from disclosure provisions of applicable state and/or federal laws. As such, in order to better ensure that the mortality review process is conducted with the full candor of all participants, as well as to increase the likelihood of protecting such documents from future disclosure, it is strongly recommended that each mortality review be initiated at the request of the agency's legal counsel. In addition, any documents generated during the mortality review should *not* be kept in an inmate's institutional or medical file. Rather, the documents should be kept separately in a quality assurance file and each page clearly labeled as follows: "Attorney-Client Privilege: This Quality Assurance Document was Attorney-Requested and Prepared in Anticipation of Possible Litigation."

GUIDING PRINCIPLES FOR SUICIDE PREVENTION

More times than not, we do an admirable job of safely managing inmates who have been identified as suicidal and placed on suicide precautions. After all, few inmates successfully commit suicide on suicide watch. What we continue to struggle with is the ability to prevent the suicide of an inmate who is not easily identifiable as being at risk for self-harm. Kay Redfield Jamison, a prominent psychologist and author, has best articulated the point by stating that if "suicidal patients were able or willing to articulate the severity of their suicidal thoughts and plans, little risk would exist" (Jamison 1999, p. 150). With this in mind, the following guiding principles to suicide prevention are offered:

1. *View the assessment of suicide risk* not *as a single event but as an ongoing process.* Because an inmate may become suicidal at any point during confinement, suicide prevention should begin at the point of arrest and continue until the inmate is released from the facility. In addition, once an inmate has been successfully managed on, and discharged from, suicide precautions, he or she should remain on a mental health caseload and assessed periodically until released from the facility.

2. *View screening for suicide during the initial booking and intake process as something similar to taking one's temperature: it can identify a current fever, but not a future cold.* The shelf life of behavior that is observed and/or self-reported during intake screening is time-limited, and we often place far too much weight on this initial data collection stage. Following an inmate suicide, it is not unusual for the mortality review process to focus exclusively on whether the victim threatened suicide during the booking and intake stage—a time period that could be far removed from the date of suicide. If the victim had answered in the negative to suicide risk during the booking stage, there is often a sense of relief expressed by participants of the mortality, as well as a misguided conclusion that the death was not preventable. Although the intake screening form remains a valuable prevention tool, the more important determination of suicide risk is the *current* behavior expressed and/ or displayed by the inmate.

3. *Determine the inmate's prior risk of suicide.* Prior risk of suicide is strongly related to future risk. If an inmate was placed on suicide precautions during

a previous confinement in the facility or agency, that information should be accessible to both correctional and health care personnel when determining whether the inmate might be at risk during their current confinement.

4. *Do not rely exclusively on the direct statements of an inmate who denies being suicidal and/or having a prior history of suicidal behavior, particularly when his or her behavior, actions, and/or history suggest otherwise.* Often, despite an inmate's denial of suicidal ideation, the inmate's behavior, actions, and/or history speak louder then his or her words. Consider the two examples below:

In Washington State, an inmate, on being booked into a county jail, informed the intake officer that she had a history of mental illness and had attempted suicide 2 weeks earlier, but "will not hurt herself in jail." Jail records indicated that the inmate had threatened suicide during a recent prior confinement in the facility. The inmate attended a court hearing 2 days later, and the escort officer noticed that she appeared despondent, was crying, and appeared worried about her children. She was not referred to mental health staff or placed on suicide precautions. The inmate committed suicide the following day.

In Michigan, police were called to the home of a man who accidentally shot and killed a friend during a domestic dispute with his estranged wife. On arrival of the police, the suspect placed a handgun to his head and clicked the trigger several times. He also encouraged the officers to shoot him. Following 5 hours of negotiations, the suspect surrendered without incident. He was transported to the county jail and denied being suicidal during the intake screening process. The inmate was not referred to mental health staff or placed on suicide precautions. He committed suicide the following day.

It is not all that surprising that these preventable deaths often escape our detection. Take, for example, the booking area of a jail facility. It is traditionally both chaotic and noisy—an environment where staff feel pressure to process a high number of arrestees in a short period of time. Two key ingredients for identifying suicidal behavior—time and privacy—are at a minimum. The ability to carefully assess the potential for suicide by asking the inmate a series of questions, interpreting their responses (including gauging the truthfulness of their denial of suicide risk), and observing their behavior is greatly compromised by an impersonal environment that lends itself to something quite the opposite. As a result, the clearly suicidal behavior of many arrestees, as well as circumstances that may lend themselves to potential self-injury, is lost to detection.

In yet another example, a suicidal inmate may appear to be stable in front of a mental health clinician, and even deny suicide risk, only to be discharged from suicide precautions and returned to the correctional facility from a hospital, where they revert to the same self-injurious behavior that prompted the initial referral. Given such a scenario, correctional staff should not assume that the clinician was cognizant or even appreciative of this cyclical behavior. On the contrary, regardless of what the clinician might have observed and/or recommended, as well as the inmate's denial of risk, whenever correctional staff hear an inmate verbalize a desire or intent to commit suicide, observe an inmate engaging in suicidal behavior, or otherwise believe an inmate is at risk for suicide, they should take immediate steps to ensure the inmate's safety.

5. *Promote and maintain communication among correctional, medical, and mental health staff.* As previously offered, many preventable suicides result from poor communication among correctional, medical, and mental health staff. Communication problems are often caused by lack of respect, personality conflicts, and other boundary issues. Simply stated, facilities that maintain a multidisciplinary approach avoid preventable suicides. As aptly stated by one clinician:

> The key to an effective team approach in suicide prevention and crisis intervention is found in throwing off the cloaks of territoriality and embracing a mutual respect for the detention officer's and mental health clinician's professional abilities, responsibilities and limitations. All of us, regardless of professional affiliation, need to make a dedicated commitment to come forward and acknowledge that suicide prevention and related mental health services are only effective when delivered by professionals acting in unison with each other. Just as the security officer alone can not ensure the safety and security of the jail facility, neither can the mental health clinician alone ensure the safety and emotional well-being of the individual inmate. (Severson 1993, p. 3)

6. *Avoid creating barriers that discourage an inmate from accessing mental health services.* Often, certain management conditions of a facility's policy on suicide precautions (e.g., automatic clothing removal/issuance of safety garment; lockdown; limited visiting, telephone, and shower access) appear punitive to an inmate, as well as excessive and unrelated to their level of suicide risk. As a result, an inmate who becomes suicidal and/or despondent during confinement may be reluctant to seek out mental health services, and may even deny there is a problem, if he or she knows that loss of these and other basic amenities are an automatic outcome. As such, these barriers should be avoided whenever possible, and decisions regarding the management of a suicidal inmate should be based solely on the individual's level of risk.

7. *Be especially vigilant about suicide risk when inmate is not on formal suicide precautions, such as in "special housing units" of the facility.* As previously noted, few suicides take place when inmates are managed on suicide precautions.

Rather, most suicides take place in various forms of (often locked down) "special housing units" (e.g., intake/booking, classification, disciplinary/ administrative segregation, mental health) of the facility. One effective prevention strategy is to create more interaction between inmates and correctional, medical, and mental health personnel in these housing areas by 1) increasing rounds of medical and/or mental health staff, in which these personnel walk up to each cell, attempt to briefly converse with the inmate, and observe his or her behavior; 2) requiring regular follow-up of all inmates released from suicide precautions; 3) increasing rounds of correctional staff; and 4) avoiding lockdown due to staff shortages (and the resulting limited access of medical and mental health personnel to the units).

8. *Create and maintain sound suicide prevention programming.* Such programming should include the eight essential components described earlier in this chapter. It also should include a comprehensively written suicide prevention policy that is reviewed and adhered to by all correctional, medical, and mental health personnel in the correctional facility.

9. *Avoid obstacles to prevention.* Experience has shown that negative attitudes often impede meaningful suicide prevention efforts. These obstacles to prevention often embody a state of mind that unconditionally implies that inmate suicides cannot be prevented (e.g., "If someone really wants to kill themselves there's generally nothing you can do about it.") There are numerous ways to overcome these obstacles, the most powerful of which is to demonstrate prevention programs that have effectively reduced the incidence of suicide and suicidal behavior within correctional facilities. As one administrator has offered: "When you begin to use excuses to justify a bad outcome, whether it be low staffing levels, inadequate funding, physical plant concerns, etc., issues we struggle with each day, you lack the philosophy that even one death is not acceptable. If you are going to tolerate a few deaths in your jail system, then you've already lost the battle" (Hayes 1998, p. 6).

CONCLUSION

Hundreds of inmates continue to commit suicide in jail and prison facilities each year. Despite increased general awareness of the problem, research that has identified precipitating and situational risk factors, emerging correctional standards that advocate increased attention to suicidal inmates, and demonstration of effective strategies, prevention remains piecemeal and inmate suicides continue to pose a serious public health problem within correctional facilities throughout the county. Although not all inmate suicides are preventable, many are, and the challenge for those who work in the correctional system is to conceptualize the issue as demanding a continuum of comprehensive suicide prevention services aimed at the collaborative identification, continued assessment, and safe management of inmates at risk for self-harm.

SUMMARY POINTS

- Suicide assessment is an ongoing process.
- Suicide risk screening at intake is important, but *current* behavior is more significant.
- Prior suicide risk is strongly related to future risk.
- Do not rely *exclusively* on an inmate's denial of suicidality. Behavior, actions, and history are extremely important.
- Communication among correctional, medical, and mental health staff is crucial.
- Mental health services must be accessible to inmates.
- Most suicides occur in "special housing units" and not while inmates are on suicide precautions.
- Comprehensive suicide prevention programming must be in place.
- Negative attitudes often impede meaningful suicide prevention efforts.

REFERENCES

American Correctional Association: Standards for Adult Local Detention Facilities, 3rd Edition. Lanham, MD, American Correctional Association, 1991

American Heart Association, Emergency Cardiac Care Committee and Subcommittees: Guidelines for cardiopulmonary resuscitation and emergency cardiac care. JAMA 268:2172–2183, 1992

American Psychiatric Association: Psychiatric Services in Jails and Prisons, 2nd Edition. Washington, DC, American Psychiatric Association, 2000

Anno B: Patterns of suicide in the Texas Department of Corrections, 1980–1985. J Prison Jail Health 5:82–93, 1985

Appelbaum K, Dvoskin J, Geller J, et al: Report on the Psychiatric Management of John Salvi in Massachusetts Department of Corrections Facilities: 1995–1996. Worcester, University of Massachusetts Medical Center, 1997

Atlas R: Reducing the opportunity for inmate suicide: a design guide. Psychiatr Q 60: 161–171, 1989

Aufderheide D: Conducting the psychological autopsy in correctional settings. Journal of Correctional Health Care 7:5–36, 2000

Bonner R: Isolation, seclusion, and psychological vulnerability as risk factors for suicide behind bars, in Assessment and Prediction of Suicide. Edited by Maris R, Berman A, Maltsberger J. New York, Guilford, 1992, pp 398–419

Bonner R: Correctional suicide prevention in the year 2000 and beyond. Suicide Life Threat Behav 30:370–376, 2000

Bureau of Justice Statistics, Office of Justice Programs: Correctional populations in the United States, 1997 (NCJ 177613). Washington, DC, Bureau of Justice Statistics, U.S. Department of Justice, November 2000

Clark D, Horton-Deutsch S: Assessment in absentia: the value of the psychological autopsy method for studying antecedents of suicide and predicting future suicides, in Assessment and Prediction of Suicide. Edited by Maris R, Berman A, Maltsberger J. New York, Guilford, 1992, pp 144–182

Cox J, Morschauser P: A solution to the problem of jail suicide. Crisis: The Journal of Crisis Intervention and Suicide Prevention 18:178–184, 1997

Davis M, Muscat J: An epidemiologic study of alcohol and suicide risk in Ohio jails and lockups, 1975–1984. Journal of Criminal Justice 21:277–283, 1993

DuRand C, Burtka G, Federman E, et al: A quarter century of suicide in a major urban jail: implications for community psychiatry. Am J Psychiatry 152:1077–1080, 1995

Felthous A: Preventing jailhouse suicides. Bull Am Acad Psychiatry Law 22:477–488, 1994

Goss J, Peterson K, Smith L, et al: Characteristics of suicide attempts in a large urban jail system with an established suicide prevention program. Psychiatr Serv 53:574–579, 2002

Hanser R: Inmate suicide in prisons: an analysis of legal liability under 42 USC sec 1983. The Prison Journal 82:459–477, 2002

Hayes L: National study of jail suicides: seven years later. Psychiatr Q 60:7–29, 1989

Hayes L: Prison suicide: an overview and guide to prevention. The Prison Journal 75:431–456, 1995

Hayes L: Jail standards and suicide prevention: another look. Jail Suicide/Mental Health Update 6:9–11, 1996

Hayes L: Model suicide prevention programs, Part III. Jail Suicide/Mental Health Update 8:1–6, 1998

Hayes L: A jail cell, two deaths, and a telephone cord. Jail Suicide/Mental Health Update 11:1–8, 2003a

Hayes L: Suicide prevention and protrusion-free design of correctional facilities. Jail Suicide/Mental Health Update 12:1–5, 2003b

Hayes L: Juvenile Suicide in Confinement: A National Survey. Washington, DC, Office of Juvenile Justice and Delinquency Prevention, U.S. Justice Department, 2005

He X, Felthous A, Holzer C, et al: Factors in prison suicide: one year study in Texas. J Forensic Sci 46:896–901, 2003

Hughes D: Can the clinician predict suicide? Psychiatr Serv 46:449–451, 1995

Jamison K: Night Falls Fast: Understanding Suicide. New York, Knopf, 1999

Marcus P, Alcabes P: Characteristics of suicides by inmates in an urban jail. Hosp Community Psychiatry 44:256–261, 1993

Maris R: Overview of the study of suicide assessment and prediction, in Assessment and Prediction of Suicide. Edited by Maris R, Berman A, Maltsberger J. New York, Guilford, 1992, pp 3–22

Meehan B: Critical incident stress debriefing within the jail environment. Jail Suicide/Mental Health Update 7:1–5, 1997

Mitchell J, Everly G: Critical Incident Stress Debriefing: An Operations Manual for the Prevention of Traumatic Stress Among Emergency Services and Disaster Workers, 2nd Edition. Ellicott City, MD, Chevron Publishing, 1996

National Commission on Correctional Health Care: Correctional Mental Health Care: Standards and Guidelines for Delivering Services. Chicago, IL, National Commission on Correctional Health Care, 1999

National Commission on Correctional Health Care: Standards for Health Services in Jails. Chicago, IL, National Commission on Correctional Health Care, 2003

New York State Department of Correctional Services: Inmate Suicide Report, 1995–2001. Albany, New York State Department of Correctional Services, 2002

Quinton R, Dolinak D: Suicidal hangings in jail using telephone cords. J Forensic Sci 48:1151–1152, 2003

Salive M, Smith G, Brewer T: Suicide mortality in the Maryland state prison system, 1979 through 1987. JAMA 262:365–369, 1989

Sanchez H: Inmate suicide and the psychological autopsy process. Jail Suicide/Mental Health Update 8:3–9, 1999

Sanville v Scaburdine, U.S. District Court, Eastern District of Wisconsin, Case No 99-C-715, 2002

Severson M: Security and mental health professionals: a (too) silent partnership? Jail Suicide Update 5:1–6, 1993

Stephan J: Census of Jails, 1999 (NCJ 186633). Washington, DC, Office of Justice Programs, Bureau of Justice Statistics, U.S. Department of Justice, August 2001

Tittle v Jefferson County Commission, 966 F.2d 606 (11th Cir. 1992)

White T, Schimmel D: Suicide prevention in federal prisons: a successful five-step program, in Prison Suicide: An Overview and Guide to Prevention. Edited by Hayes L. Washington, DC, National Institute of Corrections, U.S. Department of Justice, 1995, pp 46–57

Winkler G: Assessing and responding to suicidal jail inmates. Community Ment Health J 28:317–326, 1992

Woodward v Myres, U.S. District Court, Northern District of Illinois, Case No 00-C-6010, 2003

CHAPTER 5

Psychopharmacology in Correctional Settings

Kathryn A. Burns, M.D., M.P.H.

Since the early 1990s, the use of psychotropic medications in correctional settings has undergone a profound transformation. In the not so distant past, there was a tendency to use psychotropic medications, and in particular antipsychotic medications, for their sedating side effects as a means of managing undesirable behavior. Courts presiding over correctional litigation cases viewed psychotropic medications as "dangerous drugs" prescribed to control thinking and behavior (Ruiz v. Estelle 1980). Scientific advances in understanding serious mental illnesses as biologically based brain disorders and prescriptive advances in targeting psychotropic medication toward amelioration or elimination of specific symptoms have reformed psychopharmacological practice in both civilian and correctional populations. Subsequent class-action correctional litigation has underscored that the availability of psychotropic medication is a necessary component of inmate mental health care. Inmates with serious mental illness have a constitutional right to treatment of their condition. Withholding treatment of serious mental illness constitutes cruel and unusual punishment, a violation of the U.S. Constitution's Eighth amendment (Cohen 1998). Psychotropic medication is the medically accepted standard of care or treatment of choice for certain of the serious mental illnesses.

In this chapter, I address psychopharmacological principles in correctional settings, highlighting those aspects of care that are unique or deserving of special consideration in the correctional environment. I do not intend to imply that treatment with psychotropic medication is the sole requirement for appropriate mental health care of inmates; but rather, psychotropic medication is one component of a comprehensive treatment plan. Other treatment plan components are based on the clinical condition being treated and the duration and conditions of confinement but will not be discussed as they are outside the scope of this chapter. Underlying this chapter are two assumptions: that psychotropic medications will only be prescribed when they are clinically indicated and will not be used for disciplinary purposes, and that the correctional facility will have appropriately trained staff in sufficient numbers to periodically monitor clinical response and potential side effects when psychotropic medications are used.

PSYCHOPHARMACOTHERAPEUTIC PRINCIPLES REQUIRING SPECIAL CONSIDERATION IN CORRECTIONAL FACILITIES

Informed Consent

Correctional facilities, by their very nature, are inherently coercive environments. Nevertheless, the principles of informed consent remain applicable to inmates. The nature and purpose of treatment and the risks and benefits of potential types of treatment, including the risks and benefits of no treatment, should be explained such that the inmate can make an informed choice. The discussion itself and the inmate's consent to treatment should be documented in the medical record. As in civilian populations, this documentation may take the form of a detailed progress note or a specialized form that the inmate is asked to sign. Inmates also have a right to refuse treatment. Facility policies concerning their right to refuse treatment should conform to the rules and procedures of the jurisdiction in which the facility is located (American Psychiatric Association 2000).

Involuntary Medication: Ability to Force Medication

As in the civilian world, forcible administration of medication during an emergency is permissible if it is administered for medical reasons and for a limited duration of time. An *emergency* is defined as an imminent threat to the life or safety of the inmate or others or significant property destruction. Emergency administration of medication may prevent the need for the application of physical restraints or may be used to assist the inmate in regaining control of their thoughts and behavior if physical restraint is used. Procedures for the administration of medication during an emergency should conform to the pertinent requirements of the jurisdiction in which the facility is located.

In other, "nonemergency" situations, correctional settings also have the capacity to administer psychotropic medication to competent but refusing inmates, provided that the correctional facility follows certain procedural requirements. Correctional facilities have an obligation to protect the safety of other inmates in their custody, their own staff, and visitors, and they have an interest in maintaining order in the facility. Therefore, under certain circumstances, correctional facilities may override medication refusals when an inmate has a mental disorder and poses a likelihood of serious harm to self or others or is gravely disabled (Washington v. Harper 1990).

In 1990, the U.S. Supreme Court upheld a prison policy in Washington State that provided the following rights to inmates facing involuntary medication: the right to a hearing on the issue; the right to notice of the hearing; the rights to attend the hearing, present evidence, and cross-examine witnesses; the right to representation by a lay advisor; the right to appeal the decision; and the right to periodic review of ongoing administration of involuntary medication (Washington v. Harper 1990). Under the Washington State statute, the involuntary medication hearing is presided over by a small committee, composed of medical/mental health professionals with no current treatment relationship with the inmate, who must render a medical decision regarding the necessity of treatment with medication. Security factors may be considered, but the decision is primarily medical (Cohen 1998). Individual state laws may impose additional procedural requirements beyond these rights that were accepted as adequate by the *Harper* court.

Medication Administration

Virtually all psychotropic medication doses are individually administered in correctional settings. Medication administration is the act in which a single dose of an identified medication is given to an inmate. Correctional systems have devised several different mechanisms to accomplish this goal. This process can include "pill call" or centralized "med pass," medication "delivery" processes, or a combination of different systems.

Larger correctional facilities that permit inmate movement (alone or with correctional escorts) have a centralized medication administration area in the medical clinic or infirmary. At scheduled medication administration times, inmates walk or are escorted to the centralized administration area to receive their medications. In this model, inmates generally wait in a single-file line under the supervision of a correctional officer until called up to a medication administration "window" by a health care worker, most often a nurse. The nurse checks the inmate's identity by looking at his or her identification; reviews the medication administration record (MAR) to be certain which medications, their doses and form (liquid, pill, injectable) are to be administered at the time of the pill call; and visually inspects the medication before handing it to the inmate. Medication ingestion is observed during this process, usually accomplished by the correctional officer's supervising the inmates in line. The nurse who administers the medication makes the appropriate notation on the MAR, documenting the transaction at the time the medication is administered.

Facilities using this mechanism of medication administration must be mindful of the impact of the location, duration, and efficiency of the pill-call line administration process on medication compliance. For example, if inmates are required to wait out of doors for medication and the weather is inordinately hot or otherwise inclement, some inmates will be tempted to skip one or more doses of medication to avoid the unpleasant weather. Similarly, if receiving each dose of medication requires standing in line for more than 15–20 minutes, many inmates may opt to forgo their medication. Some facilities have attempted to address these potential problems by building an awning over the pill-call line or by issuing medications indoors to provide protection from the elements for inmates waiting in line. Others have staggered the times at which small groups of inmates are called over to the pill-call line. This may involve calling inmates over according to their assigned housing unit at staggered 5- to 10-minute intervals so that the line is never longer than 10–15 people in length.

In facilities where security concerns do not permit inmate movement to a centralized medication administration area, in segregation units, or in facilities that do not have a centralized medication administration area, medications are taken to the inmates' cells, pods, or cell blocks. Medications are administered in this delivery method by nursing staff or by correctional staff trained to do so. Certainly, it is preferable to have nursing staff administer all doses of prescription medication. Nurses can provide brief medication education during the administration process, are better able to answer questions posed by the inmate receiving the medication, and can make skilled observations of the effectiveness or potential side effects of the medication prescribed. However, some correctional facilities do not have round-the-clock nursing coverage and must use correctional officers to deliver medications. In this instance, the officers delivering medications must receive training in the basics of medication delivery to ensure that the right inmate receives the right medication at the right time, and that the process is appropriately documented. In addition, the state pharmacy and nursing boards should be consulted to ensure that the prescription medications are appropriately packaged and labeled for delivery by nonmedical personnel to be consistent with state law.

Some facilities have developed a self-carry or keep-on-person (KOP) medication administration procedure. This procedure allows some inmates to be given a specified amount of certain medications (generally medications for treatment of physical conditions) to maintain on their own and take as directed by prescription. Although any medication may be subject to a KOP procedure, psychotropic medication prescriptions are generally not subject to self-carry programs. The purpose of this limitation is to reduce the possibility of potential hoarding, overdose, trading, and/or noncompliance that might not become evident until an adverse effect on mental state or adverse incident occurs. Inmates on self-carry medication programs pick up their supply of medication from the infirmary or clinic area at proscribed intervals (often 30 days) and turn in any unused medication and/or the empty blister pack when the new supply is given to them.

Many correctional facilities, and particularly large ones, often use a combination of medication administration practices such as delivery to inmates in lock-down settings, centralized administration for general population, and a self-carry program for certain medications and/or for inmates who may not be available to participate in a centralized pill-call process because of their involvement in work details where schedules conflict with the posted pill-call times.

Since essentially all psychotropic medication is administered by staff in correctional settings (nursing staff or correctional officers trained in the appropriate delivery of medication) and recorded in real time, this represents a distinct advantage over practicing in a community outpatient setting. This practice provides valuable information about inmate medication compliance and staff observations of medication effectiveness not generally available in the community, where the only source of medication compliance information is self-report, and where observations of effectiveness are more limited to infrequent contacts. *Medication compliance* is the degree of patient adherence to taking all doses of medication as prescribed. Effectiveness of psychotropic medication is difficult, if not impossible, to assess unless the patient has been 100% compliant with taking all doses of the medication as prescribed.

These major advantages are not without some challenges, however. Medication administration records are most often maintained for the current month (and sometimes recent past month) in a location separate from the inmate medical/mental health files and, therefore, are not always immediately or readily available during mental health clinic appointments with the inmate. In addition, the time involved and staff intensiveness of some medication administration processes may limit the number of "med passes" or "pill calls" that may be accomplished during the day.

Fortunately, most psychotropic medication may be taken in once- or twice-daily doses based on their metabolism or half-life. Some medications may require more frequent delivery times, but this should be the exception, as it is often unnecessary based on metabolism, reduces inmate compliance due to the added burden of frequent dosing, and creates added work for nursing and correctional staff. Prescribers' capacity to order "stat" (emergency) medications and/or "prn" (as needed) medications may be limited.

It is imperative that prescribers of psychotropic medication be familiar with the correctional facility's medication processes, procedures, and administration times. Such familiarity may assist in choosing among various alternative medications on the basis of recommended dosing schedules, be of assistance to medication administration staff, and permit accurate orders for laboratory testing, particularly trough serum levels of medications. It is also necessary that psychotropic medication prescribers advocate for appropriate medication administration times, consistent with medication pharmacodynamics and actions. For example, administration of hs (hour of sleep) medications at 3:00 P.M. in the afternoon is problematic in terms of lithium pharmacodynamics if trough medication serum levels are drawn at 9:00 A.M. the next morning. Similarly, if medication that is sedating is prescribed at bedtime to avoid daytime sedation, afternoon administration, rather than hs administration, defeats this purpose. Some correctional facilities have attempted to eliminate hs medication administration times for budgetary reasons. Physicians must remain aware of these administrative decisions and provide appropriate education and advocacy to decision-makers when necessary so as not to compromise patient care.

Heat Sensitivity

Persons taking many of the psychotropic medications, and particularly antipsychotic and antidepressant medications, demonstrate an increased sensitivity to sunlight and are at higher risk of heat-induced syndromes: heat stroke, hyperthermia, and heat prostration. Heat stroke is a very serious and potentially fatal medical condition. Heat stroke develops with muscle cramps, weakness, nausea, vomiting, dehydration, increased heart rate, hyperventilation, hot skin (usually flushed, possibly ashen in severe cases), and agitation. Sustained high body temperatures that occur in untreated heat stroke may result in brain or muscle damage, kidney failure, coma, and even death. The occurrence of heat-related problems for inmates taking psychotropic medications may be exacerbated in correctional facilities where inmates may be assigned to work details out of doors and where many correctional facilities have very limited (or nonexistent) means of cooling the temperature in living areas of the facility.

When psychotropic medications are prescribed, appropriate precautions to prevent the development of heat-related problems should be exercised. When outdoor temperatures are elevated, excessive exhausting activities should be avoided, and when under direct sunlight, inmates should wear protective clothing and sunscreen. This has implications both for inmate outdoor work assignments and outdoor recreation activities. Additional water and break times must be provided. Inmate patients should be encouraged and permitted an adequate intake of fluid (8–12 glasses of liquid per day). Indoor temperatures of housing units should be monitored during periods of warm or hot weather and when the indoor temperature exceeds 90°F, consideration must be given to increasing ventilation (moving fans into the area), providing increased fluids and ice to the inmates, permitting additional showers to provide cooling, and even possibly transferring the patient to another area of the institution more compatible with clinical status.

It is imperative that correctional security, administrative, medical, and mental health staff be aware of the increased sensitivity of inmates taking psychotropic medication to heat-related problems, be able to recognize the signs and symptoms of heat stroke, and be able to respond rapidly to lower body temperature. Clinical Case 5–1 illustrates some of these important points.

Clinical Case 5–1

Mr. Smith is a 40-year-old inmate with a diagnosis of schizophrenia who is serving a 15-year sentence for assault. The symptoms of his schizophrenia have responded well to treatment with haloperidol 5 mg/day taken at bedtime. Mr. Smith's illness had been very stable for the past 4 years: He had a job assignment in his housing unit as an aid to another inmate, his roommate, who was wheelchair bound. He fulfilled his job assignment responsibly and was very attentive to his fellow inmate. Security staff often asked Mr. Smith to run errands for them relaying information between housing units or to other areas of the prison.

One summer evening, Mr. Smith suddenly began to behave in a bizarre manner: he stripped off all of his clothing and began yelling incoherently. He was noted to be sweating profusely. He did not respond to officers' attempts to get him to calm down, and his roommate became frightened. Medical staff had gone off-duty for the evening. Correctional staff moved Mr. Smith out of his cell into an observation area—a different cell in which he was housed alone. The cell did not contain a sink or commode, but officers permitted Mr. Smith to come out of the cell regularly for bathroom breaks and water. Medical staff were consulted and believed the problems were secondary to an exacerbation of mental illness. They did not see Mr. Smith but recommended consultation with the psychiatrist. No vital signs were taken, and the inmate was not physically assessed. The psychiatrist ordered an increased dosage of haloperidol, with which Mr. Smith was compliant.

Over the course of the next 2 days, Mr. Smith became increasingly confused and disoriented. His responses to questions were incoherent. He had great difficulty following instructions from correctional staff during bathroom breaks. He displayed difficulty operating the water fountain, and his fluid intake was nil. Similarly, officers noted his meal trays were returned untouched.

Neither medical nor mental health staff were notified of Mr. Smith's condition or lack of food and water intake. Cell block room temperatures were recorded as being between 90 and 94°F consistently throughout this time period. On the evening of the third day, Mr. Smith was discovered lifeless in his cell during routine rounds. Although CPR was initiated and EMS was summoned, Mr. Smith could not be revived. An autopsy revealed dehydration as the cause of death.

Use of Benzodiazepines

Benzodiazepine use in correctional facilities should be restricted to medical detoxification from alcohol and/or benzodiazepines and prevention of withdrawal syndromes. Intake facilities should have time-limited access to benzodiazepines for these purposes only. Benzodiazepine use is strongly discouraged in all other types of correctional facilities because of their high abuse potential in a population estimated to have a prevalence rate for substance use disorders of 70%–90% (American Psychiatric Association 2000). Use of benzodiazepines in correctional facilities raises the possibility of drug seeking or manipulation to obtain the medication and may set up serious security problems with bartering, selling, or trading the medication. Inmates with legitimate need may become targets of intimidation or assault by others seeking the benzodiazepine. Therefore, alternative, effective, but nonaddicting medications are more appropriate choices for managing anxiety in the correctional environment. (Specific suggestions for the treatment of documented anxiety disorders may be found later in this chapter.)

Medication Algorithms and Expert Consensus Guidelines

Psychotropic medication prescribing practices are becoming increasingly standardized through the issuance of expert consensus and evidence-based practice guidelines and the development of medication algorithms for the treatment of specific psychiatric disorders. *Medication algorithms* specify the conditions for which certain types of medications may be used, specify appropriate dosage levels, and provide alternative stepwise directions for changing or augmenting medication as clinically appropriate. One such medication algorithm project, the Texas Medication Algorithm Project (TMAP), was started in 1996. TMAP includes treatment algorithms for schizophrenia, major depression, and bipolar disorder. A prospective comparison of the clinical outcomes and economic costs of using the medication algorithms versus "treatment as usual" within the public mental health outpatient system in Texas has been undertaken, and the results are currently under analysis (Rush et al. 2003).

Correctional facilities may wish to consider adopting formal practice guidelines. Evidence-based expert consensus treatment guidelines offer a scientific and clinically sound basis for making treatment decisions and is consistent with the evolving community standard of care. Another potential advantage for correctional systems is treatment consistency across institutions. In addition, evidence-based treatment algorithms are likely to result in short- and long-term cost savings, both of which result from improved patient outcomes and less need of more intensive (expensive) crisis and inpatient care. If formal treatment guidelines are not adopted, consideration should be given to development of a mechanism to access consultation if psychotropic medications are being prescribed above recommended dosing guidelines or for indications not formally approved by the U.S. Food and Drug Administration (FDA).

CORRECTIONAL FORMULARY CONSIDERATIONS

In this section, I discuss major classes of psychotropic medication. The discussions are not intended to be exhaustive. In general, the classes and types of psychotropic medication that should be available in the facility's formulary are highly dependent on the facility's size and mission, the psychiatric illnesses encountered in the inmate population, and the inmate length of stay. However, if a correctional facility houses inmates with serious mental illnesses, antipsychotic, antidepressant, and mood-stabilizing medications must be included in the medication formulary. In addition, correctional policy should permit access to nonformulary medications on a case-by-case basis to ensure access to appropriate treatment for serious mental illness.

Antipsychotic Medications

Antipsychotic medications must be available for use in the treatment of schizophrenia, psychotic disorders, and psychotic symptoms accompanying other diagnoses. Antipsychotic medications are not physically addicting and have no "street value" as a desirable commodity in correctional settings. In fact, medications of this type are sometimes refused by people in need of them and are rarely sought by those without serious mental illness.

Antipsychotic medications fall into two large classes: conventional (older or "first generation") antipsychotics and "next generation" (formerly called "atypical" or "second generation") antipsychotic medications. Conventional antipsychotic medications include chlorpromazine (Thorazine), haloperidol (Haldol), fluphenazine (Prolixin), trifluoperazine (Stelazine), loxapine (Loxitane), thiothixene (Navane), and thioridazine (Mellaril). These medications were developed and released in the United States during the late 1950s through early 1970s. All of them have a high affinity for blockade of dopamine receptors in the brain, which is believed to be responsible for their ameliorative effects on hallucinations. However, the blockade of dopamine receptors throughout the brain also interferes with neurological processes involved in normal movement and is responsible for the side effects on movement observed when conventional medications are prescribed.

Side effects on movement include severe, involuntary, and painful muscle spasms (dystonia); tremors and rigidity (drug-induced parkinsonism); profound restlessness (akathisia); and the possible development, usually over time, of involuntary, uncontrolled movement of various muscle groups, most often those around the face and mouth (tardive dyskinesia). Some of these movement disorders are preventable or responsive to the concomitant administration of antiparkinsonian medications, including benztropine (Cogentin), amantadine (Symmetrel), and trihexyphenidyl (Artane). Unfortunately, particularly benztropine and trihexyphenidyl have some abuse potential in the correctional environment, as they reportedly produce a type of "high" when ingested, and inmate access to other drugs of abuse is severely limited in this controlled environment. The potential for abuse and/or "dealing" of these medications can be minimized through the use of liquid preparations, but this leads to additional problems in storage, nursing preparation, administration times, and so forth. Not all patients require antiparkinsonian medication, but it is often prescribed prophylactically to prevent the occurrence of a painful dystonic reaction that would negatively impact future medication compliance. Akathisia is poorly responsive to administration of a second medication and may require discontinuation of the conventional antipsychotic medication. Tardive dyskinesia is similarly poorly responsive to treatment but may be ameliorated or resolve with discontinuation of the conventional antipsychotic medication. Other cases of tardive dyskinesia are permanent.

In any event, when conventional antipsychotic medications are prescribed, antiparkinsonian medications for the prevention or reversal of dystonia and treatment of drug-induced parkinsonism must be readily available. In addition, use of conventional antipsychotic medications requires the adoption and utilization of an instrument at regular intervals to examine for and document either the presence or absence of involuntary movements. One such instrument is the Abnormal Involuntary Movement Scale (Munetz and Benjamin 1988). The examination and documentation should occur at the initiation of treatment with antipsychotic medications and at 6-month intervals thereafter for the duration of treatment.

Advantages for including conventional antipsychotic medications on correctional formularies include that they are all available in generic, and hence relatively inexpensive, preparations and that many are available in multiple forms (tablets, liquid, short-acting injectable, and long-acting injectable preparations).

Next generation, or "atypical," medications were developed and introduced during the 1980s to the present. Antipsychotic medications in this group include clozapine (Clozaril), risperidone (Risperdal), olanzapine (Zyprexa), quetiapine (Seroquel), ziprasidone (Geodon), and aripiprazole (Abilify). As a group, these medications do not have as high an affinity for dopamine receptors in the brain and consequently much less potential to impact normal movement or lead to the development of irreversible movement disorders. The exception is risperidone which does have some dose-dependent impact on movement; larger doses are more likely to cause movement side effects than smaller doses.

Clinically, a growing body of evidence suggests that these medications are at least as effective as the older medications on some psychotic symptoms and may be more effective than older medications on other symptoms such as expressed aggression, hostility, and social withdrawal. Studies on the use of some of the next-generation antipsychotic medications in hospitalized patients have demonstrated a decreased use of seclusion and restraint, decreased expression of aggression and hostility, and a decreased risk of suicide in patients treated with clozapine (Pinals and Buckley 1999). Although not replicated specifically in correctional settings, there is no reason to believe the results are not generalizable to institutionalized populations. A decreased use of seclusion and restraint in correctional populations is clearly desirable from the standpoint of decreasing the possibility of staff and inmate injury both in the application of the restraint and/or seclusion and in the precipitating incidents for which restraint and/or seclusion may be an appropriate response. Suicide prevention is an especially important health concern for correctional facilities (Burns 2003).

One obvious advantage of next-generation antipsychotic medication is that fewer undesirable side effects may enhance medication compliance and lead to better symptom management and less need for transfer to more intensive (and hence more expensive) mental health care such as infirmary placement, specialized treatment units, or psychiatric inpatient care. There is also less need for the concomitant prescription and administration of antiparkinsonian agents. A reduction in the use of such agents results in the dispensing of fewer meds at fewer times, which has an impact on nursing preparation and medication administration time as well as security staff time.

Although next-generation antipsychotic medications demonstrate fewer side effects on normal movement, epidemiological studies have demonstrated an increased risk of treatment-emergent hyperglycemia-related adverse effects in patients treated with these medications. In response to this observation, the U.S. Food and Drug Administration (FDA) has requested that all manufacturers of atypical antipsychotic medications include a warning regarding hyperglycemia and diabetes mellitus in their product labeling. This step has obligated prescribers of these medications to monitor all patients for symptoms of hyperglycemia, with particular attention paid to patients with preexisting diabetes and those patients with risk factors for the development of diabetes, such as obesity and/or a positive family history. In patients with coexisting diabetes or with risk factors for the development of diabetes, fasting blood glucose testing is recommended before the next-generation medication is initiated and at periodic intervals thereafter during treatment. All other patients require regular monitoring for symptoms of hyperglycemia (e.g., polydipsia, polyuria, weight gain, weakness). If symptoms develop, fasting blood glucose testing must be undertaken. In some cases, hyperglycemia resolves with discontinuation of the atypical antipsychotic agent, but some patients require continued treatment of diabetes despite discontinuation of the medication.

Other serious side effects include the development of agranulocytosis (a potentially fatal decrease in white blood cell count) in persons taking clozapine. The administration of clozapine requires a weekly, and later biweekly, complete blood count (CBC) with differential to monitor for the potential development of agranulocytosis. In addition to the cost of the medication, weekly blood work presents an added expense to correctional systems and additional procedural challenges with respect to drawing the blood, sending and receiving results, and ensuring their availability to both the pharmacy and the prescribing physician. Nevertheless, in certain cases, access to clozapine is an absolute clinical necessity: it remains the only medication with demonstrated efficacy in treatment of persons with symptoms that have been refractory to other antipsychotic medications.

Ziprasidone use has been associated with the potential to prolong the QT interval in cardiac conduction beyond the interval prolongation noted with several other antipsychotic medications. The QT interval is the interval from the beginning of the QRS complex to the end of the T wave of one heartbeat on an electrocardiogram (EKG). Ziprasidone is therefore contraindicated in patients with a known history of QT prolongation, recent acute myocardial infarction, or uncompensated heart failure, or in patients who are receiving other QT-prolonging drugs. Prolongation of the QT interval may lead to cardiac arrhythmias and death (Burns 2003).

Most correctional facilities have older, conventional antipsychotic medications available, but some have either severely restricted or not added next-generation, newer antipsychotic medications to their formulary because of the cost, particularly as compared with the conventional generic medications. Next-generation medications are far more expensive. This position is no longer defensible in light of a growing body of scientific evidence demonstrating that the newer medications make a substantial difference in symptom reduction and improved cognition, resulting in far less utilization of costly crisis and inpatient services. The medically accepted standard of care dictates that next-generation antipsychotic medications be made available in correctional formularies. It is permissible, and perhaps even desirable, for correctional systems or facilities to implement some clinical prescribing guidelines or protocols to monitor and/or contain next-generation medication expense. For example, reserving the use of olanzapine for inmates already taking it with good clinical results at the time of admission to the facility, or prescribing it only after the inmate has had a poor response to one or two other next-generation antipsychotic medications, is both a clinically and a fiscally sound recommendation. A potential disadvantage to offering *only* next generation antipsychotic medications in correctional formularies is related to the limited number of non–pill form preparations available. Only three alternative preparations are currently available. Olanzapine is available as a tablet immediately dissolvable in the mouth (Zyprexa Zydis); ziprasidone is available in a short-acting injectable form in addition to tablets; and risperidone was recently released in a long-acting injectable form (Risperdal Consta). Clinical Case 5–2 illustrates the use of next-generation antipsychotics inside a correctional facility.

Clinical Case 5–2

A 34-year-old man with a history of schizophrenia and adult-onset diabetes mellitus was booked into the county jail. At the time of screening, he reported that his psychotropic medications were olanzapine 20 mg by mouth twice a day, quetiapine 50 mg by mouth twice a day, and aripiprazole 15 mg by mouth at nighttime. He was also prescribed an oral hyperglycemic agent for his diabetes. The medications and dosages of antipsychotic medications were confirmed via facsimile from his community mental health provider when a signed release of information form was sent from the jail. Initially, all three antipsychotic medications were continued.

When the community mental health chart was received several weeks later, a review of the progress notes revealed that the patient was initially receiving olanzapine monotherapy but continued to report refractory auditory hallucinations. Subsequently, a second antipsychotic medication (aripiprazole) was added, and later a third (quetiapine). In jail, while receiving all three medications, the inmate reported experiencing occasional auditory hallucinations, particularly at night. He said that he was able to ignore the hallucinations for the most part and was not troubled by either the experience or the content of the "voices." Over the course of the next several weeks, olanzapine and aripiprazole were tapered and discontinued, while the dosage of quetiapine was increased to 300 mg by mouth twice a day. The patient reported experiencing a substantial decrease in the frequency with which he experienced auditory hallucinations, and his blood sugar improved to the extent that the dosage of his oral hyperglycemic agent was able to be reduced.

Antidepressant Medications

Accessibility to antidepressant medications for the treatment of major depression and other serious mental illnesses with an affective component is a must for correctional facilities housing inmates with serious mental illness. Many classes of antidepressant medication are available, and multiple medications are available within each class. Unlike antipsychotic medications for which clinical evidence exists to mandate the availability of medications in both conventional and atypical classes, such evidence is not available for all classes of antidepressant medication. Some classes of antidepressant medication are contraindicated in correctional facilities.

Tricyclic antidepressants (TCAs), so named because of their biochemical structure, are the oldest class of antidepressant medication. They include amitriptyline (Elavil), desipramine (Norpramin), clomipramine (Anafranil), doxepin (Sinequan), imipramine (Tofranil), and nortriptyline (Pamelor). Although clinically efficacious, TCAs have fallen out of favor in civilian populations because of the risk of death in overdose and the availability of many other efficacious and safer antidepressants. In correctional settings, TCAs carry an additional risk: potential abuse based on their anticholinergic properties in a setting where other substances of abuse are more difficult to obtain. The abuse potential and the risk of death in overdose are therefore relative contraindications for use of TCAs in correctional settings. If TCAs are used, intensive monitoring to prevent stockpiling or hoarding for purposes of overdose is required. TCAs are inexpensive (a favorable asset for inclusion in correctional formularies) and may be considered for treatment of patients who have failed to respond to adequate trials of other classes of antidepressant medication with appropriate monitoring safeguards.

A second class of antidepressant medications, the monoamine oxidase inhibitors (MAOIs), so named for their mechanism of action on the enzyme monoamine oxidase, are also contraindicated in correctional settings. The MAOIs include isocarboxazid (Marplan), phenelzine (Nardil), and tranylcypromine (Parnate). Inhibition of monoamine oxidase can precipitate hypertensive crisis if certain foods containing tyramine are ingested. Hypertensive crisis can also be precipitated by the ingestion of certain over-the-counter medications for cold and flu symptoms. Because use of the MAOIs requires fairly rigid dietary monitoring and avoidance of some common over-the-counter medications, and because a plethora of other types of equally or more efficacious antidepressants are available, the use of MAOI antidepressants in correctional settings is contraindicated.

Selective serotonin reuptake inhibitors (SSRIs) are a newer class of antidepressant medication that are very effective and have much lower toxicity than either TCA or MAOI antidepressants, even in overdose. SSRIs include fluoxetine (Prozac), citalopram (Celexa), escitalopram (Lexapro), fluvoxamine (Luvox), paroxetine (Paxil), and sertraline (Zoloft). SSRIs are generally more expensive than TCAs because many of the SSRIs are still under patent and thus generic forms are not available. However, the cost differential in procuring the medication is far outweighed by their lower toxicity. For example, the cost of one completed suicide by TCA overdose is far more than the cost of procuring and administering an SSRI (Burns 2003).

Several other available antidepressant medications do not fit neatly into any of the preceding classifications in that they are biochemically distinct. These medications include amoxapine (Asendin), bupropion (Wellbutrin), mirtazapine (Remeron), venlafaxine (Effexor), nefazodone (Serzone), and trazodone (Desyrel). In general, these antidepressants also have good safety profiles and are efficacious in the treatment of depression and in sustaining remission. One side effect worthy of mention is male priapism associated with trazodone. Priapism is a sustained, painful erection of the penis that may result in permanent sterility and which sometimes requires surgical intervention. Given the number of other antidepressant medication choices available, trazodone is generally not recommended for use with male inmates. In addition, it may be worthwhile to restrict or limit the use of bupropion in correctional settings, as there have been reports of inmates crushing and snorting it to attain a "high" not otherwise readily available to them in confinement.

In addition to treatment of depressive and other affective disorders, antidepressants have demonstrated efficacy in the treatment of anxiety disorders, including posttraumatic stress disorder. Paroxetine (Paxil), venlafaxine (Effexor), and nefazodone (Serzone) are particularly helpful in this regard. Using antidepressant medications for the treatment of anxiety disorders reinforces the recommendation to severely restrict the use of benzodiazepines for this purpose in correctional facilities.

Many inmates without psychiatric illness are prescribed low doses of antidepressant medication because of the sedating side effects and for complaints of trouble sleeping. Prescribing for side effect rather than targeted action is to be avoided primarily because of the limited psychiatric time resources available in most correctional facilities. These inmates still require periodic examination for medication review and renewals, making less time available for treatment of the seriously mentally ill. In addition, the abuse potential of some antidepressant medications in correctional facilities has previously been noted. Correctional settings are difficult places to sleep, but this problem should be managed in other ways: reducing or eliminating caffeine consumption, increasing exercise, limiting sleep to total of 6–10 hours in any 24-hour period, teaching relaxation exercises, and making earplugs available in commissary for inmate purchase and use to block out loud snoring and other disruptive noise (Burns 2003).

Mood-Stabilizing Medications

Mood-stabilizing medications must be available on correctional formularies for the treatment of serious mental illnesses: bipolar disorder, schizoaffective disorder, and other disorders with a recurrent or cyclical affective component. Lithium and some anticonvulsant medications fall into this classification. This class of psychotropic medication is the most intensive in terms of requirements for laboratory monitoring of serum levels of the medications themselves, as well as for monitoring for the development of untoward effects on other systems (liver metabolism, bone marrow production, etc.).

Lithium's efficacy in the treatment of bipolar disorder has been long recognized. It is very inexpensive. The administration of lithium requires monitoring for therapeutic blood level (monthly for 3 months, then quarterly) and periodic monitoring of renal and thyroid functioning. In addition, a baseline EKG is recommended before lithium treatment is instituted. Lithium can be fatal in overdose and also has a significant incidence of gastrointestinal distress as a side effect.

Anticonvulsants used in the treatment of bipolar and other disorders include divalproex (Depakote), valproic acid (Depakene), carbamazepine (Tegretol), gabapentin (Neurontin), clonazepam (Klonopin), lamotrigine (Lamictal), oxcarbazepine (Trileptal), and topiramate (Topamax). It is important to note that, as of this writing, only divalproex, valproic acid, and carbamazepine are approved by the FDA for treatment of bipolar disorder, though the others are widely used "off label" for this purpose (Bezchlibnyk-Butler and Jeffries 2003).

Divalproex and valproic acid are much less toxic in overdose situations than lithium but are not without potential complications on other body systems, namely, the liver and bone marrow. Use of these agents requires baseline and quarterly liver function tests and a CBC with platelets. Serum levels of valproic acid may be monitored to check on medication compliance and potentially determine dosage adequacy, although the established therapeutic window is for seizure control rather than bipolar disorder.

Carbamazepine has also been widely used in the treatment of acute mania and prophylaxis of mood cycling. It requires baseline and periodic liver function tests, CBC with platelets, and serum drug level monitoring. Carbamazepine induces its own hepatic metabolism and the hepatic metabolism of other drugs metabolized by the cytochrome P450 system. The other anticonvulsant medications noted above would best be reserved for use in cases that are refractory to adequate trials of FDA-approved medications or as adjuncts to the other medications if necessary. Because clonazepam is a benzodiazepine, its use in the treatment of bipolar disorder in correctional populations is not recommended, for all of the reasons previously stated.

Olanzapine, previously discussed as a second-generation antipsychotic, is FDA approved for the treatment of bipolar disorder. Appropriate precautions noted with respect to hyperglycemia are equally relevant when olanzapine is prescribed for bipolar disorder. The rapidly dissolving preparation of olanzapine may be particularly useful in ensuring medication ingestion and compliance, particularly since all other mood stabilizers with the exception of lithium (which is available as a liquid) are available only in tablet or capsule forms that are easy to "cheek" (intentionally not swallow).

In some instances, disorders that may not be considered "serious mental illness," such as certain personality disorders (borderline and antisocial), may nevertheless manifest symptoms amenable to psychopharmacological intervention. High degrees of impulsivity leading to aggression and potential violence may be appropriately treated with medications discussed for the treatment of bipolar disorder.

Other Psychotropic Medications

Benzodiazepines have a limited use for inclusion in correctional formularies as previously noted. Sedative/hypnotics should not be prescribed. Symptoms of anxiety may be treated with antidepressant medications (particularly the SSRIs). Other nonaddicting medications, such as buspirone (Buspar) and hydroxyzine (Vistaril), are also viable alternatives for the treatment of anxiety in correctional populations.

Lastly, it may be appropriate to include sympathomimetics on the formulary in juvenile facilities for the treatment of attention-deficit/hyperactivity disorder (ADHD) when prescribed in accordance with FDA-approved indications and doses. None of the sympathomimetics are approved for use in adult patients, and their availability on the formulary of adult facilities is strongly discouraged given the challenges presented in correctional facilities because of their addictive potential and security concerns (Zil 2000). If ADHD is suspected in an adult, obtaining a second-opinion consultation and securing either documentation of outside treatment or corroboration of symptoms are recommended. If treatment is indicated, a trial of atomoxetine (Strattera), a newer medication approved for use in adults as well as children for ADHD, should be considered before a nonformulary request for a sympathomimetic is undertaken. Atomoxetine is not a controlled substance and may therefore be a viable alternative to sympathomimetics in adult (as well as juvenile) correctional facilities.

CONCLUSION

Psychotropic medications are a necessary component of correctional mental health care. Correctional facilities are mandated to provide treatment for serious mental illnesses. Failing to do so constitutes a violation of the Eighth Amendment's prohibition of cruel and unusual punishment. In general, psychotropic medication use in correctional settings should follow the same standard of care as that found in other community settings. Nevertheless, some unique factors must be considered when practicing in correctional settings. Among these factors are securing informed consent in an environment that is inherently coercive; balancing an inmate's right to refuse medication with legitimate correctional interests of maintaining order in the institution and preventing harm to other inmates and staff; and understanding correctional medication administration processes. Factors requiring special consideration in correctional facilities include the very high prevalence rate of substance use disorders occurring in correctional populations, which dictates that formularies limit or exclude medications that have high abuse potential, and the environmental and other conditions (work details) that may exacerbate the already increased risk of malignant heat-related conditions occurring in persons taking some psychotropic medications.

Formulary considerations should be based on the facility's population characteristics as well as the duration and conditions of confinement. In facilities containing inmates with serious mental illnesses, psychotropic medication formularies must contain both classes of antipsychotic medications (conventional and next-generation), antidepressant, and mood-stabilizing medications. Prescribing practices are becoming increasingly standardized in the psychiatric community with the issuance of expert consensus medication guidelines and treatment algorithms. Correctional facilities may wish to consider adoption and implementation of these practices, in that they demonstrate adherence to the community standard of care, evidence-based medically accepted and defensible treatment rationales, uniformity in the provision of treatment, and improved clinical outcomes.

SUMMARY POINTS

Persons with serious mental illness are entitled to

- Treatment for their condition when confined in correctional facilities.
- Access to and appropriate utilization of psychotropic medication for the treatment of serious mental illness.
- Informed consent and right to refuse treatment under specified circumstances.

Prescribers in a correctional environment should

- Be familiar with the correctional facility's medication administration procedures as they may impact medication choice, frequency of dosing, timing of laboratory studies, and inmate medication compliance.
- Recognize environmental risks (e.g., heat-related problems) associated with psychotropic medication and educate inmates and medical and security administrative staff on these issues.
- Limit the use of benzodiazepines to detoxification protocols because of the development of dependence, high abuse potential, and security issues regarding illegitimate use of these drugs in a population with high prevalence of substance use.
- Consider implementation of expert consensus, evidence-based treatment guidelines or medication algorithms for the treatment of certain psychiatric disorders.
- Develop a mechanism to access consultation if psychotropic medications are being prescribed above recommended dosing guidelines or for indications not formally approved by the FDA.

Correctional administration should

- Include representative medications from the following classes of medication: antipsychotic medications (both conventional and next-generation), antidepressant medications, and mood-stabilizing medications.
- Provide access to other types of psychotropic medication on a case-by-case basis to ensure that inmates are not denied appropriate treatment of serious mental health needs.

REFERENCES

American Psychiatric Association: Psychiatric Services in Jails and Prisons, 2nd Edition. Washington, DC, American Psychiatric Association, 2000

Bezchlibnyk-Butler KZ, Jeffries JJ (eds): Clinical Handbook of Psychotropic Drugs. Seattle, WA, Hogrefe & Huber, 2003

Burns KA: Jail diversion and correctional psychotropic medication formularies, in Management and Administration of Correctional Health Care. Edited by Moore J. Kingston, NJ, Civic Research Institute, 2003

Cohen F: The Mentally Disordered Inmate and the Law. Kingston, NJ, Civic Research Institute, 1998

Munetz M, Benjamin S: How to examine patients using the Abnormal Involuntary Movement Scale. Hosp Community Psychiatry 39:1172–1177, 1988

Pinals DA, Buckley PF: Novel antipsychotic agents and their implications for forensic psychiatry. J Am Acad Psychiatry Law 27:7–22, 1999

Ruiz v Estelle 503 F.Supp. 1265 (S.D. Tex. 1980)

Rush AJ, Crismon ML, Kashner TM, et al: Texas Medication Algoithm Project, Phase 3 (TMAP-3): rationale and study design. J Clin Psychiatry 64:357–369, 2003

Washington v Harper 494 U.S. 210 (1990)

Zil JS: Psychotropic principles for correctional settings, in Playbook 2000: Guidelines for Correctional Care. Edited by Benson SG, Burrows L. Walnut Creek, CA, Registry Foundation, 2000, pp 32–33

CHAPTER 6

Mental Health Interventions in Correctional Settings

Shama B. Chaiken, Ph.D.

Christopher R. Thompson, M.D.

Wendy E. Shoemaker, Psy.D.

In *Estelle v. Gamble* (1976), the U.S. Supreme Court held that prisons cannot be "deliberately indifferent" to the serious medical needs of their inmates. To do so would be a violation of the Eighth Amendment's prohibition on cruel and unusual punishment. *Estelle* did not involve psychiatric care, but it is clear that psychiatric care is within its reach. Additionally, *Estelle* has been specifically extended to psychiatry by several lower courts. In *Newman v. Alabama* (1977), the Fifth Circuit Court of Appeals found that lack of psychiatric care was a critical deficiency in general medical care that violated prisoners' right to be free from cruel and unusual punishment. Similarly, in *Bowring v. Godwin* (1977), the Fourth Circuit Court of Appeals equated mental health treatment with medical treatment, stating, "We see no underlying distinction between the right to medical care for physical ills and its psychological counterpart."

The types of treatment that must be offered were directly addressed in the significant *Ruiz v. Estelle* (1980) decision, when a U.S. District Court in Texas provided general guidelines for planning mental health treatment services. Nine years later, in *Langley v. Coughlin* (1989), a New York judge described the deficiencies in mental health services provided to inmates at a New York state prison and indicated that medication alone was not sufficient treatment for mentally ill prisoners. Rather, medication must be part of an overall program of therapy, which might include individual and group therapy (when appropriate), as well as crisis intervention services. The court noted that "failure to provide any meaningful treatment other than medication" would violate prisoners' Eighth Amendment rights (Langley v. Coughlin 1989).

The U.S. District Court for Northern California came to a similar conclusion in *Madrid v. Gomez* (1995) in finding constitutional violations in a correctional facility, Pelican Bay State Prison, where "[t]reatment for seriously ill inmates is primarily limited to medication management through use of antipsychotic or psychotropic drugs, and intensive outpatient treatment is not available" (Madrid v. Gomez 1995). Perhaps more importantly, in *Madrid,* the court concluded that when punishing inmates, prison officials must consider the possible mental health effects that such punishment could have. In applying this standard, the court ordered mentally ill inmates removed from the Security Housing Unit, finding that sensory deprivation would likely exacerbate their symptoms of mental illness.

California correctional facilities were scrutinized by the courts again the following year. In *Coleman v. Wilson* (1995), a U.S. District Court in California found that the mental health treatment provided by the California Department of Corrections (CDC) was inadequate and that prisoners' rights under the Eighth and Fourteenth Amendments had been violated. In its decision, the court noted multiple deficiencies in the mental health treatment provided by the CDC. These included inadequate screening mechanisms, chronic understaffing, poor access to supported care and medication management, and inappropriate use of punishment for mentally ill inmates.

More recent court decisions, such as *Brad H. v. City of New York* (2001) and *Wakefield v. Thompson* (1999), have indicated that inmates and parolees, respectively, are also entitled to discharge planning and discharge medications "at least until such time as is reasonably necessary for the parolee to consult a doctor and arrange for his own supply" (Wakefield v. Thompson 1999).

States affected by these court mandates and other states with proactive legislatures have been required to develop and implement an extensive system for assessment, placement, and implementation of mental health treatment in the corrections setting. Levels of care that are similar to hospitalization, crisis intervention, day treatment, outpatient services, and drop-in clinics have been developed to meet the needs of the diverse incarcerated population. In effect, mental health programs in correctional settings have been challenged with the mission to meet or exceed community standards for treatment of mentally ill patients.

States and municipalities have generally used a variety of modalities to treat mentally ill inmates. Some, such as pharmacotherapy, group therapy, and other correctional education programs (which teach social and vocational skills), are almost ubiquitous. Others, such as sex offender treatment programs, are less available but still not uncommon. Offenders with mental illness often have a coexisting substance abuse disorder, and substance abuse treatment is offered in many correctional settings. Recently, some states have implemented novel correctional mental health programs and paradigms, the efficacy of which is, at this point, unclear:

1. New York State has established two "Behavioral Health Units" in state correctional facilities (one at a maximum security prison in Sullivan County) that serve as placement alternatives to the Security Housing Units (i.e., they house inmates who would otherwise be confined to disciplinary cells). These units are the first alternative to solitary confinement being offered to disruptive mentally ill prisoners in New York State.
2. Ohio has established the Oakwood Correctional Facility, which houses only inmates in need of intensive psychiatric care. In addition, Ohio has divided the state's 31 prisons into 12 separate catchment areas and assigned a Residential Treatment Unit (RTU) to each one. The RTUs provide care and supervision for mentally ill inmates who require special housing on a graduated basis (i.e., as active symptoms of their mental illness diminish, more privileges and movement are permitted) and offer a continuum of care ranging from outpatient to residential services.
3. California has developed a Behavioral Incentive Program (BIP) for mentally ill inmates who require a maximum security setting.

In this chapter, we review nonpharmacological mental health interventions that have been successfully implemented in the corrections setting, focusing on challenges specific to the development of correctional mental health treatment programs and evaluation of the success of these programs. A more comprehensive examination of some of these therapies can be found elsewhere (Schwartz 2003).

PROGRAM MISSION STATEMENTS

Correctional mental health programs usually employ an interdisciplinary treatment team whose members work together to assess, treat, and discharge patients. The purpose of implementing treatment team procedures is to facilitate communication between psychiatrists, psychologists, social workers, primary care physicians, nurses, psychiatric technicians, recreational therapists, custody staff, and any other staff who may interact with the patient or the patient care system. Supervisors of each discipline must be clear about mental health program admission and discharge criteria and about the mission of each program.

The mission statement of a mental health program in the corrections setting should identify ways that providing treatment improves the safety and security of the institution and enhances public safety. Successful mental health programs focus on treating serious mental illness and reducing patients' destructive, disruptive, assaultive, and self-injurious behavior, thereby increasing staff and public safety as well as reducing the cost of incarcerating mentally ill inmates. The goals of treatment and the available interventions vary in different settings, according to the patient population, the political climate, and relevant court mandates. Clearly defined quality assurance and peer review guidelines help staff to focus on the goals of the specific program and to maintain a high-quality professional work environment.

Staff morale and treatment team unity in the corrections environment are only possible when correctional, medical, and mental health staff are clear about the priorities of each program. Differences in values and beliefs about mental health treatment based on education, training, and cultural differences are inevitable in any interdisciplinary treatment team. One of the most difficult tasks of a correctional mental health program supervisor is to cultivate an environment of respect for differences in opinion. Staff conflict regarding which inmates are appropriately placed in the mental health programs can be divisive without an established forum for conflict resolution. Regular interdisciplinary discussion and cross-training enhance patient treatment and improve staff satisfaction. Adequate input and participation from both clinical and custody staff and supervisors are important factors in interdisciplinary training and team building.

One common factor that influences the efficacy of assessment and treatment is the language used to describe inmate patients' behaviors. Supervisors should encourage staff to replace generic terms with specific details. For example, the word *manipulation* can easily be used to describe many antisocial behaviors. Instead of saying that a patient is "manipulating," it is more helpful for staff to obtain a clear understanding of the patient's goal and how the patient is acting in order to achieve that goal. Clinical Case 6–1 provides an example of an inmate's behavior designed to meet his needs. (All of the clinical case examples in this chapter are fictional and are not based on any one person.)

Clinical Case 6–1: Manipulating

In two similar situations, patients who had newly arrived to a mental health treatment unit spoke to correctional officers and requested that they receive their legal paperwork. When the property officer had not arrived with the requested paperwork in the patients' expected time frame, each patient broke his food tray and stated that he would kill himself with a sharp piece of the tray. In each case, the mental health clinician arrived on the unit and was told that the patient was "manipulating."

Assessment of the first situation revealed that the patient had created reams of incomprehensible psychotic writing focused on delusional beliefs about his legal situation. Several times in the past he had seriously attempted suicide when he was not allowed to pursue his delusional legal goals through writing. In the second case, the patient had a long history of violent behavior when his perceived rights were not met, but he had no history of any self-injurious behavior.

Understanding the history, current functioning, and motivation of the patients led to slightly different interventions. In the first case, the staff assessed that developing rapport was equally as important as setting limits. While waiting for the officer to find the patient's property, clinical staff stayed at the patient's cell front and engaged in rapport building conversation. The patient was told that he could have the materials when he gave up the broken tray and agreed to attend an individual session with his assigned clinician. Then the team created a treatment plan focused on reducing psychotic symptoms, as well as self-injurious threats, ideation and behavior. In the second case, the staff felt that setting limits was the overriding treatment need. While observing for the purpose of suicide prevention, staff interacted with the patient as briefly as possible to tell him that he would not receive any property or attention to his other requests until he gave up the broken tray. The treatment plan for this patient was designed to reinforce appropriate problem solving and decrease destructive and threatening behavior.

Another term used loosely in correctional environments is *malingering*. Only after appropriate assessment should this diagnosis be given. Even then, the evaluating professional should describe the symptoms that the patient has likely exaggerated along with the suspected motivation for the malingering, rather than merely labeling the patient as a "malingerer." Malingering must also be clearly differentiated from factitious disorder and somatoform disorders (see Chapter 7, "Assessment of Malingering in Correctional Settings"). Use of any uninformed generalizations, slang, or derogatory language in describing mental health patients degrades the quality of the treatment setting. The mission statement of correctional mental health programs should therefore encourage professional and respectful language.

Table 6–1 outlines important components of a mental health program mission statement.

TABLE 6–1. Mental health program mission statements: recommended contents

- Admission and discharge criteria
- Treatment goals
- Available interventions
- Quality assurance and peer review guidelines
- Contribution to safety and security of the institution and public safety
- Methods of enhancing staff morale
  - Respect for differences of opinion
  - Focus on conflict resolution
  - Regularly scheduled discussion and cross-training
  - Input and participation from all disciplines
- Language that promotes a professional work environment

ASSESSMENT

Decisions about the type of treatment each patient needs (level of care) in a correctional environment require careful interdisciplinary treatment team review. Clinical staff must first synthesize environmental, cultural, historic, and present information before they can generate accurate diagnoses and treatment plans. Even after careful review of prior records, inmates who are referred for mental health treatment can rarely be assessed accurately in a single clinical interview. Because many inmates have learned to use deceptive measures for personal gain, historical data may be flawed, and the patient's presentation may be purposefully engineered.

Inmates may experience significant secondary gain from being identified as mentally ill, receiving medication, or being placed in a mental health services delivery system. Personal gains may include access to specialized housing, transfer to less restrictive environments, perceived or real protection from violence, reduction of pressure to conform to gang-based or other racially based prison norms, increased involvement in stimulating activity, increased access to property or other behavioral reinforcements, ability to traffic psychotropic medications, "insanity" defense for criminal/disciplinary behavior, and access to legal aid. Some inmates also try to gain access to vulnerable mentally ill patients in order to extort, abuse, or otherwise control members of this inmate population. Inmates treated in mental health programs who are scheduled for parole may have access to increased financial aid once they are released.

Severely mentally ill patients in a correctional setting may deny and cover symptoms in order to escape treatment or affect placement. Patients with subacute mania may be able to appear calm and goal directed even in extensive interviews. Psychotic patients with some insight may be able to mask thought disorder and to display increased affect for short periods of time. Patients who are adequately treated with medication on arrival in a mental health treatment program may appear symptom free and may be convincing that documentation of past symptoms was not accurate. Patients with a documented history of mental illness may falsely report that they malingered symptoms or contrived behavior in order to appear mentally ill for secondary gain.

Cultural issues often play an important role in the expression of symptoms in the correctional setting. Inmates recently incarcerated for the first time are particularly challenged with the task of adjusting to the unique prison or jail culture. Any inmate changing correctional settings faces similar stressors. Adaptation to new roles, rules, and living conditions may be exacerbated if the inmate feels he or she is not safe or is actually at risk of being physically harmed. These issues, combined with complicated issues related to race, ethnicity, gang affiliation, commitment offense, educational level, socioeconomic status, religion, and other politics, may make adjustment to the correctional environment overwhelmingly difficult. Symptoms related to adjustment may be difficult to differentiate from other diagnoses and may exacerbate other mental health symptoms.

Only after an assessment period during which information from the interdisciplinary team is gathered and discussed can an accurate diagnosis be established. Investigation of possible secondary gains is often useful. Observation of the patient's interactions with peers, custody, medical, and mental health staff is crucial to the assessment process. Level of program participation, daily living skills, and problem solving ability can also be gauged with more accuracy during the assessment period.

Diagnostic Dilemmas

Patients who isolate themselves and refuse treatment pose a particularly difficult diagnostic dilemma. Differentiation between schizoid personality traits, oppositional behavior, response to trauma, depression, paranoid or other psychotic symptoms, negative symptoms, and other potential secondary gain may require an extended observational period to assess.

Self-injurious behavior poses a treatment challenge to practitioners in any setting. Determining whether the behavior is due to psychosis, compulsion, organic impairment, impulsivity, personality disorder, or a combination of factors requires careful assessment of internal and external motivations. Patients who repeatedly ingest or insert objects for the purpose of self-injury or requiring treatment are fairly unique to the incarcerated population. Often the inmate states that the purpose of the behavior is to affect placement, receive narcotics, gain attention, protest policy or conditions, cause inconvenience to staff, or incur costly treatment. In these cases, the behavior is usually attributed to antisocial or borderline personality disorder. However, some inmates with this behavior harm themselves so severely or regularly that they cause a life-threatening condition. In these cases, it is important to consider the possibility of an Axis I disorder that may respond to psychotropic medication. Ideally, a clear and consistent policy would be present throughout the correctional system that reduces reinforcement for the behavior while providing necessary treatment.

Inmates who meet the full criteria for antisocial personality disorder, especially those who score 30 or higher on the Psychopathy Checklist–Revised (PCL-R; Hare 1991), indicating psychopathy, are generally considered poorly responsive to treatment. Some clinicians have suggested that a cutoff score on the PCL-R be used to determine appropriateness for treatment in the incarcerated population. However, others have found that even in some psychopathic inmates with a history of planned, deliberate, predatory, and sadistic behavior, a coexisting Axis I disorder may be present and can be treated. Treatment may be particularly indicated when the Axis I disorder contributes to higher scores on PCL-R items such as impulsivity, poor behavioral controls (i.e., intermittent explosive disorder), grandiose sense of self-worth (i.e., delusional disorder), need for stimulation, or promiscuous sexual behavior (i.e., bipolar disorder). More research is needed to develop successful preventative and rehabilitative programs for impulsive offenders and violent psychopaths (Hart and Dempster 1997). Table 6–2 summarizes key components of a mental health assessment.

LEVELS OF CARE

Types of mental health treatment in correctional settings generally parallel those available in the general population. Levels of care include crisis intervention, hospitalization, "day treatment" programs, outpatient programs, and walk-in clinics.

Crisis intervention and hospitalization are required for patients who are likely to harm themselves or others or who are gravely disabled because of mental illness. Psychiatric evaluation and treatment, 24-hour nursing care, assistance with daily living skills, suicide watch, medical collaboration, and a full range of individual and group therapies are used in inpatient settings. Patients who do not improve may require long-term hospitalization. Some correctional facilities send these patients to state mental health hospitals or contract with private inpatient mental health facilities.

TABLE 6–2. Mental health assessment

- Determine accuracy of historical data when possible.
- Assess secondary gain.
- Be aware that some patients may try to hide mental illness or may be stable on current medication.
- Consider cultural issues.
- Observe for an adequate assessment period.
- Accept input from all disciplines.
- Allow more time for assessment of diagnostic dilemmas.

Mentally ill inmates who are intermittently at risk of harming themselves or others, or who decompensate without a structured environment, require day-treatment-type care. These patients should be housed in units with other severely mentally ill patients in order to create a therapeutic treatment environment that is separate from the general prison environment and its stressors. Careful consideration should be given to the risks and benefits of housing patients together or in single cells. Recommendations from the interdisciplinary treatment team should be considered as part of housing determination. Although some patients may display increased symptoms related to the stress of forced cohabitation, others might benefit from social interaction. Some inmates have been prevented from successful suicide due to intervention from their cell mates.

Because isolation often exacerbates symptoms of mental illness (Grassian 1983, 1986; Kupers 1999), court mandates have required that severely mentally ill inmate patients be offered a full range of therapeutic activities. In the *Coleman* case in California, the federal court's order required the "day treatment"–type program (in this case, called the Enhanced Outpatient Program) to offer structured therapeutic activities at least 10 hours per week, yard/exercise time at least 10 hours per week, confidential individual sessions at least once a week, and psychiatric consultation at least once a month (Coleman v. Wilson 1995).

Patients who are generally stable but require medication for psychiatric symptoms, or who have mild impairment in functioning due to mental illness, may be treated on an "outpatient" basis. In the correctional environment, this means that they are housed with the general inmate population at their designated security level. These patients may be offered psychiatric consultation and group therapy as clinically indicated. Facilities often use a case-management approach, in which a primary clinician assesses the patients' level of functioning and mental health needs on a scheduled basis. Some patients may require weekly individual therapy on a short term basis for adjustment issues or insight oriented therapy. Other patients may require as little as one mental health clinician contact every 90 days in order to ensure that they continue to function at a level appropriate for outpatient treatment.

Drop-in clinic care in the correctional setting consists of a request system for inmates who are on no psychotropic medications to access mental health assessment and treatment on an intermittent basis as needed. Often in correctional environments where patients receive "outpatient" or drop-in mental health care, a clinician assesses the inmates at cell front on a regularly scheduled basis in order to identify inmates who may be experiencing the onset of mental health symptoms. This type of screening, or "rounds," is especially important in high-security correctional settings, where patients have fewer activities offered and less contact with staff.

Depending on their level of functioning, some inmates are included in mental health treatment programs solely because of developmental disabilities or medical problems that may cause behavior similar to that seen in inmates with mental illness. Inmates with dementia or lasting impairment due to brain injury and/or substance abuse may also benefit from similar programs. Dual-diagnosis patients are common in the correctional setting, and provision of appropriate mental health and medical care requires a team approach focused on prioritizing the patient's most prominent treatment needs.

THERAPEUTIC INTERVENTIONS

The availability of pharmacological treatment of mental illness is crucial to the success of any correctional mental health treatment program. Other therapeutic treatments increase the likelihood of medication compliance, insight development, behavior change, and long-term remission from symptoms. Individual therapy, group therapy, recreational therapy, therapeutic community, substance abuse programs, assistance with daily living skills, and behavioral incentive programs are among the most common interventions used with mental health patients in correctional settings. Collaborative nursing and medical care are also necessary components of mental health treatment.

Individual Psychotherapy

One variable often demonstrated to affect psychotherapy treatment efficacy is the patient's subjective experience of rapport with the therapist (Joe et al. 2001). Developing therapeutic rapport in a correctional setting can be challenging. Environmental factors often limit the mental health clinicians' ability to set up consistent space, time, and appropriate conditions to facilitate rapport building. Inmates who are moved from their institution or housing unit without notice often do not experience adequate continuity of care to develop necessary rapport. Confidential interview space and consistent access to continuous care are crucial to providing ethical and effective treatment.

Mental health clinicians who are asked to provide individual psychotherapy in settings that do not support adequate rapport should notify patients of the risks of engaging in treatment that may lack confidentiality and continuity. Short-term, goal-oriented behavioral or cognitive interventions should be employed without encouraging the patient to discuss difficult or traumatic experiences. One simple and useful intervention involves identifying resources available in the corrections setting and educating the patient about how to use these resources. Regressive interventions that require interpersonal trust, development of insight, and subsequent change in coping and/or behavior can be dangerous and counterproductive without assurance of appropriate continuity and timely termination.

In institutions where patients remain in a treatment setting with appropriate treatment space for an adequate period of time, therapists can work to overcome numerous interpersonal barriers to developing therapeutic rapport that are present in correctional treatment settings. In any mental health treatment setting, regardless of theoretical orientation, gaining patients' trust is a crucial part of providing treatment. Therapeutic rapport is generally accomplished over time by fostering empathetic interaction, setting appropriate boundaries, discussing cultural barriers, defining the parameters and goals of treatment, and providing therapy at a regularly scheduled time and place. In the corrections setting, accomplishing these basic tasks can be challenging and complex. Often, the physical plant of the correctional setting does not allow for consistent confidential interactions, and many inmate patients distrust correctional employees. In the first individual therapy contacts, the mental health clinician must identify both positive and negative factors related to building rapport with the patient. These factors include motivation for treatment, prior experiences in therapy, beliefs about mental health treatment, capacity for insight, personality traits, and current symptoms.

Many patients in correctional settings have experienced few relationships with people who are consistent, honest, direct, and caring. Patients in jail or prison often perceive mental health staff as part of the bureaucracy of the correctional setting. The first task of the therapist is to differentiate himself or herself from custody staff, correctional counselors, legal consultants, and other medical personnel. The patient may initially ask the therapist to facilitate getting the patient's perceived needs met or for help communicating with corrections staff. Common requests from inmates involve accessing phone calls, legal information, property, canteen, or writing materials. Generating a sincere response that balances empathy and boundaries is an art form. To be effective in the correctional setting, the mental health clinician must develop a style that emphasizes setting limits without being punitive. One part of the therapist's role may be to facilitate the patient's knowledge about how to access resources and get his or her own needs met. However, if the patient focuses on "using" the therapist for specific personal gain, the more important focus of the therapeutic relationship can be compromised.

One specific challenge for correctional mental health clinicians involves treatment of inmates who are referred for mental health treatment because of social withdrawal and isolative behavior. When historical and interdisciplinary treatment team information indicates that mental illness may contribute to isolative behavior, mental health staff must consider legal and ethical issues regarding placement in a treatment program and the use of behavioral incentives. In most cases, the first step should be to encourage the patient to participate in treatment. If possible, the clinician should provide cell front contact on a predictable schedule. Daily contact, at a consistent time of day, is preferable for patients who may be severely mentally ill or paranoid. The clinician may be able to determine an area of interest of the patient or to engage the patient in a superficial topic of conversation. Any interaction provides an opportunity for increased observation, assessment, and reduction of isolation. Clinical Case 6–2 describes an inmate whose mental illness contributes to his isolative behavior.

Clinical Case 6–2: The Isolative Patient

A patient with symptoms of hyperreligiosity and delusions of grandeur refused to come out of his cell for 3 weeks. Each day at approximately the same time, his assigned primary clinician approached his cell front and asked if he would like to talk. He began to reveal delusional beliefs and auditory command hallucinations of a religious nature. He was encouraged by his mental health clinician to "come out of your cell and teach me about your religion." Once the patient agreed to come out of his cell and could be closely observed, the clinician realized that he had blood on the legs of his clothing. The patient soon revealed that he had carved religious codes onto his legs in response to a command from God. He admitted that he knew it would sound crazy to other people and had been trying to hide his behavior. Medical examination revealed that he had made deep cuts requiring sutures and that his wounds were infected. With skillful empathy and reality testing, the therapist was able to convince the patient that he should cooperate with a trial of antipsychotic medication.

Another challenge specific to correctional mental health staff is creating a balance between providing treatment and maintaining appropriate boundaries. In most prisons and jails, maintaining the disciplinary system is the responsibility of all staff. Mental health clinicians are often faced with complicated ethical decisions about documenting the statements and behaviors of their patients. Disciplinary reports can lead to increased time in restrictive housing units and increased incarceration time.

Decisions about whether to focus on clinical issues related to transference must be balanced with a clear understanding of regulations designed to maintain the safety and security of the institution. For this reason, it is crucial that correctional clinicians have the opportunity for clinical discussion and supervision as part of their regular work schedule and duties.

In some correctional mental health treatment programs, mental health clinicians have the unique challenge of providing treatment to patients who interact with each other on a regular basis over a long period of time. Because inmates in correctional mental health programs live in close proximity and often attend group therapy together, they have ample opportunity to impact the treatment environment by sharing information and misinformation.

Once therapeutic rapport and clear boundaries are established with a patient, the goals of treatment must be clearly defined. In an ideal situation, patients who reach their goals in treatment are transferred to a less restrictive environment or an equally desirable (in terms of safety and access to privileges) placement at a lower level of mental health care. Unfortunately, the stigma of mental illness inherent in many inmate social structures may limit the placements to which a patient may safely graduate from a mental health treatment program. Inmates who were involved in gang activity prior to entering mental health treatment may be rejected or harmed by their prior associates, mental health patients may be pressured to stop taking psychotropic medication, and the increased stress of interacting with higher functioning inmates may cause some patients to decompensate.

Many mental health programs offer a relatively safe and entertaining environment compared with the general corrections population. Progress in therapy is dependent on the inmate-patient's motivation to change. The treatment plan must therefore include expected length of stay in the mental health program and an understanding of where the patient will be placed when treatment goals are met. Goals of treatment should include both reduction of mental health symptoms and measurable behaviors that indicate a reduction in symptoms. Table 6–3 outlines behaviors that can be measured when treatment is being provided to inmates.

To encourage progress in treatment, the clinician should focus individual contact with the patient on a few measurable goals, and the treatment team should evaluate the necessity for continued mental health treatment on a regular basis. The clinician's therapeutic orientation will affect the conceptualization of the case and the interventions used to obtain the goals. However, in order to achieve cohesive treatment, the interdisciplinary team must agree to focus on the patients' progress toward specific goals.

TABLE 6–3.   Measurable patient behaviors

- Attendance and participation in treatment activities
- Medication compliance
- Improvement of cleanliness and grooming
- Appropriate interactions with staff and patients
  - Oriented
  - Goal-directed spontaneous speech (normal rate and volume of speech)
  - Appropriate expression of emotion
  - Ability to listen and participate in conversation
  - Ability to appropriately resolve conflict
- Reduction of violent behavior
- Reduction of self-destructive and suicidal behavior
- Reduction of self-report of suicide plan and/or ideation
- Reduction of disruptive and destructive behavior
- Increase in prosocial and constructive behavior
- Normal patterns of sleep/wake cycle
- Ability to participate in school, work, and/or opportunities for fitness, arts, and social activities as available
- Verbalization of insight into past symptoms and reasons for improvement
- Positive plans for future activities and behavior

Group and Recreational Therapy

Group therapy is useful in the correctional environment for several reasons. The group process may be used for peer support, peer reality testing and feedback, didactic education, improving social skills, decreasing isolation, and increasing recreational activities. Designing therapeutic group treatment for inmates requires attention to the unique correctional culture. Issues of safety and confidentiality must be addressed in general policy and with group therapy participants. Group therapy can be harmful to participants unless rules and consequences for breaking the rules are clarified from the onset. For example, in some group therapy sessions, use of profanity is allowed, and in others, similar language would lead to disciplinary action. It is especially important in the correctional setting to have clear documented rules about how inappropriate behavior and conflict between participants will be handled.

Physical safety during group sessions can be increased through group room design and early intervention when conflicts arise. Group facilitators should always have closest access to exit the room and a means to summon correctional staff. In most settings, both an alarm system and close custody presence are implemented. In high-security settings, participants may be held in individual locked cells during group treatment. When conflict begins to arise between participants, the group facilitator must quickly decide whether the interaction can be used in a therapeutic context, or whether the behavior needs to be extinguished. Facilitators who work with patients who have a history of violent behavior should be trained to summon help quickly if attempts to diffuse the situation are unsuccessful. Even in group situations that employ individual treatment cells for patients, conflict between participants can quickly lead to assaultive behavior, such as spitting or throwing urine, or to self-injurious behavior.

Informed consent requires that participants understand that the facilitator does not have the ability to protect confidentiality in the correctional setting. While encouraging participants to maintain group session confidentiality, the facilitator should lead a discussion focused on helping participants make safe decisions about disclosing personal information. In some correctional settings, certain inmates (e.g., sex offenders, informants, gang dropouts) are at risk of being physically harmed by other inmates if their history is revealed. Avoiding discussion of types of information that are better discussed in individual sessions and providing periodic reminders that confidentiality cannot be guaranteed are ethical ways of minimizing risk to the patients.

There are risks and benefits to segregating group participants by functioning level, age, term length, race, diagnosis, or prognosis. Segregation of group therapy participants by race is particularly controversial. In environments where the inmate culture prohibits interaction between racial groups, it seems to make sense to segregate patients for group therapy so that they are more likely to talk to one another and provide some peer support. At times, custody officials prohibit racially integrated groups in an effort to prevent violent interactions. However, the danger of validating and reinforcing the violent propaganda of prison gangs often overrides the benefits of racially segregated therapy.

In the California Department of Corrections, even on some of the most violent prison yards, mental health patients participate in racially integrated group therapy. Patients who are unable to participate without threatening or violent behavior are placed in higher security units where participants are held in individual locked treatment cells during group therapy. Processing issues related to the correctional culture is a part of many group therapy discussions. The only negative aspect of providing integrated treatment in this type of setting is that on discharge from the treatment setting, some patients fear that they will be targeted for assault by general population inmates (i.e., those not requiring mental health care). Housing patients carefully on discharge is therefore necessary in order to facilitate fearful mental health patients' successful transition to a lower level of care.

Most clinicians agree that some patients are not appropriate for or likely to benefit from group therapy. Patients with acute psychosis and severe personality disorders are often treated with only individual therapy. However, in some correctional settings, severely mentally ill inmates are required by court mandate to be offered group therapy. For these patients, group sessions are designed to provide structured activity and facilitate appropriate interaction. Specific group topics may be useful for providing information or for teaching skills (see Table 6–4). Some groups may help patients who have similar mental health issues, diagnoses, or interests to develop insight. Other groups may be designed to teach recreational skills. The main job of the correctional group facilitator, regardless of the group topic, is to help patients participate and interact during the group setting without aggressive, violent, destructive, or other inappropriate behavior.

Cognitive-Behavioral Therapy

Cognitive-behavioral therapy (CBT), either group or individual, is becoming a mainstay of treatment in various correctional settings by targeting problem behaviors and maladaptive patterns of thinking. Currently, this form of therapy is used by the Florida and Illinois Departments of Corrections, among others. In Florida, the CBT regimen for the correctional system is somewhat euphemistically called the "Rethinking Personal Choice" program.

Although cruder forms of behavior modification have long been employed in penal settings, the use of more formal CBT is a more recent phenomenon. CBT stresses the interaction of the three domains of human behavior: thought, emotion, and behavior. Simply put, because thinking affects behavior, by modifying thoughts, long-term behavioral changes can be effected.

In the correctional setting, clinicians have tended to use CBT to target antisocial, socially maladaptive patterns of thinking or behavior rather than disorders that may have a lesser association with criminality or disruption of the milieu (e.g., panic disorder or obsessive-compulsive disorder). This approach is both practical and effective, since CBT models have shown positive short-term effects for the treatment of violent offenders and inmates with severe personality disorders, even psychopathy (Serin 1996). CBT, in combination with social skills training, has also been shown to be an effective treatment for sexual offenders. In several studies, the treatment groups showed reduced anxiety, improved self-esteem (Seto and Barbaree 1995), and lower levels of sexual reoffending when compared with control subjects (Hanson et al. 2002; Schwartz and Cellini 1995, 1999). However, more long-term evaluations and follow-up are needed.

TABLE 6–4. Types of group therapy in the correctional setting

Informational and skill building	Peer support/Insight development
• Advanced education	• 12-step meetings
• Anger management	• Adjustment issues
• Assertiveness vs. aggression	• Coping with a life term
• Basic neurology/the human brain	• Domestic violence reduction
• Cause and effect of substance abuse	• Empathy
• Cognitive and memory rehabilitation	• Family issues
• Communication skills	• Grief/bereavement
• Cultural differences	• Parole preparation
• General education	• Reduction of impulsivity
• Human sexuality	• Sexual predators
• Life span development	• Specific mental disorder focus
• Medication education	• Spiritual growth
• Parenting	• Substance abuse prevention
• Problem solving	• Survivors of physical abuse and neglect
• Relaxation	• Survivors of sexual abuse
• Social skills	• Victimization/cycle of violence
Recreational	**Process**
• Art (drawing, painting, creative arts)	• Open discussion facilitated by the clinician[a]
• Book club	
• Current events	
• Drama	
• Exercise/yoga/physical games	
• Meditation	
• Movie discussion	
• Music appreciation	
• Origami	
• Recreational games	

[a]This type of group is patient led, and topics may vary from session to session.

Dialectical Behavioral Therapy

More recently, a variation of CBT, dialectical behavioral therapy (DBT), has been effectively used to treat serious problem behaviors in inmates (e.g., self-injurious behavior or violence toward others). This form of therapy has particularly targeted those inmates with borderline personality disorder (BPD), who constitute a significant minority of the jail and prison population.

DBT, which was pioneered by Marsha Linehan in the mid-1980s, attempts to teach patients with BPD skills to help them cope with their abnormal response to emotional stimulation (i.e., their "emotional lability"). DBT is pragmatic and hierarchical in its approach to teaching these skills. Paramount among these skills is reducing self-injurious or life-threatening behaviors. Next is reducing behaviors that interfere with the therapy. The final skill is reducing behaviors that otherwise adversely affect the patient's quality of life. These skills are taught both through once-weekly psychotherapy sessions and in weekly 2.5-hour group therapy sessions. DBT has been shown to be quite effective in reducing parasuicidal behavior, decreasing inpatient psychiatric days, and improving compliance with therapy (Linehan et al. 1991).

Although originally developed to treat outpatients, DBT has more recently been used to treat inpatients, in both correctional and noncorrectional settings. In correctional settings, DBT is generally used as part of an "intensive behavior therapy unit." Such units have been established in maximum security prisons in Georgia and Illinois, in women's federal correctional facilities in Canada, and in the United States Navy Brig in San Diego. Preliminary results are encouraging, though there are currently not ample data on outcomes, primarily because the programs were fairly recently established.

Therapeutic Communities

Although not a new concept, the therapeutic community model is a relatively recent addition to the correctional psychiatry treatment landscape. Therapeutic communities were developed to treat individuals with substance abuse problems and continue to operate in that capacity. A therapeutic community operates under a "self-help" model in which patients are taught to work with one another and become the agents of change within the treatment community (DeLeon 1997). The typical therapeutic community model uses a phase system of treatment, including orientation, primary treatment, reentry, and community-based treatment. As the patient progresses through the phases, he or she is given increasing levels of responsibility and independence. Obviously, the goal is to return the patient to the community to live substance and crime-free as quickly as is feasible and to reduce recidivism rates compared with more conventional incarceration.

Delaware was one of the first states to implement the therapeutic community model in the treatment of cocaine-dependent prisoners. The KEY/CREST program commenced in July 1988 at the Multi-Purpose Criminal Justice Facility in Wilmington, Delaware, with 20 individuals with lengthy criminal histories and long-term drug dependence. These individuals were separated from the general prison population and a therapeutic community was established inside the correctional facility. Later, some inmates were also involved in a work-release therapeutic community. At 18-month follow-up, those individuals who had been involved in both an in-prison therapeutic community and a work-release therapeutic community were significantly less likely to have been rearrested than the control group (23% vs. 44%). They were also much less likely to have relapsed on drugs as measured by self-report and urinalysis (53% vs. 84%) (Martin et al. 1999). On the basis of the success of the KEY/CREST program, Delaware obtained additional funding and now has 550 in-prison treatment beds, 530 community-residential beds, and aftercare services for another 400 patients (Hooper 2003).

In prison and jail mental health programs where patients can safely gather with staff in groups, therapeutic community–type meetings help create a setting where patients have input into program guidelines, rules, and procedures. Regularly scheduled therapeutic community meetings also work to facilitate conflict resolution, teach social skills and leadership, and help patients learn self-advocacy and prosocial behavior. Mental health and custody supervisors should intermittently be present at therapeutic community meetings to validate and resolve reasonable concerns of the patients. Keeping an official agenda and recording minutes are helpful to document issues, discussion, and decisions made.

Behavioral Incentive Programs

Behavioral incentive programs (BIPs) and token economies have long been used to help mental health patients change maladaptive behaviors. Inmates are given opportunities to earn different privileges by exhibiting appropriate behavior and participating in beneficial activities designated by their treatment teams. These types of programs are employed at various correctional facilities nationwide, including the Tamms Correctional Center in Illinois and two prisons in the California Department of Corrections.

In the corrections environment, it is important that the BIP avoid providing incentives for patients to malinger mental illness in order to be included in the program. In the California Department of Corrections, a reinforcement system was created for the super-maximum security mental health program. Staff first identified all of the privileges (as opposed to constitutional rights) allowed inmates housed in this security level. Privileges included possession of property not necessary for legal purposes; use of radios and televisions; access to canteen and packages; use of small group yards; and out-of-cell time to clean the unit (which also allows conversation with other staff and inmates). In the mental-health-unit BIP, all these privileges are initially restricted and can be earned only through appropriate behavior and participation in treatment activities designated in the treatment plan. Medication compliance is not required for acquisition of privileges. Unless a patient meets criteria for involuntary medication, the patient's behavior is a more ethical and legal measure of his progress in treatment. Patients receive an orientation handbook explaining the details of the BIP, and the mental health staff help lower-functioning patients understand the criteria required in order to earn privileges.

Residential Community Corrections Centers

Residential community corrections centers (RCCCs) are something of a variant of transitional communities and have been established in several states, most notably Colorado. RCCCs operate under the "self-help" model of TCs and serve as decentralized, residential programs that facilitate the reintegration of inmates into the community prior to parole. Generally, inmates transition from prison to these facilities prior to entering an intensive supervision program or being released. RCCCs encourage independent living and self-sufficiency through paid employment.

Although RCCCs are not specifically designed for inmates with mental illness or substance abuse problems, many of the programs offered at RCCCs target these areas. In general, RCCCs offer self-improvement opportunities including educational, counseling, and treatment programs. More specifically, for inmates with mental illness and substance abuse issues, RCCCs offer monitored medication distribution, case management, individual counseling, group CBT, random urine screening, substance abuse treatment, and other services for the chronically mentally ill.

MEASUREMENT OF PROGRAM SUCCESS

Measuring treatment outcomes is a crucial component of developing successful correctional mental health programs. Treatment outcomes illuminate a program's strengths and help identify areas that need further development. Defining and measuring program success in a correctional setting has challenges similar to other mental health programs, and some that are unique to the corrections setting. Research in all mental health programs must take into account patient confidentiality and informed consent. The ethics of including incarcerated populations in empirical research studies may limit the kind of data which can be collected in correctional mental health programs. Often, correctional mental health programs are not designed or staffed to collect consistent data or maintain standardized data entry for regular reports. Tracking outcomes in a correctional setting may also be difficult due to irregular access to patient records and changes in patient custody or housing status during treatment.

When randomized controlled studies are not feasible, program success in a correctional setting can be indicated by dependent measures related to changes in individual patient functioning. Aggregate data such as discharge locations and disciplinary behaviors can also be used to measure factors related to patient treatment success (see Table 6–5). Over time, the mentally ill patients in the identified corrections population who are successfully treated will require lower levels of care and less restrictive environments.

TABLE 6–5. Variables used to measure treatment success

Patient-dependent measures

- Disciplinary reports (number and type)
- GAF scores, diagnosis modifications (e.g., in remission)
- Frequency of crisis intervention and time required for crisis intervention
- Suicide attempts and gestures
- Participation in program activities
- Behavioral incentive program level changes
- Length of stay
- Recidivism to higher levels of care

Program-dependent measures

- Attendance in individual and group therapy
- Medication compliance
- Suicide rate
- Discharges to lower levels of care
- Discharges to less restrictive environments
- Referrals to higher levels of care
- Complaints/appeals filed by patients
- Disciplinary reports

Regional-dependent measures

- Number of mentally ill patients requiring high security
- Percentage of the population requiring higher levels of mental health care

Note. GAF=Global Assessment of Functioning.

CONCLUSION

Appropriately staffing a mental health program is the first step in creating successful treatment. The number and type of staff needed depend on the mission statement, goals of the treatment program, and relevant court mandates. Financial considerations of staffing should include indicators that successful treatment programs reduce violent and disciplinary behaviors of mentally ill inmates, thereby significantly reducing the overall cost of the corrections system. Signs of inadequate staffing include increased inmate disciplinary reports, high rate of inmate suicide or self-injurious behavior, lack of medication continuity, failure to conduct quality assurance and peer review, inability to track outcome variables, poor staff morale, high staff turnover, and lack of compliance with court mandates.

Clinical staff time and morale can be maximized by hiring office support staff responsible for administrative tasks and for collecting and distributing relevant data. The California Department of Corrections uses a statewide mental health tracking system that is networked within each institution and downloaded to a central database. To improve treatment efficacy, correctional facilities need mental health programs that have adequate staff to collect data relevant to measuring program success. Medical records staff are also key to maintaining appropriate records of treatment and ensuring access to these records.

The challenge of maintaining quality mental health care in the corrections setting requires continual interdisciplinary training. Establishing regular systems for team building and solution-focused discussion facilitate the ability of staff from different backgrounds to work toward common goals. Professionals from custody and health care backgrounds together can develop quality mental health treatment in order to create a safer correctional and public environment.

SUMMARY POINTS

- Court decisions indicate that inmates have a right to adequate mental health treatment in the correctional setting.
- Every correctional mental health program should have a clear mission statement.
- Mental health assessment by an interdisciplinary treatment team is necessary to account for the unique challenges of the population.
- Correctional settings meet constitutional requirements for adequate mental health care by providing several levels of care based on patient needs.
- Therapeutic interventions may be modified to meet the needs of the inmate population.
- Measurable treatment goals are a crucial part of treatment planning.
- Measuring treatment outcomes is necessary to develop successful mental health programs.

REFERENCES

Bowring v Godwin, 551 F.2d 44 (4th Cir. 1977)
Brad H. v City of New York, New York County Clerk's Index No. 117882/99 (2001)
Coleman v Wilson, 912 F.Supp. 1282 (1995)
DeLeon G: Therapeutic communities: is there an essential model? in Community as Method: Therapeutic Communities for Special Populations and Special Settings. Edited by DeLeon G. Westport, CT, Praeger, 1997, pp 3–18

Estelle v Gamble, 429 U.S. 97, 97 S. Ct. 285, 50 L. Ed. 2d 251 (1976)

Grassian S: Psychopathological effects of solitary confinement. Am J Psychiatry 140: 1450–1454, 1983

Grassian S, Friedman N: Effects of sensory deprivation in psychiatric seclusion and solitary confinement. Int J Law Psychiatry 8:49–65, 1986

Hanson RK, Gordon A, Harris AJ, et al: First report of the collaborative outcome data project on the effectiveness of psychological treatment for sex offenders. Sex Abuse 14:169–197, 2002

Hare RD: Manual for the Hare Psychopathy Checklist–Revised. Toronto, ON, Multi-Health Systems, 1991

Hart SD, Dempster RJ: Impulsivity and psychopathy, in Impulsivity: Theory, Assessment, and Treatment. Edited by Webster CD, Jackson MA. New York, Guilford, 1997, pp 212–232

Hooper R: Something works–therapeutic communities in the treatment of substance abuse, in Correctional Psychology: Practice, Programming, and Administration. Edited by Schwartz B. Kingston, NJ, Civic Research Institute, Inc, 2003, pp 12/1–12/17

Joe GW, Simpson DD, Dansereau DF, et al: Relationships between counseling rapport and drug abuse treatment outcomes. Psychiatr Serv 52:1223–1229, 2001

Kupers TA: Prison Madness: The Mental Health Crisis Behind Bars and What We Must Do About It. San Francisco, CA, Jossey-Bass, 1999

Langley v Coughlin, 715 F.Supp. 522 (S.D. N.Y. 1989)

Linehan MM, Armstrong HE, Suarez A, et al: Cognitive-behavioral treatment of chronically parasuicidal borderline patients. Arch Gen Psychiatry 48:1060–1064, 1991

Madrid v Gomez, 889 F.Supp. 1146, 1280 (N.D. Calif. 1995)

Martin S, Butzin C, Saum C, et al: Three year outcomes of therapeutic community treatment for drug-involved offenders in Delaware: from prison to work release to aftercare. The Prison Journal 79:294–320, 1999

Newman v Alabama, 559 F.2d 283 (1977)

Ruiz v Estelle, 503 F.Supp. 1265 (S.D. Tex. 1980)

Schwartz BK (ed): Correctional Psychology: Practice, Programming, and Administration. Kingston, NJ, Civic Research Institute, 2003

Schwartz BK, Cellini HR: Female sex offenders, in The Sex Offender: Corrections, Treatment, and Legal Developments. Edited by Schwartz BK, Cellini HR. Kingston, NJ, Civic Research Institute, 1995, pp 5/1–5/22

Schwartz BK, Cellini HR: Sex offender recidivism and risk factors in the involuntary commitment process, in The Sex Offender: Theoretical Advances, Treating Special Populations and Legal Developments. Edited by Schwartz BK. Kingston, NJ, Civic Research Institute, 1999, pp 8/1–8/22

Serin R: Violent recidivism in criminal psychopaths. Law Hum Behav 20:207–217, 1996

Seto MC, Barbaree HE: The role of alcohol in sexual aggression. Clin Psychol Review 15:545–566, 1995

Wakefield v Thompson, 177 F.3d 1160 (9th Cir. 1999)

CHAPTER 7

Assessment of Malingering in Correctional Settings

Michael J. Vitacco, Ph.D.

Richard Rogers, Ph.D., ABPP

Rogers (1997) has developed a general model for understanding why some patients are honest and forthcoming while others engage in various forms of deception. Four principles of this model are germane to the frequent deception observed in correctional settings: agency, confidentiality, social control, and value imposition.

Deception is likely to occur when referred inmates perceive the following:

- Clinicians are working more for the institution than for the patients (agency).
- Patients' disclosures can potentially be used against them (lack of confidentiality).
- Clinicians can restrict patients' freedoms and even imposing sanctions (social control).
- Clinicians do not respect patients' autonomy but seek to induce mainstream values (value imposition).

Mental health clinicians in corrections face numerous challenges posed by inmate perceptions and institutional realities based on these principles. For instance, how should psychiatrists handle the ever-present requests for sleeping medications? One option is to conform to formal or informal institutional expectations and never diagnose or treat primary insomnia. When faced with repeated requests, clinicians are confronted with more difficult choices. For instance, should they impose sanctions by routinely characterizing recurrent requests as "treatment seeking," "manipulativeness," or even "malingering"? Once the inmates' motivations are labeled, their access to future treatment is often restricted.

Psychiatrists and inmates with disorders are both involved in a tightly controlled system that does not promote trust and self-disclosure. Distortions and deceptions are commonplace. Some deceptions reflect systemic issues, such as problems with agency and confidentiality. Other deceptions are more individualized and goal oriented. A primary goal of this chapter is for mental health professionals to appreciate the complex interplay between systemic issues and personal motivations in producing feigned and distorted response styles.

This chapter has several additional goals related to correctional practice. Building on the introduction, we explore contrasting views of why inmates may distort, and even malinger, their clinical presentations. These explanatory models influence how clinicians approach malingering, especially in correctional settings. In addition, we critically examine methods of screening and evaluating response styles, such as malingering. Before undertaking these issues, we provide, in the next section, a brief review of response styles.

RESPONSE STYLES

No clinician, patient, or inmate is entirely honest all of the time. Various forms of deception are observed in most social interactions (Miller and Stiff 1993). Response styles should be classified only when they constitute a predominant and nontransient type of deception. Response styles can be grouped by DSM-IV-TR classifications and diagnostic terms, clinical descriptions, and ambiguous constructs.

DSM-IV-TR Classification and Diagnostic Terms

The *Diagnostic and Statistical Manual of Mental Disorders,* 4th Edition, Text Revision (American Psychiatric Association 2000) provides the official nomenclature for diagnosis of mental disorders. It includes the classification of malingering (V65.2) and the diagnoses of factitious disorders and somatoform disorders.

Malingering is defined by DSM-IV-TR as the "intentional production of false or grossly exaggerated physical or psychological symptoms, motivated by external incentives." Importantly, DSM-IV-TR conceptualizes malingering as a "condition" that may be the "focus of clinical attention" (American Psychiatric Association 2000, p. 739). As simply a "condition," malingering lacks the specific inclusion criteria found with formal diagnoses. Instead, mental health providers are provided with only a description of four screening indicators for when malingering should be suspected.

Factitious disorders are described by DSM-IV-TR as "physical or psychological symptoms that are intentionally produced or feigned in order to assume the sick role" (American Psychiatric Association 2000, p. 513). Cunnien (1997) provided subtypes of factitious disorders, including psychosis, posttraumatic stress disorder, bereavement, dissociative identity disorder, child abuse, and medical disorders. For the diagnosis, the following inclusion criteria (see American Psychiatric Association 2000, p. 517) must be met: a) there must be intentional production or feigning of physical or psychological symptoms, b) the motivation for the behavior is to assume the sick role, and c) external incentives for the behavior (e.g., avoiding criminal trial or financial gain) are absent.

Correctional mental health professionals should not automatically assume inmates are always motivated by external incentives. As observed by Rogers and Neumann (2003), the simple *possibility* of an incentive (e.g., desire for a single cell) cannot be taken as actual *evidence* that the incentive actually played any role in the behavior. As a further complication, patients with factitious disorders may be unaware of their motivations in light of intrapsychic issues.

DSM-IV-TR (American Psychiatric Association 2000) classifies *somatoform disorders* as a group of diagnoses related to the *unintentional* production of physical symptoms. Rogers and Vitacco (2002) differentiated somatoform disorders from malingering in that somatoform disorders are limited to medical conditions and are not under the patient's control. Additionally, psychiatrists must apply a very general exclusion criterion: somatoform disorders cannot be "fully explained" by medical conditions, mental disorders, or the direct effects of substance abuse.

Ganser syndrome was coined by a German psychiatrist, Sigbert Ganser, to describe prisoners trying to avoid prosecution through the use of hysterical reaction (Cosgray and Fawley 1989). Currently, Ganser syndrome is no longer viewed as feigning; instead, it is subsumed under dissociative disorder not otherwise specified. It was first observed in correctional settings and is defined as providing "approximate answers to questions." Ganser syndrome, which is characterized by a history of dissociation and childhood abuse (Drob and Meehan 2000), is rare in correctional and forensic settings (Andersen et al. 2001) and not well understood.

Clinical Descriptions

Evolving from the classification, several nondiagnostic terms have gained wide acceptance as useful terms to describe patients' response styles. We categorize these terms as *clinical descriptions.*

Feigning refers to the fabrication or gross exaggeration of psychological or physical symptoms (Rogers and Vitacco 2002). Importantly, psychological tests cannot identify whether the motivation is internal (factitious) or external (malingering). Therefore, the term *feigning* is used in psychological assessments to characterize fabricated symptom presentation.

Defensiveness, the opposite of malingering, is exemplified by the denial or gross minimization of psychological symptoms for the purpose of obtaining an external goal. Defensiveness occurs commonly in correctional settings to avoid stigmatization or psychiatric intervention. It occurs most commonly when evaluations consider issues such as parole or reduction in security status.

Ambiguous Constructs

Several terms should be avoided in correctional practice because of their ambiguity or potential for misinterpretation. Ambiguous constructs include secondary gain and suboptimal effort.

Secondary gain (Rogers and Reinhardt 1998) has several conflicting definitions and should be avoided. These definitions vary from psychodynamic perspective whereby the perpetuation of impairment is motivated by unmet intrapsychic needs, to behavioral models in which the caretakers unknowingly provide positive reinforcement for continuation of the sick role. Efforts to apply this term to correctional practice lack both theory and research. We view primary gain, in contrast to secondary gain, as only peripherally related to malingering.

Suboptimal effort is a catchall term for not putting forth one's best effort. It ignores situational (e.g., prison adjustment) and psychopathological (e.g., major depression) effects on performance. Unfortunately, some clinicians attempt to equate suboptimal effort with malingering. Ironically, this facile misapplication often represents a suboptimal effort on the part of the clinician. Given both confounds and potential for misinterpretation, the term *suboptimal effort* should be avoided in correctional settings.

MISCLASSIFICATION OF MALINGERING IN CORRECTIONAL SETTINGS

DSM-IV TR (American Psychiatric Association 2000) provides four screening indicators for malingering: a) medicolegal context, b) presence of antisocial personality disorder, c) uncooperativeness with assessment and treatment, and d) marked discrepancies between claimed impairment and clinical data. The DSM indicators for suspected malingering are loosely fashioned, defined more by criminal behavior than by empirical data (Rogers and Vitacco 2002), and can easily be misused. The DSM indicators were never intended to diagnose or classify malingering; such misuses can lead to a large number of false positives (Gerson 2002).

Correctional mental health providers must be alert to misuses of DSM-IV-TR screening indices for malingering. Two indices (i.e., antisocial personality disorder and medicolegal context) are extremely common in jails and prisons. Given their prevalence, these indices are unlikely to discriminate malingered from genuine presentations. *We have no empirical evidence that these indices are effective in correctional settings.* As such, misconstruing DSM-IV TR suggestions on when to suspect malingering as actual evidence of malingering produces a false-positive rate of approximately 80% (Rogers 1990).

EXPLANATORY MODELS OF MALINGERING IN CORRECTIONAL SETTINGS

Rogers (1997) described three explanatory models that attempt to explain the underlying motivation for why persons malinger. In the earliest explanation, the *pathogenic model,* underlying psychopathology is posited to be the primary motivation for malingering. As the malingerer's adjustment continues to deteriorate, the pathogenic model predicts, the voluntary feigning of symptoms will gradually be replaced by genuine involuntary symptoms. The pathogenic model has fallen into disfavor and has been replaced by two markedly contrasting perspectives: the criminological (DSM-IV-TR) and adaptational models.

The Criminological Model

The *criminological model,* consistent with DSM-IV-TR, assumes that malingering is a specific manifestation of antisocial behavior and attitudes. In other words, antisocial persons engage in a variety of deceptive practices, which may include malingering. On the basis of this model, nearly all inmates would be deemed suspicious of malingering or other forms of deception. Clearly, the criminological model promotes distrust of most inmates, but it does not discriminate between feigning and genuine presentations. Frankly, we see unwarranted distrust as an impediment to sound clinical practice.

The acceptance of the criminological model in corrections can lead to the development of an unhealthy level of cynicism or the indiscriminant dismissal of legitimate mental health complaints. We have encountered clinicians who assess feigning in correctional settings with the working premise, "I know it is there; I just have to find it." Clinicians who strongly suspect malingering in all inmates with antisocial personality disorder commit an *ad hominem fallacy* (Rogers and Vitacco 2002), whereby negative attributions about the person overshadow diagnostic and assessment data.

Despite its limitations, the criminological model does have merit in a minority of cases in which the deception appears more characterological. Such examples include chronic conning (Rogers and Cruise 2000), attempts to frustrate staff, seeking transfer to a unit where escape is more probable, or medication seeking to sell it for profit or use it to get "high." As an example of medication seeking, the first author was recently involved in a case, described below, in which a forensic patient was able to obtain at least 40 medication changes in the course of 1 month by manipulating various on-call psychiatrists with numerous physical and psychological complaints. In this instance, the patient appeared to be "messing with the system" more than seeking a positive outcome.

Clinical Case 7–1: The Criminological Model

Mr. Wallace, a 42-year-old European American male, was referred for a psychological evaluation as part of a comprehensive assessment determining his eligibility for supervised release from a medium-security forensic hospital. He was adjudicated not guilty by reason of insanity in 2002 after pointing a loaded gun at his family during a psychotic episode secondary to cocaine use. Within months of his admission to the hospital, symptoms of active psychosis were no longer observed, and he petitioned the court for a supervised release. Although staff no longer reported observing any symptoms of mental illness, the patient continued to challenge institutional rules and reported experiencing a variety of physical and emotional problems. Notably, most of his complaints were directed at weekend or on-call psychiatrists who frequently provided him with additional pain or sleeping medications; he obtained 40 medication changes in the course of 30 days.

Mr. Wallace's evaluation for conditional release included psychological testing and a thorough review of his medication changes. Results from specialized psychological measures were consistent with an individual who knowingly fabricates symptoms. In fact, when confronted with the medication review and results from the psychological testing, Mr. Wallace readily acknowledged his conscious efforts to receive medications.

After being confronted with this information, Mr. Wallace was informed that his treatment team would not recommend release until he desists in his medication-seeking behaviors. Mr. Wallace promptly enrolled in alcohol and drug abuse classes and individual psychotherapy. He demonstrated significant improvement over several months as evidenced by infrequent limit testing and less medication seeking. In June 2004, a court granted his supervised release from the forensic hospital.

The Adaptational Model

The *adaptational model* (Rogers and Cavanaugh 1983) assumes that malingering is usually an attempt to succeed when faced with adverse, if not adversarial, circumstances. In an attempt to address these circumstances (e.g., jail violence or a pending trial), an inmate may seek a more positive alternative by malingering a mental disorder. As a vivid example, a few defendants facing California's three-strikes law have attempted to feign psychosis to avert a 25-year minimum sentence (Jaffe and Sharma 1998). Faced with this future, some defendants may understandably choose to malinger. Moreover, Rogers and Shuman (2000) found many inmates malinger to avoid going to trial (i.e., competency to stand trial; see Clinical Case 7–2 below) or adjudication as not guilty by reason of insanity.

As an instructive parallel, Wynia (2003) reported that a substantial minority of physicians report "gaming the system" to provide their patients with needed treatment. They typically justify their deceptive practices (e.g., exaggerating reports of illnesses) on the basis of adversarial views of insurers (e.g., uncaring and financially motivated) and the needed outcome for their patients (e.g., lack of other viable alternatives). The adaptational model clearly applies across health care and correctional settings.

The adaptational model has empirical support in the literature as a viable alternative to the DSM model of malingering. Vitacco (2002) found that some inmates in a correctional mental health unit manifested very low levels of psychopathology and readily acknowledged fabricating symptoms because of the calming and nonviolent nature of the jail mental health unit. Likewise, research by Walters (1988) suggested that inmates can alter their test results on the basis of the desired outcome: a single cell (malingering) or opportunity for release (defensiveness). A strength of the adaptational model is a likely reduction of countertransference issues associated with malingering. Deception under the adaptational model is illustrated in the following clinical case.

Clinical Case 7–2: The Adaptational Model

Mr. Nadir, a 28-year-old Hispanic American male, was admitted to a secure forensic unit for an evaluation of his competency to stand trial. He was charged with manufacturing cocaine and possession with intent to deliver cocaine. Given Mr. Nadir's previous drug convictions, he was facing a 15-year sentence in a state penitentiary.

Almost immediately upon admission, Mr. Nadir reported extremely atypical perceptual disturbances. He insisted he was seeing ninjas, seeing people smoking on a porch, and smelling foul odors. Notes from his intake summary stated, "In short, Mr. Nadir endorsed every psychotic symptom queried." Because of concerns about the veracity of his self-report, specialized measures of malingering were administered. Results from the Structured Interview of

Reported Symptoms (SIRS), an interview-based measure of feigning, indicated that Mr. Nadir endorsed large numbers of rare symptoms and combinations of symptoms across several clinical disorders. He reported most of his symptoms were at a high level of severity. Despite telling the competency examiner he had limited knowledge of the legal system, he frequently discussed plea options and sophisticated legal concepts like "truth in sentencing" with various unit staff members.

Although it was clearly in his best interest to try and avoid a lengthy prison sentence, staff was immediately cued into Mr. Nadir's attempts to avoid prosecution by his inconsistent and bizarre presentation. He was returned to court after completion of his evaluation and is currently awaiting trial on drug charges.

DETECTION STRATEGIES FOR THE ASSESSMENT OF MALINGERED MENTAL DISORDERS

Mental health professionals, relying on clinical interviews, can apply detection strategies to their inmate evaluations. In this section, we review seven well-validated detection strategies that can be adapted to clinical interviews:

1. *Rare symptoms.* Malingerers are often unaware of which symptoms occur infrequently among patients with genuine disorders. The rare-symptoms strategy can be used to detect feigning inmates, who endorse a substantial proportion of these highly infrequent symptoms.
2. *Improbable symptoms.* Approximately one-third of malingerers dramatically overplay their presentations and present improbable symptoms that have a very bizarre or fantastic quality (Rogers 2001). For example, an inmate's report of seeing Satan and his wife as conjoined twins would be an improbable symptom.
3. *Symptom combinations.* Many malingerers do not consider which symptoms are unlikely to occur together (i.e., symptom combinations). One approach is the use of unlikely symptom pairs in which each symptom is common by itself. For example, generalized anxiety and restful sleep are unlikely to occur together.
4. *Symptom severity.* Most genuine patients experience symptoms on a continuum from mild to moderate or even extreme. Malingerers often do not appreciate this continuum and report many symptoms as severe or extreme (i.e., symptom severity). As a caution, some inmates believe (rightly or wrongly) that exaggeration of symptom severity is essential for clinical intervention. For instance, a male inmate may believe that his recurrent yet controllable thoughts about suicide will not result in treatment. Therefore, he may exaggerate the frequency and severity of suicidal ideation in order to ensure treatment.

5. *Indiscriminant symptom endorsement.* When given a structured format covering many disorders, some malingerers endorse two-thirds or more of the symptoms presented (i.e., indiscriminant symptom endorsement). Genuine patients typically do not report such an array of diverse symptoms. However, correctional staff should be cautious in using this detection strategy. As seasoned psychiatrists know, multiple diagnoses are common in correctional populations.

6. *Obvious versus subtle symptoms.* Malingerers tend to focus on "obvious" symptoms clearly indicative of a mental disorder and overlook "subtle" symptoms that are not immediately associated with that disorder. In feigning schizophrenia, positive symptoms (e.g., hallucinations) may be emphasized and negative symptoms (e.g., avolition) entirely ignored.

7. *Reported versus observed symptoms.* Many genuine patients lack insight into their own symptoms (Neumann et al. 1996); their presentations may be highly inconsistent with clinical observations. When this detection strategy (reported vs. observed symptoms) is used, both the type and the magnitude of observed inconsistencies must be evaluated. To avoid errors, the clinician must evaluate blatant inconsistencies for the current time only, since past symptoms are not directly observable. Some clinicians choose to mention these observed inconsistencies (e.g., reportedly poor concentration but the capacity to focus on an extended interview) to the patient. As a benchmark, genuine patients are unlikely to deteriorate suddenly in their functioning after a simple remark about observed inconsistencies.

Clinicians seeking more in-depth information should consult the text *Clinical Assessment of Malingering and Deception* (Rogers 1997) and several more recent reviews (Resnick and Harris 2002; Rogers and Bender 2003; Rogers and Vitacco 2002).

MODEL FOR ASSESSING MALINGERING IN CORRECTIONAL SETTINGS

Correctional staff operates in complicated, sometimes fragmented, systems that often make individualized assessment challenging. Resources in most correctional facilities are limited. Therefore, we propose a three-stage process for evaluation of malingering and defensiveness: 1) initial evaluations, 2) systematic screens, and 3) comprehensive evaluations.

Initial Evaluations

Initial evaluations consist of a brief contact with the inmate either when he or she is processed into the facility or at the first report of mental health problems. Given the high volume, especially at urban jails, the natural tendency is to make the process routine and abbreviated. Regarding inmate deception, the risk at this point is inmate defensiveness much more than malingering. Substantial numbers of serious mental disorders are denied by inmates and overlooked by staff (Teplin 1984).

Unlike the intake process, self-referrals for mental health problems are more likely to involve malingering than defensiveness. If a correctional mental health provider suspects malingering, then the inmate should be screened. *Because of its far-ranging consequences, malingering should never be determined on the basis of a brief interview alone.* Moreover, we caution against ever assuming that suicide attempts are faked simply on the basis of history. Although such attempts are sometimes clearly manipulative, the real possibility of a genuine disorder must always be considered.

Systematic Screens

Several screens have been developed to assist clinicians in identifying cases of potential malingering (Jackson et al., in press; Miller 2001). The purpose of screens is to rapidly identify potential cases of feigning and effectively rule out genuine cases. To be efficient, the primary goal is to eliminate inmates with genuine disorders from further consideration. As a result, screens are *not* effective at correctly identifying cases of malingering, and therefore malingering cannot be determined from screens. Correctional psychiatrists should be prepared to challenge clinical staff that makes improper conclusions from malingering screens.

Comprehensive Evaluations

The goal of comprehensive evaluations (Drob and Berger 1987; Rogers et al. 2003) is to clearly determine the presence or absence of malingering. Of course, the correctional mental health professional must be cognizant that mental disorders and malingering are not mutually exclusive; the presence of malingering does not rule out actual mental disorders. This process typically includes several interviews, record reviews, and the use of standardized measures.

The importance of these determinations cannot be overestimated. Correctional records are often entered into evidence at trial or postconviction hearings. For example, we have been involved in several cases in which prison records of malingering appeared pivotal to determinations of competency to be executed.

INSTRUMENTS FOR SYSTEMATIC SCREENING

In this section, we highlight three screens for feigned mental disorders. These screens were selected because of their empirical validation and ease of use by professional staff. The strengths and weaknesses of each measure are outlined.

Miller Forensic Assessment of Symptoms Test (M-FAST)

The M-FAST (Miller 2001) is a brief (25-question) structured interview designed to assess for malingered mental disorders. It consists of a total score and seven scales.

Strengths

- The M-FAST scales are primarily based on established detection strategies, which were validated with the Structured Interview of Reported Symptoms (Rogers et al. 1992a).
- The M-FAST total score has good reliability (Miller 2001) and excellent clinical utility (Jackson et al., in press).
- The M-FAST interview format eliminates problems with reading comprehension and provides clinicians with an opportunity to observe inmates.

Weakness

- Three of the seven scales only possess one item, thus limiting their measurement of the detection strategy.

Structured Inventory of Malingered Symptomatology (SIMS)

The SIMS (Smith 1997; Smith and Burger 1997; Windows and Smith 2005) is a 75-item paper-and-pencil measure designed to assess various aspects of malingering. The SIMS has five overlapping scales designed to assess facets of malingering: a) Low Intelligence, b) Affective Disorders, c) Neurological Impairment, (d) Psychosis, and (e) Amnesia.

Strengths

- The total score of the SIMS has been found to demonstrate good ability to classify malingerers (Lewis et al. 2002; Smith and Burger 1997).
- The SIMS was found useful in assessing malingering in adolescent offenders (Rogers et al. 1995).
- The SIMS is easy to read and can be administered in small groups.

Weaknesses

- The self-report format may lead to missing important interpersonal components of an inmate's presentation.
- Elevated scores may be confounded by psychopathology (Edens et al. 1999), and this may limit the instrument's clinical utility.

M Test

The M Test (Beaber et al. 1985) is a 33-item true-false test designed to detect malingered mental disorders. Originally designed for feigned schizophrenia, it has been applied to a range of Axis I disorders.

Strengths

- Extensive research is available on its validity and utility (Smith 1997).
- A revised scoring system has been found to be highly effective (Rogers et al. 1992b).

Weaknesses

- The self-report format may lead to missing important interpersonal components of an inmate's presentation.
- High false-positive rates (Smith et al. 1993) have been reported.
- Scales and utility estimates vary markedly across studies.

INSTRUMENTS FOR COMPREHENSIVE EVALUATIONS OF MALINGERING

A single chapter cannot discuss all the instruments designed to detect malingering. However, several instruments are frequently employed and warrant attention. As such, we evaluate here one structured interview (the SIRS) and three multiscale inventories. We feature the SIRS for three reasons: its superior validity, its usefulness in classifying feigned mental disorders, and its ease of administration and interpretation.

Structured Interview of Reported Symptoms

The SIRS (Rogers et al. 1992a) is a structured interview specifically designed for the assessment of feigning and related response styles. The SIRS consists of eight primary scales that form two underlying dimensions (Rogers et al., in press).

Advantages

- The SIRS can be administered and interpreted by psychiatrists.
- The SIRS is a highly reliable measure that has been extensively validated (Rogers 2001) through a variety of research designs on correctional and forensic samples.
- The SIRS scales accurately differentiate honest responders from malingerers. They are designed to have a very low false-positive rate.

Disadvantages

- The SIRS has no indices to detect cognitive feigning.
- The SIRS is designed specifically to assess for malingering; no information on genuine psychopathology is obtained.

Multiscale Inventories

Minnesota Multiphasic Personality Inventory, 2nd Edition (MMPI-2)

The MMPI-2 (Butcher et al. 1989) is a 567-item true-false instrument designed to assess psychopathology and response styles. It is the most widely researched multiscale inventory for the assessment of psychopathology and malingering. The MMPI-2 employs seven scales in the detection of feigning (Greene 1997). In a meta-analysis of 65 MMPI-2 feigning studies, Rogers and colleagues (2003) came to two general conclusions. First, a wide range of cutoff scores are reported for most validity scales. Therefore, clinicians should only use cutoff scores in the upper ranges to reduce false positives. Second, many validity scales varied in their effectiveness, depending on the specific diagnoses found in genuine patient populations.

Advantages.

- The efficacy of the MMPI-2 validity scales has been shown in an extensive database (Rogers et al. 2003).
- Many scales are based on validated detection strategies.

Disadvantages.

- Most scales are relatively ineffective at detecting feigners. Only extreme elevations can be safely interpreted.
- Validity scales have substantial overlap, thus decreasing their validity.
- The MMPI-2 requires a seventh-grade reading level, and many inmates have difficulty with its reading comprehension.
- Many psychologists have not kept abreast of new developments and may seriously misinterpret its results.

- Computerized interpretations are often inaccurate in describing response styles.

Personality Assessment Inventory (PAI)

The PAI (Morey 1991) is a 344-item multiscale inventory that rivals the MMPI-2 in terms of its clinical and forensic applications. It has two primary methods of assessing malingering. The NIM scale, based on rare symptoms, has yielded mixed results (Bagby et al. 2002; Calhoun et al. 2000; Liljequist et al. 1998; Rogers et al. 1996). When markedly elevated, the Malingering Index appears to be effective.

Advantages.

- The PAI has a simple reading level (grade 4) and is appropriate for most inmates.
- Extreme elevations are highly accurate when tested with different research designs.

Disadvantage.

- Even with extreme elevations, only a small proportion of feigners are identified.

Millon Clinical Multiaxial Inventory–III (MCMI-III)

The MCMI-III (Millon 1994) is a 175-item multiscale inventory widely employed in the evaluation of personality disorders and Axis I syndromes. The MCMI-III's usefulness in forensic and correctional settings is markedly limited by elevations on validity scales, which may reflect genuine impairment; and modest construct validity, which argues against its use in correctional and forensic settings (Rogers 2003). Recent research (Schoenberg et al. 2003) has documented important limitations of this inventory for the detection of feigning. Therefore, it is not recommended in evaluations for issues of malingering in correctional settings.

DETECTION STRATEGIES FOR THE ASSESSMENT OF MALINGERED COGNITIVE PROBLEMS

The assessment of feigning of cognitive or neuropsychological impairments is gaining importance in correctional settings. Prisoners often will malinger cognitive deficits to feign incompetence to stand trial (Heinze and Purisch 2001) or to avoid further punishment (Brodsky and Galloway 2003). Although malingered cognitive impairment does not occur as frequently as malingered mental disorders, mental health providers in corrections should be aware of the potential for malingered cognitive impairment and basic strategies for its detection.

Assessing cognitive malingering requires different strategies than those used with mental disorders. A comprehensive model of assessing cognitive impairments should employ methods to assess both feigned and true neuropsychological impairment (Goldberg 2001). In a seminal article, Rogers and colleagues (1993) outlined different detection strategies used to assess feigned cognitive impairment. Because of the formal testing requirements, most psychiatrists will refer suspected cases for psychological consults. However, it is important to understand the following underlying detection strategies.

1. *Floor effect.* Most genuine patients with cognitive impairment can answer correctly very simple items. Some malingerers "try too hard" and miss these items. For example, asking "Which has four legs, a human or a dog?" is an example of using the floor effect. This strategy is used by a number of scales: the Rey 15-item test (Lezak 1983), the Test of Memory Malingering (TOMM) (Tommbaugh 1996), and the Hiscock Digit Memory Test (Hiscock and Hiscock 1989).

2. *Symptom validity testing (SVT).* With multiple-choice responses, SVT evaluates whether the inmate is failing at "below-chance" levels. For example, a person without any ability should still achieve close to 50% on a two-choice cognitive test. Several scales use SVT, although many feigners avoid detection by not failing on more than 50% of the items. This method can be applied to purported amnesia for a crime (Frederick et al. 1995), although great care must be taken that the alternatives have an equal likelihood of being selected (Rogers and Shuman 2000).

3. *Forced-choice testing (FCT).* Unlike SVT, FCT does not rely on probability. Instead, group differences are examined between simulators and cognitively impaired patients. This detection strategy is vulnerable to confounds and should generally not be the basis for determinations of feigned cognitive impairment.

4. *Performance curve.* Inmates malingering cognitive deficit often do not take into account item difficulty when responding to testing. For genuine patients, the proportion of correct responses decreases substantially with increases in item difficulty (i.e., the performance curve). For malingerers, this performance curve is often flattened.

5. *Magnitude of error (MOE).* The MOE evaluates the degree of inaccuracy in the responses. Patients with genuine impairment tend to make predictable mistakes. Persons feigning cognitive impairment do not take into account the

different types of incorrect answers and may be detectable by MOE. Bender and Rogers (2004) found MOE to be the most robust detector of malingering even when simulators were warned about this detection strategy.

The following two strategies have only modest validity and should be avoided:

1. *Atypical presentation.* Unusual variation of test performance (i.e., atypical presentation) has been used as an indicator of malingering (Moses et al. 1983). Because many persons with cognitive impairment evidence variable performance, this strategy is easily confounded.
2. *Psychological sequelae.* Rogers and colleagues (1993) sought to identify persons feigning cognitive impairment by focusing on their accompanying symptoms (i.e., psychological sequelae). However, naïve persons can often recognize which symptoms are typically present, thereby reducing the effectiveness of this potential strategy.

CLINICAL MANAGEMENT OF MALINGERING IN CORRECTIONAL SETTINGS

Correctional settings should establish procedures for evaluations and interventions with likely malingerers. For evaluations, a standardization of the process with formal procedures can be very helpful so that information is systematically collected and shared among health care providers. Problematic cases typically arise from an absence of standardized methods for the assessment of feigning and the lack of integrated information.

Clinical interventions for malingering are typically limited. On a programmatic level, efforts to build credibility with the inmate populations are vital. On an individual level, direct feedback to the inmate malingerer may be helpful in some cases. For example, Towers and Frederick (2002) discussed their intervention with a malingerer whom they confronted with clinical data. Subsequently, the inmate was retested and achieved valid results. The DSM-IV classification was changed from Malingering to Malingering (Resolved). They also encouraged clinicians to allow the malingerer to "save face" by externalizing the poor results.

Professional staff must remain aware that the majority of malingerers also have genuine disorders. Although treatment with malingerers is difficult, it should not be terminated. Han (1997) described a cognitive-behavioral technique in which she encouraged malingerers to engage in prosocial behaviors while demonstrating to them that their malingering was maladaptive. Her follow-up of 89 patients found no reoccurrence of malingering. As a separate intervention strategy, Chase and colleagues (1984) discussed the effective use of paradoxical techniques to treat malingerers.

Depending on the circumstances, malingering may have direct consequences to the inmate. Some facilities may impose sanctions. In cases pending trial in federal court, malingering may result in enhanced sentencing. In the landmark mental health case *U.S. v. Greer* (1993) (see Knoll and Resnick 1999), the defendant faced enhanced sentencing under federal sentencing guidelines for continuing to feign psychotic symptoms in court. Beyond clinical interventions, correctional psychiatrists may become involved with institutional or legal actions in response to malingering.

CONCLUSION

Assessment of malingering in a correctional setting is an inherently difficult task. Nonetheless, correctional psychologists and psychiatrists have a wide array of detection strategies, screens, and tests at their disposal when conducting evaluations. The choice of test utilization and interpretation should be foremost for psychologists and psychiatrists in structuring their referrals. Whether through direct use or consultation, psychiatrists should possess in-depth knowledge about malingering and related response styles and be able to utilize validated detection strategies in their assessments.

When conducting assessments of malingering, psychiatrists should consider three critical issues. First, DSM-IV-TR does not offer formal inclusion criteria, because malingering is conceptualized as a "condition," not a "mental disorder." DSM-IV-TR screening indices should not be used in correctional settings; available data suggest they are wrong four out of five times. Instead, validated screens, such as the M-FAST, are significantly more accurate and can be easily implemented. Second, comprehensive evaluations are essential for the determination of malingering. When making referrals, correctional psychiatrists must ensure that these professionals commit sufficient time to complete interviews, record reviews, and standardized assessments. Third, research on malingering and other response styles continues its rapid growth. Periodic training and educational updates are critical for both correctional psychiatrists and their consultants.

SUMMARY POINTS

- Psychiatrists and psychologists should possess in-depth knowledge about malingering and response styles.
- Psychiatrists and psychologists should be able to use validated detection strategies in assessments.

- Psychiatrists and psychologists should consider the use of validated screens such as the M-FAST (Miller Forensic Assessment of Symptoms Test) in the detection of malingering.

REFERENCES

American Psychiatric Association: Diagnostic and Statistical Manual of Mental Disorders, 4th Edition, Text Revision. Washington, DC, American Psychiatric Association, 2000

Andersen HS, Sestoft D, Lillebaek T: Ganser syndrome after solitary confinement in prison: a short review and case report. Nordic J Psychiatry 55:199–201, 2001

Bagby RM, Nicholson RA, Bacchiochi JR, et al: The predictive capacity of the MMPI-2 and PAI validity scales and indexes to detect coached and uncoached feigning. J Pers Assess 78:69–86, 2002

Beaber RJ, Marston A, Michelli J, et al: A brief test for measuring malingering in schizophrenic individuals. Am J Psychiatry 142:1478–1481, 1985

Bender SD, Rogers R: Detection of neurocognitive feigning: development of a multistrategy assessment. Arch Clin Neuropsychol 19:49–60, 2004

Brodsky SL, Galloway VA: Ethical and professional demands for forensic mental health professionals in the post-Atkins area. Ethics Behav 13:3–9, 2003

Butcher JN, Dahlstrom WG, Graham JR, et al: Minnesota Multiphasic Personality Inventory-2 Manual. Minneapolis, University of Minnesota Press, 1989

Calhoun PS, Earnst KS, Tucker DD, et al: Feigning combat-related posttraumatic stress disorder on the Personality Assessment Inventory. J Pers Assess 75:338–350, 2000

Chase JL, Shea SJ, Dougherty FI: The use of paradoxical interventions within a prison psychiatric facility. Psychotherapy: Theory, Research, Practice, Training 21:278–281, 1984

Cosgray RE, Fawley RW: Could it be Ganser's syndrome? Arch Psychiatr Nurs 3:241–245, 1989

Cunnien AJ: Psychiatric and medical syndromes associated with deception, in Clinical Assessment of Malingering and Deception, 2nd Edition. Edited by Rogers R. New York, Guilford, 1997, pp 23–46

Drob SL, Berger RH: The determination of malingering: a comprehensive clinical-forensic approach. J Psychiatry Law 15:519–538, 1987

Drob SL, Meehan KB: The diagnosis of Ganser syndrome in the practice of forensic psychology. Am J Forensic Psychol 18:37–62, 2000

Edens JF, Otto R, Dwyer T: Utility of the Structured Interview of Malingered Symptomatology in identifying persons motivated to malinger psychopathology. J Am Acad Psychiatry Law 23:387–396, 1999

Frederick RI, Carter M, Powell J: Adapting symptom validity testing to evaluate suspicious complaints of amnesia in medicolegal evaluations. Bull Am Acad Psychiatry Law 23:231–237, 1995

Gerson AR: Beyond DSM-IV: a meta-review of the literature on malingering. Am J Forensic Psychol 20:57–69, 2002

Goldberg KB: Update on neuropsychological assessment of malingering. Journal of Forensic Psychology Practice 1:45–53, 2001

Greene RL: Assessment of malingering and defensiveness on multiscale inventories, in Clinical Assessment of Malingering and Deception, 2nd Edition. Edited by Rogers R. New York, Guilford, 1997, pp 169–207

Han S: Social rehabilitation of ex-malingerers from prison. Int Med J 4:73–75, 1997

Heinze MC, Purisch AD: Beneath the mask: use of psychological tests to detect and subtype malingering in criminal defendants. Journal of Forensic Psychology Practice 1:23–52, 2001

Hiscock CK, Hiscock M: Refining the forced-choice method for the detection of malingering. J Consult Clin Psychol 46:892–900, 1989

Jackson RL, Rogers R, Sewell KW: Miller Forensic Assessment of Symptoms Test (MFAST): forensic applications as a screen for feigned incompetence to stand trial (in press)

Jaffe ME, Sharma KK: Malingering uncommon psychiatric symptoms among defendants charged under California's "Three Strikes and You're Out" law. J Forensic Sci 43:549–555, 1998

Knoll JL, Resnick, P: U.S. v Greer: longer sentences for malingerers. J Am Acad Psychiatry Law 27:621–625, 1999

Lewis JL, Simcox AM, Berry D: Screening for feigned psychiatric symptoms in a forensic sample by using the MMPI-2 and the Structured Inventory of Malingered Symptomatology. Psychol Assess 14:170–176, 2002

Lezak M: Neuropsychological Assessment. New York, Oxford University Press, 1983

Liljequist L, Kinder BN, Schinka JA: An investigation of malingering posttraumatic stress disorder on the Personality Assessment Inventory. J Pers Assess 71:322–336, 1998

Miller H: Miller Forensic Assessment of Symptoms Test (MFAST) Professional Manual. Odessa, FL. Psychological Assessment Resources, 2001

Miller GR, Stiff BJ: Deceptive Communication. Thousand Oaks, CA, Sage, 1993

Millon T: Millon Clinical Multiaxial Inventory–III (MCMI-III) Manual. Minneapolis, MN, National Computer Systems, 1994

Morey LC: Personality Assessment Inventory (PAI). Tampa, FL, Psychological Assessment Resources, 1991

Moses JA, Cardelino JP, Thompson LL: Discrimination of brain damage from chronic psychosis by the Luria-Nebraska Battery: a closer look. J Consult Clin Psychol 51:441-449, 1983

Neumann CS, Walker EF, Weinstein J, et al: Psychotic patients' awareness of mental illness: implications for legal proceedings. J Psychiatry Law 24:421–442, 1996

Resnick PJ, Harris MR: Retrospective assessment of malingering in insanity defense cases, in Retrospective Assessment of Mental States in Litigation: Predicting the Past. Edited by Simon RI, Shuman DW. Washington, DC, American Psychiatric Publishing, 2002, pp 101–134

Rogers R: Models of feigned mental illness. Professional Psychology: Research and Practice 21:182–188, 1990

Rogers R (ed): Clinical Assessment of Malingering and Deception, 2nd Edition. New York, Guilford, 1997

Rogers R: Handbook of Diagnostic and Structured Interviewing. New York, Guilford, 2001

Rogers R: Forensic use and abuse of psychological tests: multiscale inventories. J Psychiatr Prac 9:316–320, 2003

Rogers R, Bender SD: Evaluation of malingering and deception, in Handbook of Psychology, Vol 11: Forensic Psychology. Edited by Goldstein AM. Hoboken, NJ, Wiley, 2003, pp 109–129

Rogers R, Cavanaugh JL: "Nothing but the truth"…A reexamination of malingering. J Psychiatry Law 11:443–460, 1983

Rogers R, Cruise K: Malingering and deception among psychopaths, in The Clinical and Forensic Assessment of Psychopathy: A Practitioner's Guide. Edited by Gacono C. Mahwah, NJ, Lawrence Erlbaum, 2000, pp 269–284

Rogers R, Neumann CS. Conceptual issues and explanatory models of malingering, in Malingering and Illness Deception: Clinical and Theoretical Perspectives. Edited by Halligan PW, Bass C, Oakley DA. Oxford, England, Oxford University Press, 2003, pp 71–82

Rogers R, Reinhardt VR: Conceptualization and assessment of secondary gain, in Psychologist's Desk Reference. Edited by Koocher GP, Norcross JC, Hill SS. New York, Oxford University Press, 1998, pp 57–62

Rogers R, Shuman D: Conducting Insanity Evaluations. New York, Guilford, 2000

Rogers R, Vitacco MJ: Forensic assessment of malingering and related response styles, in Forensic Psychology: From Classroom to Courtroom. Edited by Van Dorsten B. New York, Kluwer Academic Press, 2002, pp 83–104

Rogers R, Bagby RM, Dickens SE: Structured Interview of Reported Symptoms (SIRS) Professional Manual. Odessa, FL, Psychological Assessment Resources, 1992a

Rogers R, Bagby RM, Gillis JR: Improvements in the M Test as a screening measure for malingering. Bull Am Acad Psychiatry Law 20:101–104, 1992b

Rogers R, Harrell EH, Liff CD: Feigning neuropsychological impairment: a critical review of methodological and clinical considerations. Clin Psychol Rev 13:255–274, 1993

Rogers R, Hinds JD, Sewell KW: Feigning psychopathology among adolescent offenders: validation of the SIRS, MMPI-A, and SIMS. Paper presented at the annual meeting of the American Psychological Association, New York, August 1995

Rogers R, Sewell KW, Morey LC, et al: Detection of feigned mental disorders on the Personality Assessment Inventory: a discriminant analysis. J Pers Assess 67:629–640, 1996

Rogers R, Sewell KW, Martin MA, et al: Detection of feigned mental disorders: a meta-analysis of the MMPI-2 and malingering. Assessment 10:160–177, 2003

Rogers R, Jackson RL, Sewell KW, et al: Detection strategies for malingering: a confirmatory factor analysis of the SIRS. Criminal Justice and Behavior (in press)

Schoenberg MR, Dorr D, Morgan CD: The ability of the Millon Clinical Multiaxial Inventory–Third Edition to detect malingering. Psychol Assess 15:198–204, 2003

Smith GP: Assessment of malingering with self-report measures, in Clinical Assessment of Malingering and Deception, 2nd Edition. Edited by Rogers R. New York, Guilford, 1997, pp 351–372

Smith GP, Burger GK: Detection of malingering: validation of the Structured Inventory of Malingered Symptomatology (SIMS). J Am Acad Psychiatry Law 25:183–189, 1997

Smith GP, Borum R, Schinka JA: Rule-out and rule-in scales for the M Test for malingering: a cross validation. Bull Am Acad Psychiatry Law 21:107–110, 1993

Teplin TA: Criminalizing mental disorder: the comparative arrest of the mentally ill. Am Psychol 39:794–803, 1984

Tommbaugh TN: TOMM: The Test of Memory Malingering. North Tonawanda, NY, Multi-Health Systems, 1996

Towers K, Frederick R: Competence to be sentenced, in Forensic Mental Health Assessment: A Casebook. Edited by Heilbrun K, Marczyk G, DeMatteo D. New York, Oxford University Press, 2002, pp 85–95

United States v. Greer, Nos 96–11433 and 96–11588, Appeal from the United States District Court for the Northern District of Texas, 1998

Vitacco MJ: Construct validity of psychopathy in mentally disordered offenders: a multi-trait multi-method approach. Unpublished doctoral dissertation, University of North Texas, Denton, 2002

Walters GD: Assessing dissimulation and denial on the MMPI in a sample of maximum-security, male inmates. J Pers Assess 52:465–474, 1988

Windows MR, Smith GP: SIMS: Structured Interview of Malingered Symptomatology. Lutz, FL, Psychological Assessment Resources, 2005

Wynia MK: When the quality of mercy is strained: US physicians' deception of insurers for patients, in Malingering and Illness Deception: Clinical and Theoretical Perspectives. Edited by Halligan PW, Bass C, Oakley DA. Oxford, England, Oxford University Press, 2003, pp 197–206

CHAPTER 8

Female Offenders in Correctional Settings

Catherine F. Lewis, M.D.

At the end of 2002, more than 2 million people were incarcerated in prisons or jails in the United States (Harrison and Beck 2003). Of those incarcerated, less than 5% were women. Although representing a minority of all prisoners, women are the most rapidly growing population within the correctional system (Beck 1993; Greenfeld and Snell 1999; Snell and Morton 1994).

The rate of incarceration for women rose 4.9% in 2002; this rate was more than twice that for men (2.4%). Additionally, women are being arrested for more serious crimes than in the past. Since 1990 the number of women convicted of felonies has grown at more than two times the rate for male offenders. In 1999, women accounted for 29% of all property crimes, 17% of all violent crimes, and 18% of all drug-related crimes (Greenfeld and Snell 1999).

Incarcerated women are a socioeconomically disadvantaged, vulnerable group with substantial physical and mental health needs. They have often experienced breakdown of their family unit and suffer from social isolation and economic hardship (Greenfeld and Snell 1999). Most incarcerated women are minorities (38.7% white, 40.4% black, 16.9% Hispanic) (Harrison and Beck 2003) in the reproductive age group and never have been married (Greenfeld and Snell 1999). The majority (70%) of these women have minor children; in state prison the average number of minor children per female inmate is 2.38 (Brooks 1993). Two out of three women in the correctional system lived with their children immediately before incarceration. Although slightly more than half of incarcerated women are high school graduates, they are less likely than their male counterparts to be employed at the time of their arrest and are more likely to have an income of less than $600 per month or to be on welfare (Greenfeld and Snell 1999). Ironically, despite significant difficulties with past trauma, addiction, and mental health and physical health problems, most women entering the correctional system do not have medical insurance at the time of their arrest (Henderson 1998; Smith 1993).

Research on incarcerated women has been a neglected area (Singer et al. 1995). There are several reasons for this oversight, including that women are a minority of all offenders, accounting for less violent crime, and that perhaps there is a more subtle tendency to give women lower priority for access to services and research (Rasche 1974). The recent surge in arrests of women has caused clinicians, policymakers, and researchers to examine the treatment needs of female offenders more closely. A consensus is emerging that incarcerated women have treatment needs that may be different from those of incarcerated men or non-incarcerated women. Research on treatment of incarcerated women is in its infancy. In this chapter, I discuss issues of specific relevance to incarcerated women and implications for mental health treatment in the correctional system.

EPIDEMIOLOGY OF PSYCHIATRIC DISORDERS IN WOMEN

Existing research on incarcerated women suggests that women arriving in the correctional system are far more likely to have psychiatric disorders than their male counterparts (DiCataldo et al. 1995; Maden et al. 1994; Teplin et al. 1996). An estimated one-third to two-thirds of all women entering correctional facilities require mental health treatment (American Correctional Association 1990; Guy et al. 1985; Singer et al. 1995; Teplin et al. 1997), and about one-fifth arrive at correctional facilities with a history of taking psychotropic medication (Beck 1993). Women use more psychiatric services than men while incarcerated (Maden et al. 1994; Steadman et al. 1991) and are extremely likely to have comorbid substance-related diagnoses and Axis I or Axis II psychopathology (Jordan et al. 1996; Lewis 2004a; Singer et al. 1995; Warren et al. 2002b).

In a study of 1,272 female jail detainees, Teplin and colleagues (1996) used the Diagnostic Interview Schedule for DSM-III-R (DIS; Robins et al. 1981) to assess psychopathology. The study assessed 6-month and lifetime prevalence of a variety of psychiatric disorders, including posttraumatic stress disorder (PTSD), antisocial personality disorder (ASPD), major depression, and drug or alcohol abuse/dependence. A comparison of Teplin et al.'s results with the results of three other studies, including the National Comorbidity Study (NCS; Kessler et al. 1994, 1995), is given in Table 8–1. The NCS data are provided to allow a comparison point to women in the community (i.e., those not incarcerated). In Teplin et al. 's sample, a high percentage of women (80%) met the criteria for a lifetime psychiatric disorder, and the majority (70%) had psychiatric symptoms at the time of incarceration. The most common diagnoses included drug abuse/dependence, alcohol abuse/dependence, and PTSD. Psychopathology was generally higher in non-Hispanic white inmates and older detainees. The majority of the women in the sample were from minority groups (33.6% white, 40.4% black, 24.7% Hispanic), and the average age was 28 years.

Jordan and colleagues (1996) studied 805 newly convicted female felons in North Carolina, using the Composite International Diagnostic Interview (Robins et al. 1988) supplemented with the DIS for assessment of ASPD. The study assessed disorders such as major depression, ASPD, borderline personality disorder (BPD), drug or alcohol abuse/dependence, and dysthymia. Jordan et al. assessed exposure to extreme traumatic events via a survey instrument used in a past national study of the prevalence of rape (Resnick et al. 1993) and reported a prevalence of PTSD based on inmate report of symptoms. The majority of the sample were from minority groups (34.8% white, 58.1% black, 3.4% Hispanic), with a mean age of 30 years. The results of the study appear in Table 8–1. Jordan et al. found a high prevalence of psychopathology in her sample, with highest lifetime prevalence for drug and alcohol abuse/dependence, PTSD, major depressive disorder, and ASPD. Six-month prevalence of BPD was also high (data not shown).

Lewis (2003) examined a sample of 125 female felons in Connecticut, using the Semi-structured Assessment for the Genetics of Alcoholism (Bucholz et al. 1994; Lewis 2004a). Unlike the Jordan and Teplin studies, the Lewis study differentiated drug and alcohol abuse from dependence and reported lifetime prevalence for dependence for a variety of drugs. The results of this study appear in Table 8–1. The mean age for the sample was 33 years, and the racial/ethnic composition was 44.1% white, 33.8% black, and 16.2% Hispanic. Lewis found high lifetime prevalence of alcohol and drug dependence, major depression, PTSD, and ASPD. The most common drugs of dependence were cocaine (49%) and heroin (35.7%). More than half of the women were dependent on more than one substance and had comorbid Axis I or Axis II psychopathology. The prevalence of ASPD was markedly higher than in Jordan's and Teplin's samples.

TABLE 8–1.   Lifetime prevalence of psychiatric diagnoses in female offenders

Disorder	Teplin et al. 1996[a] (*N*=1,272)	Jordan et al. 1996[b] (*N*=805)	Lewis 2003[c] (*N*=125)	NCS (Kessler et al. 1994, 1995)[d]
		Study		
Schizophrenia	1.4%	NR	1.6%	0.8%
Mania	2.4%	NR	3.2%	1.7%
MDD	16.9%	13.0%	38.8%	21.3%
Dysthymia	9.6%	7.1%	4.1%	8.0%
Substance abuse/ dependence	70.2%		67.3%	
Alcohol abuse	32.3%	38.0%	23.5%	6.4%
Alcohol dependence			41.8%	8.2%
Drug abuse	63.6%	44.2%	13.4%	3.5%
Drug dependence			57.1%	5.9%
Panic disorder	1.6%	5.8%	5.1%	5.0%
GAD	2.5%	2.7%	7.2%	6.6%
PTSD	33.5%	30.0%	41.8%	10.4%
ASPD	13.8%	11.9%	31.6%	1.2%

Note.   ASPD=antisocial personality disorder; GAD=generalized anxiety disorder; MDD= major depressive disorder; NCS=National Comorbidity Study; PTSD=posttraumatic stress disorder.
[a]Newly admitted female felons.
[b]Female jail detainees.
[c]Female felons serving sentence.
[d]National sample of women in community.

These three studies, drawn from three different populations and using different instruments for assessment and methods of recruitment, suggest that rates of psychopathology among female incarcerated offenders are high regardless of whether they are in jail, new arrived at the prison, or in the midst of their prison term. Lifetime prevalence rates of drug abuse/dependence, alcohol abuse/dependence, PTSD, and ASPD are particularly elevated in female inmates. The high prevalence of comorbidity among incarcerated women suggests psychiatric treatment may be challenging. The difference in prevalence of psychiatric psychopathology from the women in the NCS (Kessler et al. 1994, 1995) indicates that diagnosis and treatment of psychiatric disorders in incarcerated women may need to differ from approaches to psychiatric disorders in women in the community.

PSYCHIATRIC DISORDERS AND BEHAVIORS OF PARTICULAR IMPORTANCE

Substance Abuse/Dependence

Alcohol

Alcohol dependence is a prevalent and important problem for incarcerated women. Women who are dependent on alcohol are likely to develop physical sequelae sooner than men (Ashley et al. 1977; Schuckit et al. 1995). These sequelae include cirrhosis, hypertension, obesity, anemia, fatty liver, and malnutrition. Some sequelae (e.g., cervical cancer, HIV), while not directly caused by alcohol use, are likely related to lifestyle issues (e.g., comorbid substance abuse, including nicotine; promiscuity). Alcohol increases the likelihood of negative sequelae, including fetal alcohol syndrome, domestic violence, and marital dissolution, for future generations (Anda et al. 1988; Greenfeld 1998). Alcohol dependence also worsens the prognosis for women with other psychiatric disorders, including major depression (Drake et al. 1996; Hesselbrock et al. 1985; Kranzler et al. 1996). Women with alcohol dependence are more likely than men to develop dependence on other substances (Robins and Regier 1991). Finally, alcohol use has been linked to recidivism and reincarceration, violent behavior (including suicide and homicide), poverty, and unemployment (Greenfeld 1998).

Men are more likely than women to use alcohol daily, use alcohol in the month before incarceration, and use alcohol more often during the month before incarceration (Greenfeld and Snell 1999). Although incarcerated men score higher than incarcerated women on all of these measures, incarcerated women score higher on each measure than do men in community samples. One-quarter of women had used alcohol daily in the month before their offense, and 29% were using alcohol at the time of their offense (Greenfeld and Snell 1999). Alcohol-related disorders have a high degree of comorbidity in women (Regier et al. 1990), with elevation of rates particularly in young, uneducated women of low socioeconomic status (Kessler et al. 1997). Women with comorbid alcohol and drug dependence tend to attribute difficulties to drug use rather than to alcohol use (Weisner and Schmidt 1992).

Drugs

Women differ from men in their patterns of addiction to illegal drugs. They most commonly are introduced to substance use by men (Daly 1994; Lex 1995), and their partners are likely to use drugs (Lex 1995). Whereas men use drugs for hedonistic reasons, women tend to use drugs for escapist reasons such as numbing and comfort (Amaro 1995). Female drug abusers have more positive family history for alcohol and drug use than men and have often experienced abuse and neglect (Finkelstein et al. 1997). They also experience "telescoping" with alcohol and drug use, a phenomenon in which significant symptoms occur over a shorter period (Blume 1990; Finkelstein et al. 1997; Nespor 1990).

Women who are incarcerated are more likely than their male counterparts to have used drugs in the months preceding their incarceration. Sixty percent of women entering the correctional system had used drugs in the month before arrest, half had used daily, and 40% were using at the time of their offense (Greenfeld and Snell 1999). Incarcerated women are more likely than incarcerated men to be intravenous drug users (Hammett et al. 1999), to have partners who are intravenous drug users (Schilling et al. 1994), and to smoke rather than snort cocaine (Grella 1996; Wilsnack et al. 1997). Intravenous drug use is linked to physical illness, including hepatitis C and HIV, and psychiatric disorders, including alcohol dependence, major depression, and ASPD (Dinwiddie et al. 1992; Rounsaville et al. 1982).

Drug-addicted women are more likely than drug-addicted men to experience socioeconomic hardship and to prostitute themselves to get money for drugs (Guyon et al. 1999). Addiction is closely linked to criminality in both men and women and is associated with a more serious criminal record, earlier age at onset of criminality, and HIV risk behaviors (Guyon et al. 1999). A higher percentage of female arrestees versus male arrestees use "hard" drugs (e.g., heroin, cocaine) (Wellisch et al. 1994). The majority of incarcerated women have at least one other mental health disorder. It is possible that the emphasis on drug-related offenses by the criminal justice system is actually pushing psychiatrically impaired women into the correctional system (Chesney-Lind 1998).

Treatment Issues

Given the higher likelihood of addiction with psychiatric illness, socioeconomic hardship, and history of trauma among incarcerated women versus men, it is likely that women would benefit from treatment structured for their specific needs. It is generally less socially acceptable for women to use drugs and alcohol, and this can lead to reluctance to identify addictive problems, punitive or negative attitudes toward the female substance abuser, and treatment that fails to address addiction and focuses only on other mental health issues (Chasnoff 1989). Women are more likely than men to seek treatment when having problems with addiction, but they are less likely to receive addiction-specific treatment; most of the time they receive treatment for other mental health–related issues (see Green-Hennessy 2002; Weisner and Schmidt 1992). This can lead to inadequate recognition and treatment of addictive disorders among women.

Peters and colleagues (1997) studied a sample of 435 female and 1,220 male detainees in a Florida jail who underwent a 6-week substance abuse program. Women were more likely than men to have recent, frequent use of harder drugs. They also had more psychological impairment, including a history of requiring psychiatric medications, attempting suicide, being sexually abused, or having major depression. Female addicts were likely to suffer obstacles to employment, be unemployed, and earn less than men. Peters et al. viewed the 12-step programs, with their emphasis on personal accountability and abstinence, as potentially damaging to traumatized incarcerated women. Instead, he recommended cognitive-behavioral interventions aimed at enhancing self-esteem and social functioning.

In a study of 1,326 male and 318 female federal prisoners who volunteered for a 12-month residential program, Langan and Pelissier (2001) concurred with previous authors' assessment that addicted incarcerated women's needs were not getting met by traditionally male programs (Miller 1984; Wellisch et al. 1993). Like Peters et al., Langan and Pelissier observed that women used harder drugs, used drugs more often, and had more educational, family, mental health, and physical problems than men. Langan and Pelissier stressed the need to focus on well-being rather than self-control in treating addicted women. They also noted that the harmful effects of alcohol should be less of a focus than recovery from trauma and empowerment for incarcerated women. Specifically, women are likely to remain in negative relationships with their partners even as they try to stay abstinent (Anglin et al. 1987; Steffensmeier and Allen 1996). Treatment must therefore address interpersonal issues and issues related to reenacting past traumatic experience. Emphasis should be placed on strengthening competencies rather than emphasizing deficits (Langan and Pelissier 2001).

The first step in treating substance-dependent incarcerated women is recognition of acute medical and psychiatric issues. Detoxification should be provided when necessary, preferably in a special unit. Because of the medical sequelae of alcohol and drug dependence, women should undergo careful physical examination and testing when appropriate. Sociocultural and psychopathological issues are of critical importance to addicted incarcerated women. General clinical considerations include recognition of and sensitivity to trauma-related issues and depressive symptoms, and recognition of the importance of interpersonal relationships to sobriety for women. Treatment matching should occur (Farabee et al. 1999), in which women with the most serious dependence are placed in the most intensive treatment setting (hospital or therapeutic community) and women with less serious dependence are placed in less intensive settings. This approach is rarely taken in correctional settings, which tend to view addiction as a yes/no phenomenon and fail to recognize the gradation of addictive disorders (Farabee et al. 1999).

Farabee and colleagues (1999) recommend the model of the therapeutic community for incarcerated women with severe addiction (see De Leon 1995). Therapeutic communities assist inmates with the social learning process. Once the inmate has completed the program, follow-up treatment and transition to aftercare are critical. During incarceration, motivational interviewing could be used with inmates to assist them in entry to the therapeutic community; it has been found effective in other populations to have more individual sessions during the beginning of treatment and to demonstrate the success of previous program graduates (De Leon 1995; Miller 1984). Once an inmate has completed treatment in the therapeutic community and is released, he or she optimally would have continuity of care to minimize the risk of treatment dropout (Prendergast et al. 1996; Singer et al. 1995).

Cognitive-behavioral interventions, both on group and on individual levels, have been used with some success in incarcerated populations. In a study of male and female detainees at the Baltimore City Jail, Peyrot and colleagues (1994) found that a cognitive-behavioral intervention emphasizing concepts such as consequential thinking, anger management, and stress management led to better outcomes than traditional substance abuse education programs. The outcome measures involved information retained by the participants rather than long-term assessments of sobriety.

Contingency management (a therapy in which desired behaviors are reinforced with rewards while negative behaviors are discouraged through withholding of rewards) is often paired with traditional cognitive-behavioral therapy and has proved effective in HIV-positive, antisocial, and drug-addicted populations (Higgins et al. 1991; Messina et al. 2003). Despite its success in treating addiction in community settings, contingency management has had limited application in correctional settings. Further research is needed on integrated cognitive-behavioral and contingency-based treatment in secure settings.

Treatment of underlying depressive illness is particularly important in addicted incarcerated women. This treatment has been shown to decrease relapse risk and compromise from depressive symptoms in non-incarcerated populations (Greenfield et al. 1998; Mason et al. 1996). Psychopharmacological treatment for symptoms of major depression should not be withheld because of a recent history of substance abuse or dependence. Care must be taken, however, to avoid creating iatrogenic drug dependence (e.g., benzodiazapines), given the comorbid history of addiction, and to avoid prescribing multiple medications at subtherapeutic levels. Clinical Case 8–1 provides practical guidelines when assessing a woman who presents with substance use issues in a correctional setting.

Clinical Case 8–1

A 28-year-old mother of two was incarcerated for armed robbery and possession of heroin and crack cocaine. Shortly after booking, correctional officers called mental health services because she was agitated and appeared "hyper." When assessed, she stated she had been drinking a quart of vodka a day and using intravenous heroin and cocaine daily up to the time of her arrest. She also said she has bipolar affective disorder but had stopped taking her medication about 10 days ago. She recognized that she needs mental health treatment but expressed concern that she did not want any medication metabolized by her liver because she has hepatitis C. This was, in fact, the reason why she stopped taking the medication previously prescribed for her. She expressed no desire to harm herself or others but conceded she feels like she is "thinking too fast" and feels very nervous.

This case illustrates the complexity of the presentation of polysubstance-dependent women in correctional settings. Consider the following when treating women such as the one in the clinical example:

- Conduct a physical examination, including vital signs, to assess for signs of withdrawal. Even if there are no active signs at the time of booking, the patient should be monitored for withdrawal and placed on a detoxification protocol for alcohol and heroin.
- Obtain relevant laboratory work. A liver function panel can be drawn to assess the patient's degree of liver impairment. HIV and hepatitis B and C testing should also be performed.
- Provide education about the risks and benefits of medication, including the possibility of using medication not metabolized by the liver or using hepatically metabolized medication at lower doses.
- Consider admission to a detoxification unit, where the patient's mental health needs, as well as her impending withdrawal, could be addressed.

Trauma and Posttraumatic Stress Disorder

Prevalence and Comorbidity

Incarcerated women are likely to have experienced physical abuse, sexual abuse, and exploitation before arriving at correctional facilities (Lewis 2003, 2004b; Singer et al. 1995; Zlotnick 1997). PTSD is the most common diagnosis other than substance abuse in multiple studies involving incarcerated women (Hutton et al. 2001; Jordan et al. 1996; Lewis 2003, 2004b; Teplin et al. 1996). In a study of 805 convicted felons, Jordan and colleagues (1996) found that 30% of the women had been exposed to trauma severe enough to cause symptoms of PTSD. Zlotnick (1997) noted that 78%–85% of incarcerated women have experienced at least one traumatic event and that this percentage is higher for women in the general population (69%) (Jordan et al. 1996; Lake 1993; Resnick et al. 1993; Zlotnick 1997). Zlotnick (1997) also found high prevalence of current PTSD (48.2%), lifetime PTSD (20%), childhood sexual abuse (40%), childhood physical abuse (55%), adult physical abuse (63%), and rape in adulthood (53%) in a study of 85 randomly selected incarcerated women. These findings are similar to those of Hutton et al. (2001), who interviewed 177 female prisoners and found a 33% lifetime prevalence of PTSD and a 15% prevalence of current PTSD, as well as a 36% lifetime prevalence of major depression and a 10% prevalence of current depression. Lewis (2004b) found a similar prevalence of lifetime PTSD in a sample of 125 female felons but a higher prevalence of lifetime PTSD (72%) in a sample of 81 HIV-positive inmates (Lewis 2003). These findings suggest HIV-positive incarcerated women may be a group at particular risk for PTSD.

What is clear from the existing literature is that traumatic experiences are common among incarcerated women and that the prevalence of PTSD among incarcerated women is two to three times that of women in the general population (Kessler et al. 1995). PTSD and trauma history are associated with suicidal ideation and attempts (Brodsky et al. 2001; Kotler et al. 2001; Lewis 2004b), HIV high-risk behavior (Kimmerling and Goldsmith 2000; Logan and Leukefeld 2000), and substance abuse (Brady et al. 1994; Brown et al. 1998).

The traumas experienced by incarcerated women are diverse and repetitive and occur early in their lives. A Bureau of Justice survey of 38,978 women in prison found 43% had been assaulted, 34% had been physically abused, and 34% had been sexually abused before their incarceration. Of the women reporting sexual abuse, 56% had had a completed rape (Snell and Morton 1994). A second survey, involving 1,720 women, conducted by the American Correctional Association found that 53% had experienced physical abuse and 36% had experienced sexual abuse. Of those sexually abused, one-third had been abused between 5 and 14 years of age (American Correctional Association 1990). Other authors, using more detailed question strategies, found a higher prevalence of abuse. Bloom and colleagues (1994) found that 29% of the female inmates interviewed had been physically abused by a parent, 31% had experienced childhood sexual abuse, 60% had been physically abused as an adult, and 23% had been sexually abused as an adult. Browne and colleagues (1999) reported a high prevalence of childhood physical abuse (70%), childhood sexual abuse (59%), and physical abuse in adulthood by an intimate (75%) among incarcerated women. These prevalences are far higher than those recorded for the general population for childhood sexual (Finkelhor 1994) or physical (Tjaden and Thoennes 1992) abuse. Women are more likely to develop PTSD than are men exposed to similar trauma (Kessler et al. 1995).

The interrelationships with PTSD and other psychiatric disorders, including addiction, are complex, and there is substantial comorbidity (Bremner et al. 1992; Kessler et al. 1994; van der Kolk et al. 1996). PTSD has been associated with higher preference for "hard" drugs, such as heroin and cocaine (Najavits et al. 1996). PTSD is also associated with development of other psychiatric disorders, including BPD, major depressive disorder, and substance abuse (Shalev et al. 1998; Zlotnick 1997). Symptoms of PTSD worsen during early abstinence (Brady et al. 1994), and PTSD worsens comorbid psychiatric conditions (Shalev et al. 1998). Childhood trauma is associated with a variety of psychiatric symptoms, including dissociation, somatization, affect dysregulation, and persistent hyperarousal (van der Kolk et al. 1996).

Treatment Issues

PTSD is often underdetected by medical and mental health treatment providers (Grossman et al. 1997). A critical first step in the treatment of PTSD in incarcerated female offenders is recognition of the disorder in affected inmates. Evaluation of past trauma history and ongoing symptoms should be considered for inclusion in mental health screening for newly incarcerated inmates. Screening questionnaires (e.g., Najavits et al. 1998a) for trauma can be used in initial assessments when available. The treatment of PTSD ideally would address issues related to low self-esteem, physical and sexual abuse, depression, anxiety, self-abuse, and addiction (Gil-Rivas et al. 1996; Najavits et al. 1996).

Research on therapy for incarcerated women with PTSD is limited. Zlotnick and Najavits evaluated a cognitive-behavioral intervention, "Seeking Safety," through a pilot study of 17 incarcerated women with PTSD and addiction who were on a residential unit (Najavits et al. 1998b; Zlotnick et al. 2003). The treatment was manual-based and addressed cognitive, behavioral, and interpersonal aspects of treatment over eight sessions each. Seeking Safety combines educational intervention, cognitive-behavioral therapy for addiction, and treatment for PTSD (Herman 1992). The program goals are abstinence and personal safety. Women participating in the program had a decrease in PTSD symptoms that was maintained at 3 months and decreased substance abuse at 6 weeks. The likelihood of relapse with substances after 6 weeks, however, remained high. Given the prevalence of addiction among incarcerated women and the comorbidity of addiction with PTSD, continued development of services addressing victimization and drug abuse is critical (Austin et al. 1992; Henderson 1998; Prendergast and Wellisch 1995).

Pomeroy and colleagues (1998) studied 13 incarcerated women who underwent a psychoeducational group intervention that focused on numerous topics, including low self-esteem, victimization, depression, symptoms of PTSD, and basic life skills. Participants met three times a week for 90 minutes over 5 weeks. At the end of the study, the participants self-reported greater improvement in symptoms of anxiety and depression than in symptoms of stress and trauma.

Bradley and Follingstad (2003) compared a small sample of incarcerated women who participated in dialectical behavior therapy (DBT) (Linehan et al. 1999) and writing assignments with a matched sample of women who received treatment as usual (i.e., supportive therapy and psychopharmacological interventions where appropriate). DBT focused on skills training related to self-esteem, management of trauma, anxiety and depressive symptoms, and development of trust and self-control. Participating inmates self-reported reduction in PTSD, mood, and interpersonal symptoms.

The implications of these trials are not clear because of their small sample size and the absence of control groups. The treatment of PTSD in incarcerated women remains a largely unexplored field. Nonetheless, preliminary results suggest an integrated approach, including psychoeducational, interpersonal, and cognitive-behavioral interventions, would be of likely benefit. Psychopharmacological interventions can also be used to treat depressive or anxiety symptoms related to underlying traumatic experience.

Personality Disorders

Prevalence

Personality disorders are prevalent among incarcerated women, and comorbidity between Axis I and Axis II disorders is high. In a study of 261 female felons, Warren and colleagues (2002a) found, using the Structured Clinical Interview for DSM-IV (SCID-II) (First et al. 1997), 200 women who screened positive for Cluster B personality pathology (e.g., antisocial, borderline, histrionic, or narcissistic personality traits). The most common personality disorder was ASPD (43%), followed by paranoid personality disorder (27%) and BPD (24%). Warren et al. suggested that paranoid personality disorder may be overdiagnosed in correctional populations, because women responding affirmatively to questions targeting paranoid symptoms may, in fact, be accurately reporting reasonable feelings and experiences, given their traumatic and dangerous environments. Most women in Warren et al.'s sample evidenced more than one personality disorder. For example, 43% of the women with ASPD also met criteria for BPD, and there was high co-occurrence between Cluster A disorders and ASPD (e.g., schizoid 54%, schizotypal 56%). An earlier study of male and female offenders (Coid 1992) had found a similarly high degree of comorbidity between ASPD and BPD and a high number of mean personality disorders per offender (3.6). Coid (1992) suggested that given the high comorbidity of personality disorder diagnoses in inmates, personality pathology should be viewed as a recurring pattern of covariant traits versus a single unified diagnosis.

Zlotnick (1999) found a high prevalence of personality disorders, including ASPD (40%) and BPD (49%), in a group of 85 female prisoners in Rhode Island. There was a strong association with poor anger modulation and ASPD, even after BPD and PTSD were controlled for. This elevated state of arousal was not associated with past childhood abuse, contrary to previous reports of association of abuse with ASPD (Windle et al. 1995). Additionally, self-mutilation was not associated with ASPD in the absence of BPD.

Treatment Issues

Female inmates with severe personality pathology who attempt to harm themselves pose a unique challenge to the correctional system. *Parasuicidal behavior,* defined as self-harm whose intent is not death but improvement in one's emotional state, (e.g., cutting, burning), is a particular problem in correctional settings for women. The Intensive Healing Program was developed by the Canadian Correctional System to specifically address parasuicidal behavior among female inmates (Roth and Presse 2003). The program uses Linehan's model for DBT (Linehan et al. 1999). DBT has been shown to be effective in reducing parasuicidal behavior in noncorrectional populations (Alper and Peterson 2001; Linehan et al. 1999). The therapeutic environment is critical to treatment; women are housed in a specified unit where adaptive behaviors are reinforced and crisis management is readily available. Components of the program include a therapeutic community, individual counseling, group activities (e.g., anger management, DBT, relapse prevention, psychoeducation on violence, parenting, empathy), and educational and vocational training. Primary therapists are based on the inmate's housing unit, and therapeutic protocol exists to handle parasuicidal behavior. Examples of the protocol include giving no additional psychoactive medications after a parasuicidal act, making verbal contracts not to engage in self-harm, and conducting behavioral chain analysis of the incident of self-harm. Evaluation of this program with a control group has not yet been reported.

Anger management is a second problem often seen in female inmates with personality disorders, particularly those with Cluster B pathology. Warren and colleagues (2002a) noted that the combination of narcissistic psychopathology and paranoid psychopathology seen in Cluster A disorders (e.g., paranoid, schizoid, schizotypal) may be particularly associated with violent behavior both before and during incarceration, while ASPD is associated with violence during incarceration. Interventions targeting anger management and impulsivity are likely to benefit women with affect dysregulation (Zlotnick 1999). A constant tension exists between the need for institutional sanctions and the need for psychiatric interventions. The optimal treatment consists of collaborative efforts with custody and mental health staff. Such collaboration sets reasonable limits while ensuring physical safety and treatment of comorbid psychopathology (e.g., addiction, major depression). Potential interventions for incarcerated women with personality pathology are noted in the following case.

Clinical Case 8–2

A 23-year-old single woman serving a 6-year sentence for drug possession with the intent to distribute and prostitution was referred to mental health services by correctional officers who reported she had been scratching herself with her fingernails until her arms and legs bled. The woman was well known to mental health and had been on the inpatient unit at least six times. When questioned about her symptoms, the woman reported feeling "empty, like a shell," "very, very sad like I wished I was gone," and "alone." She reported feeling "relaxed" and "free" when she hurts herself. She described a history of severe childhood sexual abuse beginning at age 4. Although she said she would not mind if she were to die, she adamantly denied thoughts or intent to kill herself. She had a history of two suicide attempts before incarceration (by drug overdose) and one attempt (labeled a gesture by some staff members) in which she placed a sheet around her neck, tied it to her bed, and lay on her cell floor. Correctional staff believes she is not safe in her own cell and needs mental health intervention.

This case illustrates the nuances of dealing with a patient who self-mutilates, has a suicide history, and yet denies suicidal intent/thoughts within the correctional system. A challenge of cases such as this is to provide a safe environment for the patient without repeatedly hospitalizing her in the inpatient unit for brief periods in a "revolving door" scenario. Interventions that may be considered include the following:

- Transfer to a unit for housing mentally ill inmates who are not ill enough to require inpatient hospitalization. Such a unit would optimally have a variety of groups that could address issues such as learning anger management, surviving trauma, achieving abstinence from substances, and avoiding revictimization.
- Referral to a psychiatrist to consider medication to assist with depressive symptoms, impulsivity, affective lability, and anxiety.
- Enrollment in treatment involving manualized therapy such as DBT to assist in the management and treatment of symptoms related to trauma and the urge to self-harm.

TABLE 8–2. Suicide history in sample of 125 female prisoners

	N	% of sample
Have you ever thought of suicide?	87	69.4
% reporting thoughts lasted for a full week		44.1
% reporting having had a plan		82.1
Have you ever tried to kill yourself?	65	52.0

Suicide

Epidemiology

Suicide is an important but understudied topic among incarcerated women. Data from the general population suggest that women are more likely to attempt but less likely to complete suicide than men (Moscicki 1994). Incarcerated women have multiple risk factors for suicidal behavior, including mood disorders, high total numbers of psychiatric disorders (Kessler et al. 1999), comorbid Axis I and II disorders (Hawton et al. 2003; Kessler et al. 1999), drug and alcohol dependence (Hesselbrock et al. 1988; Roy 2003; Schuckit 1986), and childhood trauma (Canetto and Lester 1995; Kingree et al. 1999). Additional risk factors include low social support and socioeconomic status (Murphy and Robins 1967), and younger age (Gomberg 1989).

In a study of 81 incarcerated HIV-positive women, Lewis (2003, 2004a) found lifetime history of suicide attempts was more strongly associated with lifetime PTSD than lifetime history of affective disorder, ASPD, BPD, and addiction. Childhood sexual abuse was even more strongly associated with suicide attempts than was PTSD. A history of childhood sexual abuse may therefore be important in identifying HIV-positive women at heightened risk for suicide attempts. In a second study of 125 incarcerated female felons, Lewis (2004b) found a high number of women with positive histories for suicidality when in the community (Lewis 2004b). The majority of women (69.4%) had thought of suicide; of those who had thought of suicide, most (82.1%) had a plan and had actually tried (52.0%) to take their lives. Tables 8–2 and 8–3 summarize findings on suicide thoughts and suicide attempts in a sample of female offenders.

What is salient is the severity of attempts (e.g., proportion of women requiring medical treatment, hospitalization) and reported desire and intent to die. About one-third of the women had attempted suicide when using drugs, and one-quarter had attempted suicide when using alcohol. The most common methods of suicide attempts in this sample were cutting and overdose; hanging becomes more prevalent during actual incarceration. In this study, suicide attempts were associated with depressive symptoms, alcohol

TABLE 8–3.   Characteristics of 125 female prisoners with actual suicide attempt history

Required medical treatment	56.9%
Admitted to hospital	31.4%
Really wanted to die	84.3%
Sorry did not die	60.8%
Depressed at time	94.1%
Using alcohol at the time	29.4%
Using drugs at the time	23.5%
Had severe intent to die	54.9%

dependence, and PTSD. Further research is needed to assess patterns of suicide attempts and successful suicide attempts during incarceration.

Treatment Issues

The strong association between suicide attempts and affective illness and/or past trauma is not surprising (Brodsky et al. 2001; Kingree et al. 1999). Treatment prevention strategies should implement screening for suicide that includes assessment of trauma history, addiction, and ongoing affective symptoms. Depressive symptoms are closely associated with attempted and completed suicide (Kessler et al. 1999; Roy 2003). As such, these symptoms should be treated aggressively from a psychopharmacological perspective. This treatment should occur even when recent substance abuse or dependence is present. Comorbidity heightens the risk of suicide (Hawton et al. 2003; Kessler et al. 1999; Roy 2003; Schuckit 1986). Multiple suicide attempts are themselves a risk factor for completed suicide (Roy 2003). For these reasons, aggressive pharmacotherapy for depressive and traumatic symptoms in incarcerated women can be an important component of suicide prevention. Aggressive treatment of withdrawal symptoms is also critical. Specialized housing units, such as group housing for inmates with suicidal ideation, have also shown potential benefit in correctional settings (Goss et al. 2002).

MEDICAL ISSUES OF PARTICULAR IMPORTANCE

General Medical

Incarcerated women often have physical illness, including HIV, cervical dysplasia, obesity, hypertension, asthma, hepatitis B and C, and other sexually transmitted diseases (De Groot 2000; Lewis 2004b; Onorato 2001). An initial physical examination accompanied by appropriate testing helps place psychiatric symptoms in context for effective treatment. Initial medical evaluation would optimally include a physical examination (including an obstetric-gynecological examination with pregnancy testing and assessment of hormonal levels where appropriate; Papanicolaou's test; HIV testing; testing for tuberculosis; testing for sexually transmitted diseases; and testing for hepatitis B and C), review of HIV risk factors, and mental health assessment, including assessment of trauma, depressive symptoms, and neurocognitive functioning. Other disorders, such as heart disease and osteoporosis, while less common in younger women, are likely to become more prevalent as the correctional population ages. Consideration should be given to medical issues with specific impact on psychiatric well-being in women (e.g., postpartum depression, perimenopausal depression, premenstrual dysphoric disorder). Effective and appropriate psychopharmacological intervention in the treatment of psychiatric symptoms is critical in optimizing both psychiatric and physical health.

HIV and AIDS

Epidemiology

HIV is an important problem for the correctional system; currently close to 30,000 incarcerated people are HIV-positive (Hammett et al. 1999; Maruschak 2001). HIV infection is more prevalent in incarcerated women than in incarcerated men. An estimated 3.5% of incarcerated women are HIV-positive, compared with an estimated 2.3% of incarcerated men or 0.15% of women in the general community (Farley et al. 2000; Hammett et al. 1999; Maruschak 2001; Singleton et al. 1990; Vlahov et al. 1991). The gender disparity is more striking in the Northeast, where 13% of incarcerated women, versus 7% of incarcerated men, are HIV positive (Hammett et al. 1999). Minority women are the group in which HIV infection is rising most rapidly in the United States (De Groot 2000; Onorato 2001); in 1986, women represented 6.7% of all cases of HIV, and by 1999, the percentage was 18% (Harris et al. 2003). Nearly three-quarters of these new cases of HIV in women are in minority groups (Maruschak 2001; Wish et al. 1990).

Incarcerated women are at particular risk for infection with HIV because of high-risk lifestyles, which can include prostitution (Guyon et al. 1999), sexual abuse (Klein and Chao 1995), homelessness (Shlay et al. 1996), involvement with regular sexual partners who are at high risk for HIV (Berman and Brown 1990), and intravenous drug use (Guyon et al. 1999; Vlahov et al. 1991). HIV-positive incarcerated women are socioeconomically disadvantaged and lack necessities such as food, clothing, housing, transportation, and health insurance (Lewis 2003; Sheu et al. 2002). Most HIV-positive incarcerated women are mothers, never married, unemployed, with less than a high school education (Lewis 2003). The vast majority are injection drug users (84%) (Brewer and Derrickson 1992; Farley et al. 2000), and about one-third of these injection drug users have engaged in prostitution. HIV-positive women are particularly likely to have experienced sexual (67.0%) abuse and have a lifetime history of major depression (46.1%), antisocial personality disorder (18.5%), PTSD (72.1%), alcohol dependence/abuse (81.5%), and drug dependence (95.1%) (Lewis 2003).

Treatment Issues

HIV-positive incarcerated women are likely to suffer from complex medical and psychiatric pathology. Incarceration offers a unique opportunity to influence the lives of HIV-positive women through testing, counseling, and treatment of HIV and comorbid medical and psychiatric disorders (Hammett 2001). Women who are at risk for infection with HIV or who are HIV-positive are hard to reach in the community (Lubelczyk et al. 2002). Most women who are incarcerated are asymptomatic at the time they test positive for HIV, so their diagnosis may come as a surprise or shock (Farley et al. 2000). Pre- and posttest counseling are critical for inmates regardless of their serostatus. Medical issues are also important and can affect mental health. For example, women with HIV are more likely than non-HIV-positive women to have hepatitis C and other sexually transmitted diseases (Onorato 2001). Consideration should be given early in treatment to the possibility that women are pregnant to allow treatment with antiretrovirals to minimize transmission of HIV to the child.

Effective mental health treatment for HIV-positive incarcerated women should include HIV intervention (e.g., education about risky behaviors, education about illness, testing), treatment for addiction, and treatment for comorbid psychiatric conditions such as PTSD, major depression, and personality disorders. The high-risk behavior often seen in individuals with personality disorders has been linked to increased likelihood of transmission of HIV (Brooner et al. 1993; Jacobsberg et al. 1995). Programs designed to reduce risky behavior in incarcerated populations have been shown to be effective and motivational interviewing for soon-to-be-released inmates has also shown potential efficacy (Lubelczyk et al. 2002). el-Bassel and colleagues (1997) developed a cognitive-behavioral intervention designed to increase social support among incarcerated women at high risk for HIV. The intervention included support groups with former inmates, educational sessions, and cognitive-behavioral therapy to enhance coping and social support. Women participating in the program were almost four times as likely as those who participated in an HIV information group only to maintain safe sexual practices (el-Bassel et al. 1997).

Continuity of care is an important concept in treating incarcerated women with HIV. Programs in which the same physician follows the HIV-positive inmate in prison and after discharge in the community have been shown to increase treatment retention, decrease recidivism, and provide social support (Farley et al. 2000; Guyon et al. 1999). Because of the complexity of psychopathology, socioeconomic hardship, and medical issues of HIV-positive women, case management is an important intervention for this population. Ideally, interventions would start for women jailed even for minor offenses, because these women exhibit high-risk behavior and are likely to return to the community soonest (McClelland et al. 2002). Ultimately, services for HIV-positive incarcerated women should integrate medical treatment, psychiatric treatment (including treatment for substance use, traumatic symptoms, and personality disorders), and psychosocial interventions (vocational counseling, use of entitlements) with as much continuity of care as is feasible.

Pregnancy and Motherhood

Pregnancy

Services and outcome.   One in four women entering prison has been pregnant in the year before her incarceration (Fogel 1993; Safyer and Richmond 1995), and 6% are pregnant at the time of incarceration (Snell and Morton 1994). Incarcerated women are at high risk for late entry into prenatal care, sexually transmitted diseases, HIV, substance abuse (including nicotine), and interpersonal violence (Snell and Morton 1994). Fewer than half of existing correctional facilities have programs for prenatal care, special prenatal diets, light work duty for pregnant women, or policies regarding pregnant women's control or travel; fewer than one in five offers instruction in birthing (e.g., Lamaze) (Siefert and Pimlott 2001). A survey of wardens identified multiple institutional limitations in dealing with pregnant inmates, including programs that were inadequate to deal with the trauma of miscarriage, unavailability of maternity clothes, institutional requirements that inmates wear belly chains, no separate visiting area for newborns, and necessity of placing minimum-security pregnant inmates in maximum-security facilities to receive adequate care (Siefert and Pimlott 2001).

Data on the outcome of pregnancies in inmates are conflicting. Early work suggested that pregnant inmates have more frequent complications, including anemia, urinary tract infections, and bleeding (Fogel 1993; Shelton and Gill 1989). Later studies have suggested that length of incarceration is linked to pregnancy outcome; specifically, women with short incarcerations are more likely to have complications, including low birth weight in their babies. Women with longer incarcerations have fewer complications (e.g., stillbirths, low APGAR scores, anemia) and higher-birth-weight babies than women on parole (Cordero et al. 1991; Elton 1985; Martin et al. 1997) or in methadone maintenance programs (Kyei-Aboagye et al. 2000). The association with better physical outcomes for longer incarcerations may be linked to decreased access to substances of abuse, decreased exposure to sexually transmitted disease (including streptococcus B), access to food and shelter, and decreased exposure to domestic violence (Cordero et al. 1991; Elton 1985; Martin et al. 1997). There is little information about the mental health of incarcerated pregnant women or their babies. The prevalence of depression may be higher in pregnant inmates than in nonpregnant inmates (Fogel 1993), but further study is needed on the effect of the mental health of pregnant inmates on their children. Nicotine abuse remains an issue in some prison settings for pregnant women, even when they are participating in prenatal care within the facility (Cordero et al. 1991); this suggests smoking cessation programs may benefit pregnant female inmates.

Although the prison environment may offer a certain type of stability that, on paper, enhances pregnancy outcomes, many variables remain unexplored. The impact of familial separation and loss of privacy on long-term maternal child bonding has not been explored in a correctional population. Very few facilities exist where mothers can stay with their babies after birth, and visiting with newborns is often limited (Wooldredge and Masters 1993). The effect of this separation is not known.

Treatment issues.   Research on treatment of pregnant offenders has focused primarily on community-based interventions as alternatives to incarceration (Barkauskas et al. 2002; Siefert and Pimlott 2001). Barkauskas and colleagues (2002) described a community-based residential program in which women are provided with family planning, prenatal and postpartum services, rehabilitation for addiction, job training, health care from conception through the fourth month, on-site child care, lactation consultation, labor assistance, and infant rooming-in. Such programs, while they have reportedly good outcomes, are limited by cost and complexity of administration. The central concepts of community programs are transferable to correctional facilities that house pregnant women. Specifically, programs in correctional facilities would benefit from having nurse midwives to coordinate care, education on nutrition and spacing pregnancies, prenatal care, treatment for substance abuse, smoking cessation, parenting, childbirth, and stress management (Barkauskas et al. 2002; Fogel 1993). The Federal Bureau of Prisons allows most infants to stay with their mothers for 3 months postpartum; most state facilities do not currently have this option.

In considering psychopharmacological intervention for incarcerated women with mental health disorders, the issue of pregnancy must be considered. Specific consideration should be given to the potential teratogenicity of medications being prescribed. Women should be offered a pregnancy test and counseled thoroughly on potential risks and benefits of proposed treatment on themselves and on their fetus. Similarly, nursing mothers (although rare in the correctional system) should be advised of any potentially adverse effects of psychotropic medications on their nursing babies. Treating physicians within the correctional system should be able to obtain consultation from psychiatrists with expertise in psychopharmacology in pregnancy and during lactation when complex questions about treatment arise.

Motherhood

Challenges. Most incarcerated women (70%–80%) are mothers; of these mothers, 8%–10% have children in foster care (Barry 1985; McGowan and Blumenthal 1978). Maternal grandmothers care for the majority of the children of incarcerated women (Beckerman 1994). Incarcerated women are generally concerned about their children's welfare, miss them, and want to reunite with them (Thompson and Harm 1995). While many incarcerated women value the maternal role, they are often confused about their legal rights and responsibilities in regard to their children (Beckerman 1994; McGowan and Blumenthal 1978). Children of incarcerated mothers experience loneliness, fear, and embarrassment (Hale 1988). They are at potentially increased risk for mental illness, learning disabilities, teen pregnancy, and PTSD (Moses 1995). They have a deeper drop in economic resources and are more likely to have a change in their primary caretaker, dislocation, and family dissolution than when a father is incarcerated (Brooks 1993). More than half of the children of incarcerated women never visit their mothers in prison because of difficulty scheduling visits, remote location of prisons, and difficulties negotiating the complexities of the child welfare system (Hufft 1999). Although contact between the incarcerated mother and the caseworker for her children is critical, such contact is often strained and infrequent (McGowan and Blumenthal 1978). Incarcerated mothers experience difficulty getting and making phone calls at specified times, difficulty coordinating family court visits, and difficulty receiving, understanding, and responding to correspondence about their children.

Treatment issues. Incarcerated mothers with children would benefit from the assistance of a dedicated legal educator and advocate helping negotiate the child welfare system (Beckerman 1994). Given the high number of incarcerated mothers, it is possible that a specific caseworker or caseworkers should be assigned this role. Interventions aimed at enhancing parenting skills are also of benefit. A fundamental focus of treatment should be addressing substance abuse and dependence, both of which can interfere with parenting ability (Kemper and Rivara 1993). Psychoeducational interventions can focus on enhancing self-esteem, increasing empathy, assisting with developing effective strategies for discipline, decreasing risk factors for child abuse, understanding the maternal role, decreasing recidivism, and addressing addiction (Browne et al. 1999; Thompson and Harm 1995). A second approach is to provide interventions for both children and mothers. Such interventions can include supervised visitation or programming that emphasizes providing appropriate adult role models, helping parents and children develop structured goals they can meet, and enhancing communication between parent and child (Hairston 1991; Hufft 1999).

CONCLUSION

In this chapter, I have reviewed issues of particular relevance to the treatment of women in the correctional system. Relationships between past traumatic experiences, substance abuse and dependence, and personality pathology have been emphasized. The complex psychopathology seen in incarcerated women worsens their prognosis and makes them a challenging treatment population.

Studies of treatment for incarcerated women with mental illness are few in number and rarely contain control groups to assess efficacy. It is difficult to assume treatment outcomes for incarcerated women on the basis of studies of men and women in the community or incarcerated men because of variation among the samples. Indeed, incarcerated women represent a unique population, which has just begun to be researched from an epidemiological and treatment efficacy perspective.

Future research should address delineating epidemiology of psychiatric illness further among incarcerated women, assessing efficacy of treatment interventions, and gaining knowledge about factors associated with treatment entry, retention, and completion. More studies on incarcerated women with dual diagnoses are needed, and further development of modalities to treat substance abuse/dependence within this population is critical. The inexorable rise in the number of women incarcerated in the United States underscores the timeliness and critical nature of this research agenda.

In 1994, Camp and Camp (1994) reported that there were 422 psychiatrists and 1,900 psychologists to cover 48 correctional facilities housing 1.1 million inmates. The burgeoning population of female inmates with complex psychopathology is taxing an already stressed system. Health care budgets can be twice as high for female versus male correctional facilities, and facilities providing care for women with HIV are among the most expensive programs in the country (De Groot 2000).

While integrative treatment and holistic approaches are likely to benefit incarcerated women, funding for such programs is a serious limitation to program implementation. Correctional mental health services will need to expand to meet the increasing demands of this heterogeneous population (Marquart et al. 2001; Morash et al. 1994); this expansion will almost certainly require additional funding and optimization of health services delivery. Incarceration represents a unique opportunity to access a hard-to-reach population with complex medical and psychiatric needs. Successful interventions enhancing medical and psychiatric well-being of female inmates are likely to benefit not only the inmates but also their families, partners, and communities (Hammett et al. 2001).

SUMMARY POINTS

- Most women in the correctional system have a history of drug and/or alcohol addiction.
- Psychiatric disorders, including PTSD, ASPD, and major depression, have a high prevalence in incarcerated women.
- HIV is more highly prevalent in incarcerated women than in incarcerated men.
- Mental health treatment for incarcerated women should include the following:
  - Coordinated and closely linked services for mental health and addiction, with emphasis on dual diagnosis
  - Assessment of trauma history and treatment of trauma-related symptoms
  - Psychopharmacological management of symptoms where appropriate
  - Treatment matching for severity of disorder and therapeutic setting
  - Coordination and close linkage to HIV services and other medical services
  - Counseling regarding pregnancy, motherhood, and familial interactions
  - Vocational/educational training
  - Assistance in transitioning to community/continuity of care

REFERENCES

Alper G, Peterson SJ: Dialectical behavior therapy for patients with borderline personality disorder. J Psychosoc Nurs Ment Health Serv 39:38–45, 2001

Amaro H: Love, sex, and power: considering women's realities in HIV prevention. Am Psychol 50:437–447, 1995

American Correctional Association: The Female Offender. Washington, DC, St Mary's Press, 1990

Anda RF, Williamson DF, Remington PL: Alcohol and fatal injuries among U.S. adults. findings from the NHANES I Epidemiologic Follow-up Study. JAMA 260:2529–2532, 1988

Anglin MD, Hser YI, Booth MW: Sex differences in addict careers. Am J Drug Alcohol Abuse 13:253–280, 1987

Ashley MJ, Olin JS, Le Riche WH, et al: Morbidity in alcoholics: evidence for accelerated development of physical disease in women. Arch Intern Med 137:883–887, 1977

Austin J, Bloom B, Donahue T: Female Offenders in the Community: An Analysis of Innovative Strategies and Programs. Washington, DC, National Institute of Corrections, 1992

Barkauskas VH, Low LK, Pimlott S: Health outcomes of incarcerated pregnant women and their infants in a community-based program. J Midwifery Womens Health 47:371–379, 2002

Barry E: Children of prisoners: punishing the innocent. Youth Law News 6:12–17, 1985

Beck AJ: Survey of state prison inmates 1991 (NCJ 136949). Washington, DC, Office of Justice Programs, Bureau of Justice Statistics, U.S. Department of Justice, March 1993

Beckerman A: Mothers in prison: meeting the prerequisite conditions for permanency planning. Soc Work 39:9–14, 1994

Berman J, Brown D: AIDS knowledge and risky behavior by incarcerated females: IV and non-IV drug users. Sociology and Social Research 75:8–16, 1990

Bloom B, Chesney L, Owen B: Women in California Prisons: Hidden Victims of the War on Drugs. San Francisco, CA, Center on Juvenile and Criminal Justice, 1994

Blume SB: Chemical dependency in women: important issues. Am J Drug Alcohol Abuse 16:297–307, 1990

Bradley RG, Follingstad DR: Group therapy for incarcerated women who experienced interpersonal violence: a pilot study. J Trauma Stress 16:337–340, 2003

Brady K, Killeen T, Saladain M, et al: Comorbid substance abuse and posttraumatic stress disorder: characteristics of women in treatment. Am J Addict 3:160–164, 1994

Bremner JD, Southwick S, Brett E, et al: Dissociation and posttraumatic stress disorder in Vietnam combat veterans. Am J Psychiatry 149:328–332, 1992

Brewer T, Derrickson J: AIDS in prison: a review of epidemiology and preventive policy. AIDS 6:623–628, 1992

Brodsky BS, Oquendo M, Ellis SP, et al: The relationship of childhood abuse to impulsivity and suicidal behavior in adults with major depression. Am J Psychiatry 158:1871–1877, 2001

Brooks MK: Working With Children of Incarcerated Parents: Serving Special Children, Vol 1. New York, Osbourne Association, 1993

Brooner RK, Greenfield L, Schmidt CW, et al: Antisocial personality disorder and HIV infection among intravenous drug abusers. Am J Psychiatry 150:53–58, 1993

Brown PJ, Stout RL, Gannon Rowley J: Substance use disorder–PTSD co-morbidity: patient's perception of symptom interplay and treatment issues. J Subst Abuse Treat 15:445–448, 1998

Browne A, Miller B, Maguin E: Prevalence and severity of lifetime physical and sexual victimization among incarcerated women. Int J Law Psychiatry 22:301–322, 1999

Bucholz KK, Cadoret R, Cloninger CR, et al: A new, semi-structured psychiatric interview for use in genetic linkage studies: a report on the reliability of the SSAGA. J Stud Alcohol 55:149–158, 1994

Camp G, Camp C: The Corrections Yearbook 1993. Middletown, CT, Criminal Justice Institute, 1994

Canetto S, Lester D: Women and Suicidal Behavior. New York, Springer, 1995

Chasnoff IJ: Drug use and women: establishing a standard of care. Ann N Y Acad Sci 562:208–210, 1989

Chesney-Lind M: Women in prison: from partial justice to vengeful equity. Corrections Today 60:66–73, 1998

Coid J: DSM-III diagnosis in criminal psychopaths: a way forward. Criminal Behavior and Mental Health 2:78–94, 1992

Cordero L, Hines S, Shibley KA, et al: Duration of incarceration and perinatal outcome. Obstet Gynecol 78:641–645, 1991

Daly K: Gender, Crime and Punishment. New Haven, CT, Yale University Press, 1994

De Groot AS: HIV infection among incarcerated women: an epidemic behind the walls. HIV Education Prison Project 3:1–4, 2000. Available at: http://www.aegis.com/pubs/hepp/2000/HEPP2000–0401.html. Accessed December 27, 2004.

De Leon G: Therapeutic communities for addictions: a theoretical framework. Int J Addict 30:1603–1645, 1995

DiCataldo F, Greer A, Profit WE: Screening prison inmates for mental disorder: an examination of the relationship between mental disorder and prison adjustment. Bull Am Acad Psychiatry Law 23:573–585, 1995

Dinwiddie SH, Reich T, Cloninger CR: Psychiatric comorbidity and suicidality among intravenous drug users. J Clin Psychiatry 53:364–369, 1992

Drake RE, Mueser KT, Clark RE, et al: The course, treatment, and outcome of substance disorder in persons with severe mental illness. Am J Orthopsychiatry 66:42–51, 1996

el-Bassel N, Ivanoff A, Schilling R, et al: Skills building and social support enhancement to reduce HIV risk in women in jail. Crim Just and Behavior 24:205–223, 1997

Elton P: Outcome of pregnancy among prisoners. J Obstet Gynaecol 5:241–244, 1985

Farabee D, Prendergast M, Cartier J, et al: Barriers to implementing effective correctional drug treatment programs. The Prison Journal 79:150–162, 1999

Farley JL, Mitty JA, Lally MA, et al: Comprehensive medical care among HIV-positive incarcerated women: the Rhode Island experience. J Womens Health Gend Based Med 9:51–56, 2000

Finkelhor D: The international epidemiology of child sexual abuse. Child Abuse Negl 18:409–417, 1994

Finkelstein N, Kennedy C, Thomas K, et al: Gender-Specific Substance Abuse Treatment. Washington, DC, National Women's Resource Center for the Prevention and Treatment of Alcohol, Tobacco and Other Drug Abuse and Mental Illness, 1997

First MB, Gibbon M, Spitzer RI, et al: Structured Clinical Interview for DSM-IV Axis II Personality Disorders (SCID-II). Washington, DC, American Psychiatric Press, 1997

Fogel CI: Pregnant inmates: risk factors and pregnancy outcomes. J Obstet Gynecol Neonatal Nurs 22:33–39, 1993

Gil-Rivas V, Fiorentine R, Anglin MD: Sexual abuse, physical abuse, and posttraumatic stress disorder among women participating in outpatient drug abuse treatment. J Psychoactive Drugs 28:95–102, 1996

Gomberg ES: Suicide risk among women with alcohol problems. Am J Public Health 79:1363–1365, 1989

Goss JR, Peterson K, Smith LW, et al: Characteristics of suicide attempts in a large urban jail system with an established suicide prevention program. Psychiatr Serv 53:574–579, 2002

Greenfeld LA: Alcohol and crime: an analysis of national data on the prevalence of alcohol involvement in crime (NCJ 168632). Washington, DC, Office of Justice Programs, Bureau of Justice Statistics, U.S. Department of Justice, April 1998

Greenfeld LA, Snell TL: Special report: women offenders (NCJ 175688). Washington, DC, Office of Justice Programs, Bureau of Justice Statistics, U.S. Department of Justice, December 1999

Greenfield SF, Weiss RD, Muenz LR, et al: The effect of depression on return to drinking: a prospective study. Arch Gen Psychiatry 55:259–265, 1998

Green-Hennessy S: Factors associated with receipt of behavioral health services among persons with substance dependence. Psychiatr Serv 53:1592–1598, 2002

Grella C: Background and overview of mental health and substance abuse treatment systems: meeting the needs of women who are pregnant and parenting. J Psychoactive Drugs 28:319–343, 1996

Grossman LS, Willer JK, Stovall JG, et al: Underdiagnosis of PTSD and substance use disorders in hospitalized female veterans. Psychiatr Serv 48:393–395, 1997

Guy E, Platt J, Zwerling I, et al: Mental health status of prisoners in an urban jail. Crim Justice Behav 12:29–53, 1985

Guyon L, Brochu S, Parent I, et al: At-risk behaviors with regard to HIV and addiction among women in prison. Women Health 29:49–66, 1999

Hairston C: Family ties during imprisonment: important to whom and for what? Journal of Sociology and Social Welfare 18:87–104, 1991

Hale DC: The impact of mothers' incarceration on the family system: research and recommendations. Marriage and Family Review 12:143–154, 1988

Hammett TM: Making the case for health interventions in correctional facilities. J Urban Health 78:236–240, 2001

Hammett TM, Harmon P, Rhodes W: The burden of infectious disease among inmates and releasees from correctional facilities. Prepared for the National Commission on Correctional Health Care–National Institute of Justice, Chicago, IL, June, 1999

Harris RM, Sharps PW, Allen K, et al: The interrelationship between violence, HIV/AIDS, and drug use in incarcerated women. J Assoc Nurses AIDS Care 14:27–40, 2003

Harrison PM, Beck AJ: Prisoners in 2002 (NCJ 200248). Washington, DC, Office of Justice Programs, Bureau of Justice Statistics, U.S. Department of Justice, July 2003

Hawton K, Houston K, Haw C, et al: Comorbidity of Axis I and Axis II disorders in patients who attempted suicide. Am J Psychiatry 160:1494–1500, 2003

Henderson DJ: Drug abuse and incarcerated women: a research review. J Subst Abuse Treat 15:579–587, 1998

Herman JL: Trauma and Recovery. New York, Basic Books, 1992

Hesselbrock MN, Meyer RE, Keener JJ: Psychopathology in hospitalized alcoholics. Arch Gen Psychiatry 42:1050–1055, 1985

Hesselbrock MN, Hesselbrock V, Syzmanski K, et al: Suicide attempts and alcoholism. J Stud Alcohol 49:436–442, 1988

Higgins ST, Delaney DD, Budney AJ, et al: A behavioral approach to achieving initial cocaine abstinence. Am J Psychiatry 148:1218–1224, 1991

Hufft AG: Girl Scouts Beyond Bars: a unique opportunity for forensic psychiatric nursing. J Psychosoc Nurs Ment Health Serv 37:45–51, 1999

Hutton HE, Treisman GJ, Hunt WR, et al: HIV risk behaviors and their relationship to posttraumatic stress disorder among women prisoners. Psychiatr Serv 52:508–513, 2001

Jacobsberg L, Frances A, Perry S: Axis II diagnoses among volunteers for HIV testing and counseling. Am J Psychiatry 152:1222–1224, 1995

Jordan BK, Schlenger WE, Fairbank JA, et al: Prevalence of psychiatric disorders among incarcerated women, II: convicted felons entering prison. Arch Gen Psychiatry 53:513–519, 1996

Kemper KJ, Rivara FP: Parents in jail. Pediatrics 92:261–264, 1993

Kessler RC, McGonagle KA, Zhao S, et al: Lifetime and twelve-month prevalence of DSM-III-R psychiatric disorders in the United States: results from the National Comorbidity Survey. Arch Gen Psychiatry 51:8–19, 1994

Kessler RC, Sonnega A, Bromet E, et al: Posttraumatic stress disorder in the National Comorbidity Survey. Arch Gen Psychiatry 52:1048–1060, 1995

Kessler RC, Crum RM, Warner LA, et al: Lifetime co-occurrence of DSM-III-R alcohol abuse and dependence with other psychiatric disorders in the National Comorbidity Survey. Arch Gen Psychiatry 54:313–321, 1997

Kessler RC, Borges G, Walters EE: Prevalence of and risk factors for lifetime suicide attempts in the National Comorbidity Survey. Arch Gen Psychiatry 56:617–626, 1999

Kimmerling R, Goldsmith R: Links between exposure to violence and HIV-infection: implications for substance abuse treatment. Alcoholism Treatment Quarterly 18: 61–70, 2000

Kingree JB, Thompson MP, Kaslow NJ: Risk factors for suicide attempts among low-income women with a history of alcohol problems. Addict Behav 24:583–587, 1999

Klein H, Chao BS: Sexual abuse during childhood and adolescence as predictors of HIV-related sexual risk during adulthood among female sexual partners of injection drug users. Violence Against Women 1:55–76, 1995

Kotler M, Iancu I, Efroni R, et al: Anger, impulsivity, social support, and suicide risk in patients with posttraumatic stress disorder. J Nerv Ment Dis 189:162–167, 2001

Kranzler HR, Del Boca FK, Rounsaville BJ: Comorbid psychiatric diagnosis predicts three-year outcomes in alcoholics: a posttreatment natural history study. J Stud Alcohol 57:619–626, 1996

Kyei-Aboagye K, Vragovic O, Chong D: Birth outcome in incarcerated, high-risk pregnant women. J Reprod Med 45:190–194, 2000

Lake ES: An exploration of the violent victim experiences of female offenders. Violence Vict 8:41–51, 1993

Langan NP, Pelissier BM: Gender differences among prisoners in drug treatment. J Subst Abuse 13:291–301, 2001

Lewis CF: Prevalence of psychiatric diagnoses in HIV positive incarcerated women. Paper presented at the 156th annual meeting of the American Psychiatric Association, San Francisco, CA. May 17–22, 2003

Lewis CF: Ethnicity, diagnosis and healthcare utilization in incarcerated women. Paper presented at the annual meeting of the American Psychiatric Association, New York, May 2004a

Lewis CF: HIV positive incarcerated women: trauma and suicide history. American Academy of Psychiatry and the Law Newsletter 29:10–11, 2004b

Lex BW: Alcohol and other psychoactive substance dependence in women and men, in Gender and Psychopathology. Edited by Seeman MV. Washington, DC, American Psychiatric Press, 1995, pp 311–358

Linehan MM, Schmidt H 3rd, Dimeff LA, et al: Dialectical behavior therapy for patients with borderline personality disorder and drug-dependence. Am J Addict 8:279–292, 1999

Logan TK, Leukefeld C: Violence and HIV risk behavior among male and female crack users. J Drug Issues 30:261–282, 2000

Lubelczyk RA, Friedmann PD, Lemon SC, et al: HIV prevention services in correctional drug treatment programs: do they change risk behaviors? AIDS Educ Prev 14:117–125, 2002

Maden T, Swinton M, Gunn J: Psychiatric disorder in women serving a prison sentence. Br J Psychiatry 164:44–54, 1994

Marquart JW, Brewer V, E., Simon P, et al: Lifestyle factors among female prisoners with histories of psychiatric treatment. J Crim Justice 29:319–328, 2001

Martin SL, Kim H, Kupper LL, et al: Is incarceration during pregnancy associated with infant birthweight? Am J Public Health 87:1526–1531, 1997

Maruschak LM: HIV in prisons and jails, 1999 (NCJ 187456). Washington, DC, Office of Justice Programs, Bureau of Justice Statistics, U.S. Department of Justice, July 2001

Mason BJ, Kocsis JH, Ritvo EC, et al: A double-blind, placebo-controlled trial of desipramine for primary alcohol dependence stratified on the presence or absence of major depression. JAMA 275:761–767, 1996

McClelland GM, Teplin LA, Abram KM, et al: HIV and AIDS risk behaviors among female jail detainees: implications for public health policy. Am J Public Health 92:818–825, 2002

McGowan B, Blumenthal KL: Why Punish the Children? A Study of Children of Women Prisoners. Hackensack, NJ, National Council on Crime and Delinquency, 1978

Messina N, Farabee D, Rawson R: Treatment responsivity of cocaine-dependent patients with antisocial personality disorder to cognitive-behavioral and contingency management interventions. J Consult Clin Psychol 71:320–329, 2003

Miller RE: Nationwide profile of female inmate substance involvement. J Psychoactive Drugs 16:319–326, 1984

Morash M, Haarr R, Rucker L: A comparison of programming for women and men in U.S. prisons in the 1990s. Crime and Delinquency 40:197–221, 1994

Moscicki EK: Gender differences in completed and attempted suicides. Ann Epidemiol 4:152–158, 1994

Moses M: A synergistic solution for children of incarcerated parents. Corrections Today 57:124–126, 1995

Murphy GE, Robins E: Social factors in suicide. JAMA 199:303–308, 1967

Najavits LM, Weiss RD, Liese BS: Group cognitive-behavioral therapy for women with PTSD and substance use disorder. J Subst Abuse Treat 13:13–22, 1996

Najavits L, Weiss R, Reif S: The Addiction Severity Index as a screen for trauma and posttraumatic stress disorder. J Stud Alcohol 59:56–62, 1998a

Najavits LM, Weiss RD, Shaw SR, et al: "Seeking Safety": outcome of a new cognitive-behavioral psychotherapy for women with posttraumatic stress disorder and substance dependence. J Trauma Stress 11:437–456, 1998b

Nespor K: Treatment needs of alcohol-dependent women. Int J Psychosom 37:50–52, 1990

Onorato M: HIV infection among incarcerated women. HIV and Hepatitis Education Prison Project 4: 1–4, 2001. Available at: http://www.aegis.com/pubs/hepp/2001/HEPP2001–0501.html. Accessed December 27, 2004.

Peters RH, Strozier AL, Murrin MR, et al: Treatment of substance-abusing jail inmates: examination of gender differences. J Subst Abuse Treat 14:339–349, 1997

Peyrot M, Yen S, Baldassano CA: Short-term substance abuse prevention in jail: a cognitive-behavioral approach. J Drug Educ 24:33–47, 1994

Pomeroy EC, Kiam R, Abel E: Meeting the mental health needs of incarcerated women. Health Soc Work 23:71–75, 1998

Prendergast M, Wellisch J: Assessment of and services for substance-abusing women offenders in community and correctional settings. The Prison Journal 75:240–256, 1995

Prendergast M, Wellisch J, Wong M: Residential treatment for women parolees following prison-based drug treatment: treatment experiences, needs and services, outcomes. The Prison Journal 76:253–274, 1996

Rasche C: The female offender as an object of criminological research. Crim Justice Behav 1:301–320, 1974

Regier DA, Farmer ME, Rae DS, et al: Comorbidity of mental disorders with alcohol and other drug abuse: results from the Epidemiologic Catchment Area (ECA) Study. JAMA 264:2511–2518, 1990

Resnick HS, Kilpatrick DG, Dansky BS, et al: Prevalence of civilian trauma and posttraumatic stress disorder in a representative national sample of women. J Consult Clin Psychol 61:984–991, 1993

Robins LN, Regier DA: Psychiatric Disorders in America. New York, Free Press, 1991

Robins LN, Helzer JE, Croughan J, et al: National Institute of Mental Health Diagnostic Interview Schedule: its history, characteristics, and validity. Arch Gen Psychiatry 38:381–389, 1981

Robins LN, Wing J, Wittchen H-U, et al: The Composite International Diagnostic Interview: an epidemiologic instrument suitable for use in conjunction with different diagnostic systems and in different cultures. Arch Gen Psychiatry 45:1069–1077, 1988

Roth B, Presse L: Nursing interventions for parasuicidal behaviors in female offenders. J Psychosoc Nurs Ment Health Serv 41:20–29, 2003

Rounsaville BJ, Weissman MM, Kleber H, et al: Heterogeneity of psychiatric diagnosis in treated opiate addicts. Arch Gen Psychiatry 39:161–168, 1982

Roy A: Characteristics of drug addicts who attempt suicide. Psychiatry Res 121:99–103, 2003

Safyer SM, Richmond L: Pregnancy behind bars. Semin Perinatol 19:314–322, 1995

Schilling R, el-Bassel N, Ivanoff A, et al: Sexual risk behavior of incarcerated, drug-using women, 1992. Public Health Rep 109:539–547, 1994

Schuckit MA: Primary men alcoholics with histories of suicide attempts. J Stud Alcohol 47:78–81, 1986

Schuckit MA, Anthenelli RM, Bucholz KK, et al: The time course development of alcohol-related problems in men and women. J Stud Alcohol 56:218–225, 1995

Shalev AY, Freedman S, Peri T, et al: Prospective study of posttraumatic stress disorder and depression following trauma. Am J Psychiatry 155:630–637, 1998

Shelton BJ, Gill DG: Childbearing in prison: a behavioral analysis. J Obstet Gynecol Neonatal Nurs 18:301–308, 1989

Sheu M, Hogan J, Allsworth J, et al: Continuity of medical care and risk of incarceration in HIV-positive and high-risk HIV-negative women. J Womens Health (Larchmt) 11:743–750, 2002

Shlay JC, Blackburn D, O'Keefe K, et al: Human immunodeficiency virus seroprevalence and risk assessment of a homeless population in Denver. Sex Transm Dis 23:304–311, 1996

Siefert K, Pimlott S: Improving pregnancy outcome during imprisonment: a model residential care program. Soc Work 46:125–134, 2001

Singer MI, Bussey J, Song LY, et al: The psychosocial issues of women serving time in jail. Soc Work 40:103–113, 1995

Singleton J, Perkins C, Trachtenberg A, et al: HIV antibody seroprevalence among prisoners entering the California correctional system. West J Med 153:394–399, 1990

Smith BV: Special Issues of Women in the Criminal Justice System. Washington, DC, National Women's Law Center, 1993

Snell TL, Morton DC: Survey of state prison inmates 1991: women in prison (NCJ 145321). Washington, DC, Office of Justice Programs, Bureau of Justice Statistics, U.S. Department of Justice, March 1994

Steadman HJ, Holohean EJ Jr, Dvoskin J: Estimating mental health needs and service utilization among prison inmates. Bull Am Acad Psychiatry Law 19:297–307, 1991

Steffensmeier D, Allen E: Gender and crime: toward a gendered theory of female offending. Annual Review of Sociology 22:459–487, 1996

Teplin LA, Abram KM, McClelland GM: Prevalence of psychiatric disorders among incarcerated women, I: pretrial jail detainees. Arch Gen Psychiatry 53:505–512, 1996

Teplin LA, Abram KM, McClelland GM: Mentally disordered women in jail: who receives services? Am J Public Health 87:604–609, 1997

Thompson PJ, Harm NJ: Parent education for mothers in prison. Pediatr Nurs 21:552–555, 1995

Tjaden PG, Thoennes N: Predictors of legal intervention in child maltreatment cases. Child Abuse Negl 16:807–821, 1992

van der Kolk BA, Pelcovitz D, Roth S, et al: Dissociation, somatization, and affect dysregulation: the complexity of adaptation of trauma. Am J Psychiatry 153:83–93, 1996

Vlahov D, Brewer TF, Castro KG, et al: Prevalence of antibody to HIV-1 among entrants to U.S. correctional facilities. JAMA 265:1129–1132, 1991

Warren JI, Burnette M, South SC, et al: Personality disorders and violence among female prison inmates. J Am Acad Psychiatry Law 30:502–509, 2002a

Warren JI, Hurt S, Loper AB, et al: Psychiatric symptoms, history of victimization, and violent behavior among incarcerated female felons: an American perspective. Int J Law Psychiatry 25:129–149, 2002b

Weisner C, Schmidt L: Gender disparities in treatment for alcohol problems. JAMA 268:1872–1876, 1992

Wellisch J, Anglin MD, Prendergast ML: Treatment strategies for drug abusing women offenders, in Drug Treatment and Criminal Justice. Edited by Inciardi JA. Newbury Park, CA, Sage, 1993, pp 5–29

Wellisch J, Prendergast ML, Anglin MD: Drug-abusing women offenders: results of a national survey (NCJ 149261). Washington, DC, Office of Justice Programs, Bureau of Justice Statistics, U.S. Department of Justice, 1994

Wilsnack C, Vogeltanz NDI, Klassen AD, et al: Childhood sexual abuse and women's substance abuse: national survey findings. J Stud Alcohol 58:264–271, 1997

Windle M, Windle RC, Scheidt DM, et al: Physical and sexual abuse and associated mental disorders among alcoholic inpatients. Am J Psychiatry 152:1322–1328, 1995

Wish ED, O'Neil J, Baldau V: Lost opportunity to combat AIDS: drug abusers in the criminal justice system. NIDA Res Monogr 93:187–209, 1990

Wooldredge JD, Masters K: Confronting problems faced by pregnant inmates in state prisons. Crime and Delinquency 39:195–203, 1993

Zlotnick C: Posttraumatic stress disorder (PTSD), PTSD comorbidity, and childhood abuse among incarcerated women. J Nerv Ment Dis 185:761–763, 1997

Zlotnick C: Antisocial personality disorder, affect dysregulation and childhood abuse among incarcerated women. J Pers Disord 13:90–95, 1999

Zlotnick C, Najavits LM, Rohsenow DJ, et al: A cognitive-behavioral treatment for incarcerated women with substance abuse disorder and posttraumatic stress disorder: findings from a pilot study. J Subst Abuse Treat 25:99–105, 2003

CHAPTER 9

Individuals With Developmental Disabilities in Correctional Settings

Barbara E. McDermott, Ph.D.

Kimberly A. Hardison, Psy.D.

Colin MacKenzie, M.D.

The overall mission of the U.S. correctional system is multifaceted and includes punishment and removal of the offender from society, although arguably one component is rehabilitation. Training and habilitation programs may be useful in assisting facilities in maintaining order and control (Hall 1992). With no offenders is this more relevant than those with developmental disabilities. Although the research is controversial, most studies suggest that offenders with developmental delays commit less serious offenses, yet serve more time in prison than offenders without such delays (MacEachron 1979; Petersilia 2000a). In 1975, Talent and Keldgord opined, "Less effort has been expended in the United States to rehabilitate the mentally retarded offender than any other group of offenders" (p. 39). In 2000, Petersilia noted that 25 years later this situation has remained essentially unchanged (Petersilia 2000a).

In this chapter, we outline the progress that has been made in the identification and habilitation of individuals with developmental disabilities in the criminal justice system. We discuss definitions, legal issues, and prevalence rates as well as the particular vulnerabilities individuals with developmental delays present to the criminal justice system. Finally, we address screening, management, and habilitation in corrections arising directly from these vulnerabilities and describe model programs in several states.

DEFINITIONS

Federal law has provided a definition of the term *developmental disability,* which incorporates a spectrum of disorders. The Developmental Disabilities Assistance and Bill of Rights Act of 2000 outlines the legal standard required for an individual to be designated as having a developmental disorder and includes the following:

1. The disability is attributed to a mental or physical impairment or combination of the two.
2. The disability manifested before the age of 22.
3. The disability is likely to continue indefinitely.
4. The disability results in functional limitations in three or more of the following areas:
   a. Self-care
   b. Receptive or expressive language
   c. Mobility
   d. Self-direction
   e. Capacity for independent living
   f. Economic self-sufficiency
5. Individualized support is of a lifelong or extended duration and is individually planned.

Some states, such as California, have a more narrow definition of the term *developmental disability* (Petersilia 2000a). In 1977, California adopted the Lanterman Developmental Disabilities Services Act (2004), which delineates the state's responsibility to provide services to individuals with developmental disabilities. In Welfare and Institutions Code Section 4512 (a) of the Lanterman Developmental Disabilities Services Act (2004), developmental disability is defined as "a disability that originates before an individual attains age 18 years, continues, or can be expected to continue, indefinitely, and constitutes a substantial disability for that individual." Further, the definition includes "mental retardation, cerebral palsy, epilepsy, and autism. This term shall also include disabling conditions found to be closely related to mental retardation or to require treatment similar to that required for individuals with mental retardation, but shall not include other handicapping conditions that are solely physical in nature."

According to the Centers for Disease Control and Prevention (1996), mental retardation is the most common developmental disability. For this reason, persons with mental retardation in the criminal justice system are the primary focus of this chapter. Some research has indicated that mental retardation is overrepresented within the criminal justice system (e.g., Cockram et al. 1998; Petersilia 1997; Santamour and West 1982a), although others have found no differences from the general population (Conley et al. 1992; MacEachron 1979; New York State Commission on Quality of Care for the Mentally Disabled 1991). Approximately 89% of all individuals with mental retardation have mental retardation that falls within the mild range (Ellis and Luckasson 1985), and, consistent with the general population, the majority of inmates with mental retardation have mental retardation that falls in the mild range (Noble and Conley 1992). Therefore, the particular vulnerabilities and habilitation issues present in an individual with mild mental retardation is most relevant to those working with individuals with developmental disabilities within the correctional system. Offenders with moderate to profound mental retardation are unlikely to remain in the criminal justice system (Conley et al. 1992).

The distinction between mental retardation and mental illness is especially important in a discussion of appropriate interventions in corrections, although it is arguably relevant in pretrial concerns as well. An individual with a mental illness may be amenable to treatment, and the symptoms of his or her illness can be expected to be ameliorated as a result of this treatment. In contrast, an individual with mental retardation or another developmental disability, by definition, has a condition that will continue indefinitely and is not necessarily responsive to treatment. Therefore, a discussion of interventions with such individuals must necessarily focus on habilitation rather than treatment. Additionally, identification of such inmates is of paramount importance, as many proceed through the criminal justice system undetected (Petrella 1992).

DSM-IV-TR (American Psychiatric Association 2000) requires the following criteria for an individual to be diagnosed with mental retardation:

1. Subaverage intellectual functioning (generally defined as an IQ of 70 or less)
2. Impairments in adaptive functioning
3. Onset before age 18

The severity of mental retardation is coded on the basis of the degree of intellectual impairment. DSM-IV-TR defines four categories: mild, moderate, severe, and profound. Mild includes individuals with a measured IQ of 50–55 up to 70; moderate is 35–40 up to 50–55; severe is 20–25 up to 35–40; and profound is below 20–25.

The American Association on Mental Retardation (AAMR) defines mental retardation as "a disability characterized by significant limitations both in intellectual functioning and in adaptive behavior as expressed by conceptual, social, and practical adaptive skills" (American Association on Mental Retardation 2002). The disability must originate before the age of 18. The AAMR presents five assumptions essential to the application of the above definition:

1. The context of the individuals' community environments, which are considered typical for his or her age, peers, and culture, must be considered when addressing limitations in current functioning.
2. Assessment must take into consideration cultural and linguistic diversity as well as differences in communication, sensory, motor, and behavioral factors.
3. Limitations and strengths coexist within an individual.
4. Describing limitations is useful in the development of needed supports.
5. The life functioning of an individual with mental retardation generally will improve with appropriate individualized support over a sustained period of time.

PREVALENCE

Prevalence rates of mental retardation in the general population vary depending on the definitions, method of study, and population studied. According to DSM-IV TR (American Psychiatric Association 2000), the prevalence rate of individuals with mental retardation is estimated to be about 1% of the population. The Arc of the United States (formerly the Association of Retarded Citizens of the United States) reviewed prevalence studies in the early 1980s and determined that 2.5%–3% of the general population has mental retardation (The Arc of the United States 1998).

Unfortunately, the literature reporting the prevalence rates of incarcerated individuals with mental retardation contains many methodological problems. As previously noted, most studies indicate that individuals with mental retardation are overrepresented in correctional facilities; however, reported prevalence rates vary significantly. As with the general population, differences in assessment, definition, and methodology, as well as regional differences, affect prevalence reports. Santamour and West (1982a) reported that the rate of adults with mental retardation in prison ranged from 8% to almost 30%. Specifically, the South Carolina Department of Corrections indicated a rate of 8%; Texas reported a 10% rate of offenders with mental retardation; and Georgia reported a rate of 27%. Petersilia (1997) estimated that 6,400 adult and juvenile inmates have mental retardation in the California corrections system. An estimated 4%–10% of individuals in prison or jail in California are developmentally disabled (Petersilia 2000a). However, some reports suggest that the prevalence of individuals with mental retardation in corrections is comparable to the prevalence in the general population. For example, the New York State Commission on Quality of Care for the Mentally Disabled (1991) reported that 2% of approximately 53,400 inmates are developmentally disabled. Noble and Conley (1992) reported that approximately 14,000–20,000 inmates have developmental disabilities, constituting roughly 2% of all inmates in state and federal prisons. They also noted that rates of mental retardation ranged from 0.5% to almost 20% within state and federal prisons, asserting that the differences are secondary to the methods of assessment.

LEGAL ISSUES

Although Talent and Keldgord (1975) asserted that little effort has been expended on offenders with mental retardation, the management and treatment of individuals with developmental disabilities in the criminal justice system has received substantial legal attention in the past several decades. Case law and statutes have illuminated the scope of the problem and, in some instances, provided guidance as to reparative measures. One significant problem that has hampered the development of appropriate approaches with these individuals is the confusion and/or lack of distinction in the legal system between mental illness and mental retardation or developmental disabilities. As an example of this problem, in a study of the attorneys general of the United States and four territories (McAfee and Gural 1988), the results suggest that the identification of individuals with developmental disabilities in the criminal justice system is unlikely to occur and that most protections for such individuals are contained in statutes pertaining to mental illness. In only one reporting state (South Carolina), the attorney general noted that judges routinely inquire about a defendant's IQ when a guilty plea is entered, presumably to ensure that the defendant has knowingly and intelligently entered the plea. Although many of the attorneys general described that special postconviction protections were in place for defendants with developmental disabilities, several reported that these protections were inconsistently employed. Eighty-six percent reported the use of a postconviction psychological evaluation, although no other named protection (e.g., reduced sentence, incarceration in a specialized unit, special training or education) was used in more than 50% of the respondent states.

Various courts in the United States have provided guidance to the correctional system in the management of offenders with developmental disabilities. For example, the U.S. Supreme Court, in *Estelle v. Gamble* (1976), established the constitutional right of prisoners to medical treatment by holding that inmates could not be confined with "deliberate indifference" to their serious medical needs. While individuals with developmental disabilities were not mentioned specifically, *Estelle* has been interpreted by lower courts to include psychiatric/psychological needs. One year later, the Fourth Circuit Court of Appeals, in *Bowring v. Godwin* (1977), confirmed that psychiatric needs were included in the definition of severe medical needs, opining, "We see no underlying distinction between the right to medical care for physical ills and its psychological or psychiatric counterpart." The U.S. District Court for the Southern District of Texas, in *Ruiz v. Estelle* (1980), made specific references to "retarded inmates," noting repeatedly the injustices replete in the correctional system for these offenders, although reparative measures suggested were generic to mental disorders. In *Kendrick v. Bland* (1981), the District Court for the Western District of Kentucky approved a consent decree requiring correction of conditions in Kentucky prisons, including the provision of education programs for "disadvantaged individuals under the age of 21 with learning problems and learning disabilities." This decision arose from the Education of All Handicapped Children Act of 1975 (EHA), which has been interpreted to include incarcerated individuals 21 or younger. This act requires that "free appropriate public education" be provided to all covered prisoners. The EHA was amended, with the use of "people first" language, and renamed the Individuals with Disabilities Education Act of 1990 (IDEA).

Recently, federal legislation has been interpreted to include the criminal justice system. In *Pennsylvania Department of Corrections v. Yeskey* (1998), the U.S. Supreme Court held, in a unanimous decision, that the Americans with Disabilities Act of 1990 (ADA) applies to state prisoners: inmates with disabilities cannot be excluded from prison programs on the basis of their disability. In *Clark v. State of California* (1998), a class action lawsuit was filed alleging that incarcerated individuals suffered discrimination as a result of their developmental disabilities, and sought injunctive relief under the ADA. As a result of the *Yeskey* decision, California prison officials agreed to a settlement requiring the development and implementation of a plan to screen inmates for developmental disabilities and to provide these inmates with safe housing and supportive services.

These cases illustrate that the correctional system can no longer simply house inmates with developmental disabilities without providing appropriate screening and support. As a consequence, prisons increasingly are expected to develop specialized programs for these offenders.

DISPROPORTIONATE REPRESENTATION OF INDIVIDUALS WITH MENTAL RETARDATION IN CORRECTIONAL SETTINGS

The literature is controversial regarding the disproportionate representation of offenders with mental retardation in correctional facilities. However, if such individuals are overrepresented, several factors may explain this disparity. The definitions of mental retardation and developmental disability require that the individual evidence impairments in adaptive functioning. These impairments can span numerous areas, often resulting in cognitive limitations that affect their decision-making skills, communication skills, social understanding, moral reasoning, and ability to learn from past mistakes (McGee and Menolascino 1992). Deficits in these areas may lead to increased criminal behavior. Additionally, individuals with mental retardation are more likely to come from low-income minority groups residing in areas with increased police presence, and this places them at a higher risk of arrest (Petersilia 1997).

Once arrested, offenders with mental retardation may not understand their rights. For example, studies have shown that people with mental retardation often do not understand the *Miranda* warning against self-incrimination (Cloud et al. 2002; Ellis and Luckasson 1985; Everington and Fulero 1999; Fulero and Everington 1995; Petersilia 2000a). Given this lack of knowledge, an individual with mental retardation is more likely to waive his or her rights and provide incriminating information—an outcome that increases the likelihood of conviction and incarceration. Individuals with mental retardation are more vulnerable in interrogations because they are more susceptible to suggestion, acquiesce more often, and have a desire to please authority figures (Cloud et al. 2002; Everington and Fulero 1999; Matikka and Vesala 1997; Pelka 1997; Petersilia 1997). These characteristics increase the likelihood of both false and legitimate confessions, which in turn increases the likelihood of conviction.

Santamour and West (1982a) proposed that probation is more likely given to individuals with higher intelligence, greater educational attainment, and an adequate work history. If this assertion is accurate, many people with mental retardation would not be granted probation, as they often are less educated and may not have a stable work history. Mason and Murphy (2002) studied a group of 90 probationers in southeast England and found no significant differences in two outcome measures of probation officer satisfaction for people with intellectual disability when compared with those functioning within the normal range (of intelligence). Additionally, there were no differences in number of probation violations between the two groups. The authors noted that the lack of significant differences may be accounted for by the probation officers' ability to detect and counteract the difficulties of probationers with cognitive deficits. However, if Santamour's supposition is accurate, this study suggests, the unwillingness to utilize probation is based on faulty beliefs about individuals with disabilities.

All of the above-described issues may have an impact on the number of individuals who are in prison and may explain the research that indicates that there is a disparity between the number of individuals with mental retardation in the general population and the number in prisons. Clearly the deficits described impact the ability of the offender with mental retardation to successfully navigate the criminal justice system prior to incarceration. These same vulnerabilities lead to predictable problems in the prison system.

VULNERABILITY OF INDIVIDUALS WITH MENTAL RETARDATION IN CORRECTIONAL SETTINGS

Prisoners with developmental disabilities are most often housed with the general population (Giamp and West 2003; New York State Commission on Quality of Care for the Mentally Disabled 1991; Smith et al. 1990). This housing situation places the inmate with developmental disabilities at risk for victimization by other inmates. People with developmental disabilities are 4–10 times more likely to be victims of crime than those who do not have disabilities, and this trend holds true for persons with developmental disabilities in prison as well (Petersilia 2000b). Prisoners with mental retardation are more likely to be exploited, victimized, abused, and injured secondary to the previously noted cognitive deficits (Ellis and Luckasson 1985; Giamp and West 2003; Müller-Isberner and Hodgins 2000; Petersilia 1997; Santamour and West 1982a; Smith et al. 1990; Stavis 1991). Petersilia (1997) reported that offenders with mental retardation who are housed with the general population are victimized in such ways as having their property stolen, being raped, or being manipulated by other inmates to violate the rules. They have difficulty understanding the rules, which also increases the likelihood of disciplinary action. In *Ruiz v. Estelle* (1980), the court opined, "Mentally retarded persons meet with unremitting hardships in prison. They are slow to adjust to prison life and its requirements, principally because they have almost insurmountable difficulties in comprehending what is expected of them. Not understanding or remembering disciplinary rules, they tend to commit a large number of disciplinary infractions."

Aside from the obvious consequences of such maltreatment (e.g., physical injury, emotional turmoil), there are more subtle consequences. Inmates who are developmentally disabled are likely to resolve conflicts with others by using physical aggression because of, in part, limitations in communication skills (Petersilia 1997; Smith et al. 1990). Individuals with mental retardation are more likely to have low frustration tolerance (Day 1990) and poor self-control (Benson 1994; Cullen 1993), increasing the likelihood of more disciplinary problems. Smith et al. (1990) found that youthful inmates who were mentally retarded received approximately three times as many disciplinary reports for noncompliant behavior and hygiene offenses (e.g., not showering) and assaulted other inmates or correctional staff more than twice as often as other inmates. As a result of such disciplinary problems, inmates with mental retardation may serve longer prison sentences, be denied parole, or be transferred to a more secure prison (Ellis and Luckasson 1985; Giamp and West 2003; Petersilia 1997; Santamour and West 1982a; Stavis 1991). In *Ruiz v. Estelle* (1980), the court noted

> It is common for mentally retarded inmates in TDC [Texas Department of Corrections] to serve longer sentences than inmates not fitting this category. Several reasons are evident. As previously noted, retarded inmates are more likely to have poor disciplinary records than their peers, which disqualify the former for early parole. They are frequently unable to succeed in institutional programs whose completion would increase their chances for parole, and they are also unlikely to be able to present well-defined employment and residential plans to the Parole Board.

Table 9–1 summarizes areas of vulnerabilities for offenders with developmental disabilities in a correctional environment.

TABLE 9–4. Vulnerabilities of offenders with developmental disabilities

---

Cognitive limitations
*   Difficulty understanding *Miranda* warning
*   Less cognizant of pleas/plea bargaining
*   Difficulty understanding/following rules

Adaptive skills deficits
*   Difficulty following guidelines/routines
*   More hygiene infractions

Impaired social understanding
*   Vulnerable to manipulation/victimization
*   Tendency to resolve conflicts with aggression

Lower educational/occupational functioning
*   Less likely to be paroled

RECEPTION AND ASSESSMENT PROCEDURES

Upon arrival to most correctional systems, inmates are subject to reception and assessment procedures to identify any circumstance that would require specialized housing. During this classification process, some correctional systems attempt to identify offenders with mental retardation. At this stage a brief psychological and educational history may be obtained or certain testing may be performed to assess intelligence and adaptive functioning. For example, Giamp and West (2003) reported that a Colorado correctional facility utilizes the Culture Fair IQ Test (Cattell and Cattell 1973) and the Reading Level score from the Test of Adult Basic Education (TABE; Test of Adult Basic Education 2005) to screen for mental retardation. If an inmate scores below a particular cut-off point, he or she is referred for further evaluation. This additional testing typically includes the Wechsler Adult Intelligence Scale–III (WAIS-III; Wechsler 1997) and an adaptive measure such as Vineland Adaptive Behavior Scale (Sparrow et al. 1984) or the Adaptive Behavior Scale–Residential and Community, 2nd Edition (Nihira et al. 1993). In California, a screening tool was developed by the Department of Corrections to assess an inmate's cognitive abilities and functioning skills. It noted several problems with the tool, most notably that, compared with the assessment used by the Department of Developmental Services, the Department of Corrections tool over-identifies offenders with developmental disabilities.

Appropriate services are dependent on the use of valid and reliable instruments. As the AAMR suggests, assessments must consider cultural and linguistic issues in addition to other sensory and communication factors. MacEachron (1979) found that the prevalence of offenders with mental retardation dropped significantly when individual (rather than group) assessments of intelligence were administered. McGee and Menolascino (1992) have argued that even screening assessments should be administered individually and only by professionals trained in such administration. They recommended using the Peabody Picture Vocabulary Test (PPVT; Dunn and Dunn 1997), a third edition of which has recently been published. Many jurisdictions (e.g., South Carolina, North Carolina) use the Revised Beta-II (Revised Beta Examination 1974) and the Wide Range Achievement Test (WRAT; Wilkinson 1993) as a screening for intellectual or academic deficits. Scores below a certain cut-off indicate the need for further assessment. As in Colorado, the most widely used test of intelligence in adults is the Wechsler Adult Intelligence Scale, which yields both Verbal and Performance IQ estimates. The Vineland Adaptive Behavior Scale is often used as the assessment of adaptive skills.

The assessments mentioned above are used primarily as a method of identifying inmates with deficits. Critical in formulating an individualized habilitation plan is use of a more comprehensive assessment that includes both strengths and deficit areas that may be most amenable to habilitation. Many jurisdictions use their own assessments to identify functional deficits (e.g., California, North Carolina); however, rarely are these assessments normed or standardized. Recently, the AAMR has published a comprehensive assessment called the Support Intensity Scale (SIS; Tasse et al. 2005). This instrument was developed over a period of 5 years and includes an extensive literature review, a Q-sort, and three field tests. It is purported to have "excellent psychometric properties." The SIS is designed to identify deficits in 57 specific life activities, 15 medical conditions, and 13 problem behaviors. Although the instrument appears promising, to date no research has been conducted documenting its use.

HABILITATION ISSUES

The management of inmates with developmental disabilities has presented correctional systems with significant problems. One controversy has been whether inmates with developmental disabilities should be housed in the general prison population. Those in favor of housing with the general prison population adhere to the principle of normalization, suggesting that individuals with mental retardation should, as much as possible, be treated like others (Santamour and West 1982a). However, as previously noted, much has been published on the disadvantages and risks to the prisoner with mental retardation when placed in the general prison population. Critics argue that normalization does not take these disadvantages into account. According to Petersilia (1997, p. 6), "The emerging consensus within the profession seems to be that there are highly unique aspects to the correctional environment and that the normalization goals for the mentally retarded should not fully apply in this setting." Her statement suggests that specialized units may be more appropriate for such individuals.

Although court cases such as *Ruiz v. Estelle* (1980) established that individuals with mental retardation or developmental disabilities have the right to treatment, Hall (1992) estimated that fewer than 10% of inmates with such deficits receive specialized services. In fact, many authors have indicated that specialized services for prisoners with mental retardation are inadequate (Giamp and West 2003; Müller-Isberner and Hodgins 2000). Although Hall (1992) noted that advocates for these offenders must be cautious in their expectations—"it is unreasonable to conceptualize prisons as care and treatment facilities"—services designed to aid the offender with mental retardation adapt to incarceration and reintegrate into society are increasingly expected of correctional facilities.

Unlike programs for offenders with mental illness, the goal of specialized programs for offenders with developmental disabilities is not remediation of their disability. The goal of most programs is education, training, and skills enhancement tailored to the specific needs of the inmate. As with any other disorder, the diagnosis of mental retardation provides no information about the needs of the specific individual. For these reasons, assessment is a critical component in any specialized program. For example, as a result of *Clark v. State of California* (1998), prison officials in California developed a "remedial plan" (known as "the Clark plan") for identifying prisoners with developmental disabilities and providing them with access to a variety of programs that would make early release more likely. This plan includes 1) screening for developmental disabilities; 2) housing inmates with developmental disabilities together on the basis of level of functioning; 3) providing additional staff to these housing units; 4) training staff on interacting with inmates with developmental disabilities; 5) providing instructors with special education credentials for each developmental disability program responsible for developing individually tailored programs as necessary; and 6) providing parole agents to ensure that inmates with developmental disabilities understand the terms of parole and are aware of services available in the community.

Programs for offenders with mental retardation generally focus on improving the functioning and adaptation of the inmate while incarcerated and upon release (Santamour 1987). The vulnerabilities outlined in the previous sections lead to logical interventions that include skills training, educational/vocational rehabilitation, and counseling/treatment specific to the needs of each offender.

Skills Training

Day (1988) designed a program in the United Kingdom for offenders with intellectual deficits. An individual treatment program was developed for each offender on the basis of a token economy system. The system consisted of a weekly grading scheme, which included both monetary and social incentives. A "practical skills training package" included skills such as maintaining a clean living area, laundering clothing, budgeting, and using community facilities. Leisure activities also were encouraged. Fifty-five percent of the participants evidenced a "good" response to treatment, with 30% rated as fair. A reported 15% of enrollees did not benefit. Follow-up after approximately 3 years indicated that 70% of the participants who completed the program were evaluated as doing well in the community, especially those offenders who had committed crimes against persons (as compared with property).

Corrigan (1991) conducted a meta-analysis of social skills training programs and found that individuals with developmental disabilities evidenced the greatest improvement. However, generalization of skills learned was lowest for this group. Social skills training was least effective for the offender group. Interestingly, although the offenders acquired the requisite skills, these skills did not translate into behavior change. This study suggests that social skills training may improve institutional behavior, at least with those individuals with developmental disabilities, but may not generalize to other settings.

Cole and colleagues (1985) evaluated the efficacy of a self-management training program with adults with mental retardation and conduct problems in a vocational setting. The participants—six adults who exhibited significant behavior problems unresponsive to alternative treatments—were taught a variety of skills, including self-monitoring, self-evaluation, self-consequation, and self-instruction. An immediate decrease in disruptive behavior occurred and was maintained in a 9-month follow-up.

Skills training for the offender with mental retardation can encompass a wide variety of areas. The assessment process will guide the areas most necessary for each individual but may include social skills training or training in areas of adaptive functioning. Although much of the literature on skills training with individuals with mental retardation is not specifically directed to the offender population, correctional programs can use this literature to guide the development of appropriate services for the offender group.

Vocational Training

Vocational training is an important aspect of a comprehensive program to treat inmates with developmental disabilities for several reasons. Vocational training teaches inmates skills and information necessary to perform a job upon release and allows the inmate to work in a sheltered environment before reentry into the community (Santamour and West 1982b). Vocational training also provides inmates with developmental disabilities the opportunity to engage in meaningful, productive work that decreases behavioral issues and increases feelings of self-worth (Shively 2004).

Harley (1996) has advocated for a "multistage vocational rehabilitation plan" that deals with vocational training both before and after release from prison. Although this plan was not developed specifically for inmates with developmental disabilities, individual needs are evaluated and conforms to the "Individualized Habilitation Plan." Harley recommended an initial vocational assessment during incarceration to identify strengths and needs, including a comprehensive evaluation, which would result in a diagnosis, a functional assessment and prognosis for outcome. The second stage is to develop a specific habilitation plan that includes both pre- and postincarceration components. She recommended that transition goals and objectives be included in the plan, as well as "exit criteria" (the level of skill required for successful completion of the program).

Anger Management Program

Anger management is an important component in a treatment program for prisoners with mental retardation (Hall 1992). As previously noted, self-control and aggression can be a problem for some inmates (Shively 2004). Lack of self-control in a prison environment can lead to negative consequences, such as increased disciplinary reports (Smith et al. 1990). The lack of communication and interpersonal skills can lead to frustration and an increased likelihood of acting out conflicts (Smith et al. 1990). However, administrators must necessarily be cautious regarding the methods of management. For example, in a study comparing the use of medication in controlling aggressive behavior, the authors found that there was increased aggressive behavior in the patients who received thioridazine compared with the patients who received placebo (Elie et al. 1980).

Benson (1994) modified an anger management program for use with adults with mental retardation. Although this program was not developed specifically for offenders, it may be useful in an overall habilitation program that includes individualized treatment. As Benson points out, self-control training may generalize more easily from one situation to another and can reduce incidents of aggression while incarcerated and enable the inmate to control his or her anger in the community. The four components of the program include 1) identification of feelings, 2) relaxation training, 3) self-instruction training, and 4) the development of problem-solving skills. Although additional research is necessary to establish its effectiveness, initial results indicate that this program can have a therapeutic effect and may increase personal control.

Denkowski and Denkowski (1985) evaluated the effectiveness of a community-based treatment program for adolescent offenders with mental retardation. The program was based on a token-economy system, although enhanced for one group by the offering of "social points." Additionally, this group was required to spend a fixed amount of time in a "timeout room" for any instance of aggression. The enhanced treatment group evidenced the greatest success in reduction of physical and verbal aggression. While this program was community based and was used with adolescents, a population likely more responsive to the use of timeouts, this study suggests that the appropriate use of social learning techniques can be effective in modifying problematic behavior in an offender population.

The foregoing discussion presents various programs designed to modify aggressive behavior in individuals with mental retardation. Most research has indicated that behavior disorders are the most common co-occurring disturbance with offenders with mental retardation (Gardner et al. 1998). However, an offender with mental retardation can be diagnosed with a major psychiatric disorder (e.g., schizophrenia, bipolar disorder). Treatment approaches for such offenders would necessarily address the psychiatric disturbance as well as the habilitative needs associated with the developmental disability. Chapter 6 ("Mental Health Interventions in Correctional Settings") provides an excellent overview of treatment approaches for offenders with mental illness.

THREE MODEL PROGRAMS FOR OFFENDERS WITH DEVELOPMENTAL DISABILITIES

The South Carolina Habilitation Unit

The South Carolina Habilitation Unit (President's Committee on Mental Retardation 1992) was established in 1975 to provide residential services to male inmates with developmental disabilities and day treatment services to female inmates with developmental disabilities. The stated goal was to improve institutional adjustment and postrelease functioning. The unit houses a maximum of 40 men and can provide services to 10 women. In general, eligibility includes individuals with intellectual or physical impairments that limit their ability to function in the general population and an expectation that they will benefit from the services. The South Carolina Department of Corrections (DOC) adheres to the PL 106-402 definition of developmental disability (Developmental Disabilities Assistance and Bill of Rights Act of 2000). In addition, the DOC requires that the inmate agree to participate and demonstrate a potential for improvement. Prisoners in maximum security are not eligible. Referrals are generally made by "regional classification coordinators" or psychologists at the Reception and Evaluation Centers. Inmates referred from the Reception and Evaluation Centers suspected of having a developmental disability are administered the Beta-II (a nonverbal, culturally fair test of intelligence), the WAIS, and the WRAT. They also are interviewed extensively. Inmates referred from other facilities are administered the Beta-II, the WRAT, and a DOC instrument designed to assess functional abilities. Entry requirements include a score of 60 or below on the Beta-II and a third-grade reading level or lower.

Each inmate has an Individual Habilitation Plan (IHP) developed by a multidisciplinary team that consists of special education, work activity, a social work program (for life skills and counseling), and recreation. Inmates are involved in scheduled activities for a minimum of 38 hours per week.

Special Education

Ongoing educational assessment, curriculum and lesson plan development, and classroom instruction (both group and individual) are included in this program. This program is approved by the State Department of Education and receives funding for qualified inmates (21 or younger) under the IDEA.

Work Activity

The South Carolina Habilitation Unit program focuses on job acquisition and retention skills in a simulated work environment. The objectives are to develop positive work behavior, attitudes, and skills to maintain a job. A vocational assessment and on-the-job experience in various prison industries are provided to simulate a real-life work setting.

Social Work Program

The social work program is responsible for the initial needs assessment and orientation as well as the development of the IHP. Each inmate is assigned a primary case manager who organizes all habilitative services. Such services might include individual counseling, group treatment, and community release planning. The life skills component focuses on behaviors that will allow the inmate to function independently postrelease.

Recreation

The recreation program is designed to promote leisure skills and to develop effective interpersonal skills. Activities include team sports and arts and crafts.

Release Planning

Most inmates are released to the community rather than transferred to another facility. Release plans include organizing residential plans, vocational/occupational issues (job placement or training), follow-up treatment, and educational services. An attempt is made to involve family members, if appropriate. Social workers can be present at parole hearings to assist the inmate.

Texas Department of Criminal Justice
Mentally Retarded Offender Program

The Texas Department of Criminal Justice (TDCJ) Mentally Retarded Offender Program (MROP) (President's Committee on Mental Retardation 1992) arose from the *Ruiz v. Estelle* (1980) decision and was formulated to integrate the offender into the community. Inmates are identified on the basis of IQ testing performed by the diagnostic unit in Huntsville. Two facilities are used to house the program—one for each gender.

All inmates are screened with the Revised Beta-II. Those scoring 70 or less are administered the Culture Fair IQ Test. A similar score leads to administration of the WAIS. The Vineland Adaptive Behavior Scale is also administered. Other additional evaluations, including a psychiatric evaluation, are performed as indicated.

The treatment team on the MROP units include a psychologist, a case manager, and rehabilitation aides. They develop an individual habilitation plan, which can include educational and vocational training and specialized services such as individual and group counseling. The program for women also includes life skills classes such as parenting, health and nutrition, and money management. A very structured disciplinary procedure is used for infractions. Each infraction leads to a "ticket," which is sent to the Disciplinary Court. Punishments can include loss of good time, cell restriction, or extra work duties.

North Carolina Division of Prisons
Mental Health Services

In the North Carolina Division of Prisons (2004), offenders are admitted to one of the ten diagnostic centers, based on where they were arrested and whether the committing offense was a felony or a misdemeanor.

Offenders committing misdemeanors are screened with the WRAT reading subtest. If the inmate scores below a third-grade level, the Beta-II is administered. A score below 69 leads to a second administration of the Beta-II. A referral to a psychologist is made if the score remains below 69. The psychologist may then decide to administer additional tests before referring to the Mental Health Tracking System. The procedure for felons is the same with the exception that low Beta-II scores lead to the administration of an individual IQ assessment (WAIS). A score below 70 leads to a referral to the Mental Health Tracking System. North Carolina differs from other programs in that the inmates remain in the general population unless protective housing is necessary.

After transfer to the assigned unit, an inmate with a developmental disability is assigned a DD case manager. This case manager is responsible for assessing adaptive functioning and developing a treatment plan and also represents the inmate at disciplinary hearings. A minimum of one monthly meeting is required. Compensatory Education and Vocational Rehabilitation services are available for some inmates, though the Division of Prisons asserts that more programs are needed. Aftercare planning is based on need and is designed to assist the inmate in transitioning back into the community. Whenever possible, this planning involves the coordination of services with local DD staff.

CONCLUSION

The habilitation of individuals with developmental disabilities in the correctional system can no longer be ignored. Although Hall (1992) noted that correctional facilities should not be viewed as treatment facilities, such institutions can no longer be deliberately indifferent to the needs of these offenders. Inmates with developmental delays may be more easily led, suggestible, and dependent. Lower levels of comprehension and poor adaptive skills can lead to more rule infractions and disciplinary action, leading to a decreased likelihood for parole. Research has indicated that these offenders serve more time for the same crime than do offenders without developmental disabilities (Petersilia 2000a).

Opinions are mixed as to whether appropriate services for such individuals should be provided on specialized units. Proponents of this approach cite the vulnerabilities of these offenders. However, all agree that specialized services must include appropriate assessment that takes into account culture and individualized approaches to habilitation. It cannot be presumed that services designed for the individual with mental illness will be appropriate for inmates with developmental disabilities.

Little research has been conducted on the efficacy of specialized services for offenders with developmental disabilities. As such, correctional facilities must necessarily draw on research based on nonoffending samples. An active collaboration between departments of corrections and agencies providing services for individuals with developmental disabilities can enhance service delivery and improve the integration of the offender into the community. As courts continue to protect the rights of offenders with developmental disabilities, correctional facilities must explore creative ways to deliver appropriate services.

SUMMARY POINTS

- Inmates with developmental disabilities have increased vulnerability secondary to cognitive and adaptive skills deficits.
- Early identification and detection is crucial in addressing the needs of these offenders.
- Legislation requires that programs be developed to address these special needs in a correctional setting.
- Programs should include 1) skills development, 2) educational opportunities/vocational training, and 3) cognitive-behavioral interventions to address specific areas of concern.

REFERENCES

American Association on Mental Retardation: Definition of mental retardation. American Association on Mental Retardation, 2002. Available at: http://www.aamr.org/Policies/faq_mental_retardation.shtml. Accessed January 20, 2005.

American Psychiatric Association: Diagnostic and Statistical Manual of Mental Disorders, 4th Edition, Text Revision. Washington, DC, American Psychiatric Association, 2000

Americans with Disabilities Act of 1990, 42 U.S.C. §§ 12101–12213

Benson BA: Anger management training: a self-control programme for persons with mild mental retardation, in Mental Health in Mental Retardation: Recent Advances and Practices. Edited by Bouras N. New York, Cambridge University Press, 1994, pp 224–232

Bowring v Godwin, 551 F.2d 44 (4th Cir. 1976)

Cattell RB, Cattell AKS: Culture Fair Intelligence Test, Third Edition. Savoy, IL, IPAT, 1973

Centers for Disease Control and Prevention: State-specific rates of mental retardation–United States, 1993. MMWR Morb Mortal Wkly Rep 45:61–65, 1996. Available at: http://www.cdc.gov/epo/mmwr/preview/mmwrhtml/00040023.htm. Accessed December 25, 2004.

Clark v State of California, U.S. District Court of Northern California, No C96–1486 FMS, 1998

Cloud M, Shepherd GB, Barkoff A, et al: Words without meaning: the constitution, confessions, and mentally retarded suspects. University of Chicago Law Review 69:495–624, 2002

Cockram J, Jackson R, Underwood R: People with an intellectual disability and the criminal justice system: the family perspective. Journal of Intellectual and Developmental Disability 23:41–56, 1998

Cole CL, Gardner WI, Karan OC: Self-management training of mentally retarded adults presenting severe conduct difficulties. Appl Res Ment Retard 6:337–347, 1985

Conley RW, Luckasson R, Bouthilet GN: The Criminal Justice System and Mental Retardation. Baltimore, MD, Paul H Brookes, 1992

Corrigan PW: Social skills training in adult psychiatric populations: a meta-analysis. J Behav Ther Exp Psychiatry 22:203–210, 1991

Cullen C: The treatment of people with learning disabilities who offend, in Clinical Approaches to the Mentally Disordered Offender. Edited by Howells K, Hollin CR. Chichester, West Sussex, UK, Wiley, 1993, pp 145–162

Day K: A hospital based treatment programme for mentally handicapped offenders. Br J Psychiatry 153:635–644, 1988

Day K: Mental retardation: clinical aspects and management, in Principles and Practice of Forensic Psychiatry. Edited by Bluglass R, Bowden P. Edinburgh, UK, Churchill Livingstone, 1990, pp 399–418

Denkowski GC, Denkowski KM: Community based residential treatment of the mentally retarded adolescent offender, Phase 1: reduction of aggressive behavior. J Community Psychol 13:299–305, 1985

Developmental Disabilities Assistance and Bill of Rights Act of 2000, 42 U.S.C. §§ 15001–15115

Dunn LM, Dunn LM: Peabody Picture Vocabulary Test–Third Edition (PPVT-3). Circle Pines, MN, AGS Publishing, 1997

Education of All Handicapped Children Act of 1975, 20 U.S.C. §1400 et seq

Elie R, Langlois Y, Cooper SF, et al: Comparison of SCH-12679 and thioridazine in aggressive mental retardates. Can J Psychiatry 25:484–491, 1980

Ellis JW, Luckasson RA: Mentally retarded criminal defendants. The George Washington Law Review 53:414–493, 1985

Estelle v Gamble, 426 U.S. 97 (1976)

Everington C, Fulero SM: Competence to confess: measuring understanding and suggestibility of defendants with mental retardation. Ment Retard 37:212–220, 1999

Fulero SM, Everington C: Assessing competency to waive Miranda rights in defendants with mental retardation. Law Hum Behav 19:533–543, 1995

Gardner WI, Graeber JL, Machkovitz SJ: Treatment of offenders with mental retardation, in Treatment of Offenders With Mental Disorder. Edited by Wettstein RM. New York, Guilford, 1998, pp 329–364

Giamp JS, West ME: Delivering psychological services to incarcerated men with developmental disabilities, in Correctional Psychology: Practice, Programming, and Administration. Edited by Schwartz BK, Kingston, NJ, Civic Research Institute, 2003, pp 8.1–8.29

Hall JN: Correctional services for inmates with mental retardation, in The Criminal Justice System and Mental Retardation Defendants and Victims. Edited by Conley RW, Luckasson R, Bouthilet GN. Baltimore, MD, Paul H Brookes, 1992, pp 167–190

Harley DA: Vocational rehabilitation services for an offender population. J Rehabil 62:45–48, 1996

Individuals with Disabilities Education Act of 1990, 20 U.S.C. § 1400 et seq

Kendrick v Bland, 541 F.Supp. 21 (1981)

Lanterman Developmental Disabilities Services Act, Welfare and Institutions Code Section 4500–4519, State of California, Department of Developmental Services, January 2004. Available at: http://www.dds.cahwnet.gov/statutes/PDF/LantermanAct_2004.pdf. Accessed January 21, 2005.

MacEachron AE: Mentally retarded offenders: prevalence and characteristics. Am J Ment Defic 84:165–176, 1979

Mason J, Murphy G: Intellectual disability amongst people on probation: prevalence and outcome. J Intellect Disabil Res 46:230–238, 2002

Matikka LM, Vesala HT: Acquiescence in quality-of-life interviews with adults who have mental retardation. Ment Retard 35:75–82, 1997

McAfee JK, Gural M: Individuals with mental retardation and the criminal justice system: the view from states' attorneys general. Ment Retard 26:5–12, 1988

McGee JJ, Menolascino FJ: The evaluation of defendants with mental retardation in the criminal justice system, in The Criminal Justice System and Mental Retardation Defendants and Victims. Edited by Conley RW, Luckasson R, Bouthilet GN. Baltimore, MD, Paul H Brookes, 1992, pp 55–77

Müller-Isberner R, Hodgins S: Evidence-based treatment for mentally disordered offenders, in Violence, Crime and Mentally Disordered Offenders. Edited by Hodgins S, Müller-Isberner R. Chichester, West Sussex, UK, Wiley, 2000, pp 7–38

New York State Commission on Quality of Care for the Mentally Disabled: Inmates with developmental disabilities in NYS correctional facilities, March 1991. Available at: http://www.cqc.state.ny.us/publications/pubinmat.htm. Accessed January 20, 2005.

Nihira K, Leland H, Lambert N: Adaptive Behavior Scale–Residential and Community (ABS-RC:2). Austin, TX, Pro-Ed, 1993

Noble JH, Conley RW: Toward an epidemiology of relevant attributes, in The Criminal Justice System and Mental Retardation Defendants and Victims. Edited by Conley RW, Luckasson R, Bouthilet GN. Baltimore, MD, Paul H Brookes, 1992, pp 17–53

North Carolina Division of Prisons Mental Health Services website http://www.
doc.state.nc.us/DOP/health/mhs/special/spec0005.htm. Accessed December 15,
2004.

Pelka F: Unequal justice: preserving the rights of the mentally retarded in the criminal
justice system. Humanist 57:28–32, 1997

Pennsylvania Department of Corrections v Yeskey, 524 U.S. 206 (1998)

Petersilia J: Justice for all? Offenders with mental retardation and the California corrections system. The Prison Journal 77:358–381, 1997

Petersilia J: Doing justice? Criminal offenders with developmental disabilities. California Policy Research Center Brief, Vol 12, No 4, University of California, August
2000a. Available at: http://www.ucop.edu/cprc/PetersiliaMR-DD.pdf. Accessed
January 20, 2005.

Petersilia J: Invisible victims: violence against persons with developmental disabilities.
Human Rights 27:9–13, 2000b

Petrella RC: Defendants with mental retardation in the forensic services system, in
The Criminal Justice System and Mental Retardation Defendants and Victims.
Edited by Conley RW, Luckasson R, Bouthilet GN. Baltimore, MD, Paul H
Brookes, 1992, pp 79–96

President's Committee on Mental Retardation: Correctional industries: background,
planning and development guide for inmates with mental retardation. Hyatts-
ville, MD, Sociometrics, March 27, 1992. Available at: http://www.nicic.org/pubs/
1992/011245.pdf. Accessed December 15, 2004.

Revised Beta Examination–Second Edition (Revised Beta-II). San Antonio, TX, Psychological Corporation, 1974

Ruiz v Estelle, 503 F.Supp. 1265 (S.D. Tex 1980), cert denied, 460 U.S. 1042, 1983

Santamour MB: The offender with mental retardation. The Prison Journal 66:3–18,
1987

Santamour MB, West B: The mentally retarded offender: presentation of the facts and
a discussion of issues, in The Retarded Offender. Edited by Santamour MB, Watson PS. New York, Praeger, 1982a, pp 7–36

Santamour MB, West B: Retarded offenders: habilitative program development, in
The Retarded Offender. Edited by Santamour MB, Watson PS. New York, Praeger, 1982b, pp 272–296

Shively R: Treating offenders with mental retardation and developmental disabilities.
Corrections Today 66:84–87, 2004

Smith C, Algozzine B, Schmid R, et al: Prison adjustment of youthful inmates with
mental retardation. Ment Retard 28:177–181, 1990

Sparrow S, Balla DA, Cicchetti DV: Vineland Adaptive Behavior Scales: Survey Form
Manual. Circle Pines, MN, American Guidance Service, 1984

Stavis PF: Doing justice? The criminal justice system and persons with mental retardation. New York State Commission on Quality of Care for the Mentally Disabled,
Quality of Care Newsletter, Issue 47, January-February 1991. Available at: http://
www.cqc.state.ny.us/counsels_corner/cc47.htm. Accessed January 21, 2005.

Talent A, Keldgord R: The mentally retarded probationer. Federal Probationer 2:39–
46, 1975

Tasse MJ, Schalock R, Thompson JR, et al: Guidelines for Interviewing People With
Disabilities: Support Intensity Scale. Washington, DC, American Association on
Mental Retardation, 2005

Test of Adult Basic Education (TABE). Monterey, CA, CTB/McGraw-Hill, 2005

The Arc of the United States: Introduction to mental retardation. September 1998. Available at: http://www.thearc.org/faqs/mrqa.doc. Accessed January 21, 2005.

Wechsler D: WAIS-III Administration and Scoring Manual. San Antonio, TX, Psychological Corporation, 1997

Wilkinson GS: Wide Range Achievement Test–3 Administration Manual. Wilmington, DE, Wide Range, 1993

CHAPTER 10

Offenders With Mental Illnesses in Maximum- and Supermaximum- Security Settings

Gary E. Beven, M.D.

The provision of mental health care in administrative segregation unit settings, including those found in maximum- and supermaximum-security prisons, presents a difficult challenge. Often the most violent and seriously behaviorally disordered offenders are housed in these facilities, and they are commonly kept for extended periods of time in solitary confinement and isolation. Arguably, these institutional settings are the most stressful areas both for inmates and for corrections staff. Significant barriers to providing adequate care can stand in the way of the mental health clinician's mission, and the provision of clinically necessary treatment is often considered to be at odds with institutional security requirements (Eshem et al. 2001).

Prolonged isolation of inmates in segregation poses an inherent risk of psychological deterioration that cannot be ignored but that becomes difficult to address effectively when it occurs. As a result, many maximum- and super-maximum-security prisons and other administrative segregation facilities have inadvertently become warehouses for aggressive inmates with serious mental illness or disorders who have received inadequate care, or none at all (Human Rights Watch 2003). This, in turn, has repeatedly invited legal scrutiny and extensive litigation. Such litigation involves the basic constitutional right to adequate mental health care for those with serious mental illness and the related legal right to avoid penal conditions so harsh that they "cause" mental illness or exacerbate an existing condition (Cohen 1988, 1998).

In this chapter, I present an overview of segregation confinement, discuss the inherent difficulties inmates housed in these settings face, and address the deleterious psychological effects of prolonged isolation, especially for the offender with mental illness. Examples of common barriers to rendering adequate mental health treatment in administrative segregation are discussed. I provide guidelines for the effective screening, monitoring, and treatment of segregated inmates so that both community standards of care and constitutional requirements are met.

SEGREGATION CONFINEMENT

Prison administrative staff use segregation—a setting in which an inmate is kept for as many as 23 hours per day in his or her cell—as a management tool for the control of prisoners deemed disruptive, dangerous, or predatory or who otherwise violate institutional rules of conduct. Long-term segregation, often called *administrative segregation,* presents a heightened risk of injury to inmates with mental illness and is the principal environmental focus of this chapter. Administrative segregation usually lasts at least 3 months and may continue indefinitely, even for many years. Offenders placed into administrative segregation have been judged as representing serious management problems who jeopardize the safe and orderly management of an institution or prison system. Inmates considered to be the most problematic and incorrigible offenders include sexual predators, gang leaders, enforcers, extortionists, drug dealers, escapees, insurrectionists, and aggressive prisoners with mental illness.

Isolation of an inmate in administrative segregation is meant to separate unruly offenders from the prison general population, insulate segregated inmates from one another, act as a deterrent to potential wrong-doers, and motivate the insubordinate inmate to conform his or her actions to institutional standards of acceptable behavior. In theory, the judicious use of segregation confinement provides a safer and more orderly correctional facility for staff and inmates. The consignment of inmates to segregation is a relatively common occurrence. In early 2001, 36 states reported a total of more than 49,000 inmates in segregation confinement (Camp and Camp 2002), and in 2000 more than 20,000 offenders were housed in supermaximum-security level facilities (Human Rights Watch 2000).

Inmates housed in administrative segregation may be kept in a discrete solitary confinement area of a prison with several security levels or in a maximum- or supermaximum-security institution designed specifically for such a purpose. Administrative segregation facilities are labeled by a variety of euphemisms, including "special housing unit," "secure housing unit," "intensive management unit," "administrative control unit," and "maximum or supermaximum security unit or prison." An inmate's administrative segregation time ends when prison administrators declare that it is over, and signs of unrepentence or continued recalcitrant behavior may prolong the sanction indefinitely. Because the decision to confine is labeled "administrative" and may not be based on a specific violation, the protections of normal due process are often lacking in placement and retention determinations.

Supermaximum-security facilities are considered to be the most isolative, incapacitating, and restrictive of penal settings (Holton 2003; Riveland 1999). Built specifically to house the most dangerous offenders, a supermaximum-security-level institution is an extreme form of administrative segregation. Unique characteristics of these facilities include prolonged lengths of stay, architectural design that relies on automation and diminished human contact as security safeguards, greatly diminished environmental stimulation, and austere privilege restrictions that require of inmates high levels of patience and submission. Partly because of these factors, some have alleged that supermaximum-security prisons are inhumane, nonrehabilitative, and psychologically injurious, especially for mentally ill offenders. Consequently these facilities have triggered controversy and considerable litigation, the most basic of which challenges the confinement of inmates with a history of mental illness in these facilities (Harrington 1997; Metzner 2002).

Life in Segregation Confinement

No matter its duration, life in a prison segregation unit is a hardship. The restrictions placed on inmates in such settings are many, and while incarceration itself is difficult, the contrast between life in general population and segregation is striking.

A jaunt through a typical correctional institution's general population often reveals a great deal of relatively normal activity, such as a baseball game in the recreation yard, inmates returning from work in the prison industry building, and religious celebration in the chapel. One may encounter a gymnasium with inmates playing basketball, a busy dining hall, and a visiting area filled with families, offenders and their children. Segregation units, in contrast, are notable for being generally devoid of any such productive activity, and living conditions are often unpleasant. The restrictions placed on offenders in these settings are burdensome, and virtually every aspect of an inmate's

TABLE 10–5. Common restrictions in segregation confinement

- In cell 23 hours per day
- Noncontact visitation
- Solitary recreation
- No work
- No religious programs
- No group programs
- No school versus self-study in cell
- Movement only while escorted and shackled
- Meals alone in cell
- Restricted shower schedule
- Clothing restriction
- No (or restricted) access to television, radio, and phone
- No library/law library access
- Restricted commissary list
- Restricted list of personal items in cell
- No art or music programs
- No privacy (sick-call, mental health staff and administrative staff visits at cellfront)
- Diminished or excessive environmental stimulation
- No social contact with other inmates except verbal communication through cell door

life is adversely affected. A walk through any segregation unit likely will reveal prisoners sleeping, reading, drawing, pacing, praying, staring out the cell door, or otherwise engaged in solitary activity. The unit may be nearly silent or deafening, as a chorus of pounding, racial epithets, insults, accusations, and profanity reveal that unceasing boredom and anger have taken their toll. Table 10–1 summarizes common segregation confinement restrictions.

Psychological Effects of Prolonged Isolation

Prolonged isolation of any kind may cause psychological deterioration. The deleterious consequences of long-term isolation have been identified in very disparate populations, including Russian cosmonauts (Kanas 2000; Kozerenko et al. 2000), Antarctic researchers (Palinkas et al. 2000), and incarcerated felons (Toch 2001). Cosmonauts participating in long-duration space missions have experienced fatigue, irritability, dysphoria, mood instability, withdrawal, territorial behavior, sleep disturbance, and cognitive performance decrements. Indeed, one of the principal human hurdles to a potential mission to Mars is the National Aeronautic and Space Administration's (NASA) ability to successfully select and then adequately monitor astronauts' ability to tolerate the extreme isolation and related psychological stress such a voyage would entail over the course of 24–36 months (Arehart-Treichel 2002).

Although some segregated offenders may remain entirely unscathed by the experience, long-term segregation confinement is potentially psychologically detrimental (Metzner 2003; National Commission on Correctional Health Care 2003; Toch 2001). Even for inmates with no previous history of a psychiatric disorder, prolonged solitary confinement may lead to a decrement in functioning and the insidious development of psychological deterioration (Grassian 1983; Grassian and Friedman 1986; Haney and Lynch 1997). Indicators of behavioral decline include 1) restlessness and agitation; 2) concentration and memory impairment; 3) irritability, anger, and frustration intolerance; 4) apathy, social withdrawal, and dysphoria; 5) mood and affective lability; 6) generalized anxiety and panic attacks; and 7) irrational suspicion and paranoia.

Over time, a mental health clinician making regular rounds on an administrative segregation unit may notice a previously "normal" inmate pacing restlessly; becoming unaware of the date or time spent in isolation; refusing family visitation and correspondence; declining meals; failing to regularly shower, clean the cell, or exercise; revealing sudden and irrational fits of anger or accusation; ignoring entreaties of therapeutic interaction; sleeping throughout the day and remaining awake during the night; mumbling or speaking to himself or herself; and refusing medical or psychiatric evaluation. It is this author's experience that in segregated inmates without preexisting mental illness, signs of psychological decline typically abate upon release and return to a general population living environment.

The degree of negative psychological impact caused by prolonged segregation is correlated with several factors, including the duration of segregation, the extent of isolation, the degree of environmental stimulation deprivation, and the inmate's premorbid psychological fitness (Grassian and Friedman 1986; Haney and Lynch 1997). Administrative segregation units also commonly produce gross sensory overstimulation (Metzner 2002). The correctional environment may turn clamorous, abusive, and chaotic, as social relationships between segregated inmates become stilted and acrimonious. In this setting, sleep deprivation and intense hostility are common.

Factors with more subtle influence on the psychological impact of segregation include the inmate's perception of the justness underlying the decision to implement his or her segregation, expectations regarding the inmate's ability to earn release, the length of the inmate's prison sentence, and the inmate's ability to use rationalization as a defense mechanism. This defense may allow the inmate to discover something uniquely positive about the segregation experience, such as freedom from fear of sexual assault in general population or the time to immerse himself or herself in religious study.

Inmates With Mental Illness in Segregation Confinement

Inmates with mental illness, as a group, are overrepresented in segregation facilities, and correctional mental health experts have asserted that the relative number of seriously mentally ill prisoners housed in segregation is a gauge of the overall quality of a prison system's mental health care (Metzner 2003). Offenders with a history of psychiatric illness are often placed into administrative segregation because of behavior that is related to their mental disorder (National Commission on Correctional Health Care 2001). Examples include a prisoner's being sent into segregation because of assaultiveness that is linked to paranoid delusions, or possessing a "weapon" such as a razor used in a suicide attempt. Other inmates with behavioral disorders who are prone to placement into segregation units include those who have genuine difficulty following rigid prison rules or whose symptoms lead to continual episodes of disruptiveness, outbursts of anger, intrusiveness, or hostility. Inmates in this category include those with mental retardation, borderline personality disorder, mania, organic mental disorders, or impulse-control disorders.

Prolonged segregation produces a more damaging effect on an inmate previously diagnosed as being mentally ill, and it is more common for this group of offenders to be harmed by the experience (Metzner 2002). The stress of long-term segregation may exacerbate preexisting symptoms of mental illness or cause symptoms previously in remission to emerge. This exacerbation or reemergence of symptoms is often compounded by the loss of previously effective multidisciplinary treatment in the general population and the subsequent inadequacy of mental health care in many administrative segregation facilities.

Inmates who deteriorate psychiatrically while in administrative segregation can become enmeshed in a cycle of futility in which behavioral dyscontrol is interpreted by custody staff as intentional disobedience or disruptiveness (Holton 2003). Such an interpretation results in further administrative intervention and prolonged segregation with even greater austerity. This scenario may produce a downward spiral of psychiatric decompensation, behavioral instability, and increasingly self-defeating, yet reflexively administered punitive sanctions that persist indefinitely.

Common Barriers to Mental Health Care in Segregation Confinement

Security and safety are the cardinal interests of segregation unit custody staff; these issues supersede all others. Consequently, mental health clinicians assigned to work within a segregation facility often have a discouraging task. Segregation unit custody staff frequently assign mental health issues low priority. Within this setting, even highly dedicated and capable mental health clinicians can experience a disquieting sense that their efforts to intercede on behalf of segregated inmates are discounted, or worse, meaningless. An awareness of common obstructions to providing adequate care is necessary to overcome them and also avoid feelings of apathy.

Barriers to the provision of mental health care in administrative segregation generally fall into two categories (Metzner 2003). The first of these comprises philosophical impediments arising from the conviction that segregated offenders manifesting behavioral problems be addressed with orthodox correctional methods, principally additional disciplinary and control measures. This approach, which is based on correctional tradition and training, is effective with inmates whose disruptiveness emanates from volitional actions unrelated to symptoms of mental illness. However, mentally ill inmates often respond poorly to greater restrictions. Subsequent therapeutic intervention by mental health clinicians, including advocacy to divert disruptive mentally ill offenders from administrative segregation into a treatment setting, may be met with derision by custody staff. An awkward scenario may then ensue, in which the correctional mental health clinician feels trapped between a professional duty to the inmate with mental disorder and an allegiance to fellow institutional staff who are responsible for ensuring the clinician's safety. A byproduct of this circumstance is a potential overreliance on the diagnosis of malingering, even in the face of significant behavioral disturbance and self-injury (Bonner 2001). The diagnosis of malingering may arise insidiously as "burned out" clinicians become desensitized by incessant exposure to abusive and indignant offenders. Such abuse can take the form of repeatedly observing disturbing scenes of psychological deterioration (e.g., fecal smearing), having their therapeutic efforts continually thwarted, and facing the concomitant indifference, or perhaps even callousness, of some segregation unit custody staff.

The second category of common hindrance to mental health treatment in segregation is resource limitations. Examples include mental health staff shortages; lack of office space for private interviews and counseling; absence of secure mental health group program facilities; segregation cells that afford inadequate observation, communication, and ventilation; unavailability of maximum security residential care facilities; and insufficient availability of acute

TABLE 10–6. Characteristics of segregation facilities with inadequate mental health care

- Long-term segregation confinement
- No (or discounted) mental health diversion efforts
- Overrepresentation of inmates with serious mental illness in administrative segregation
- Adversarial, or unduly chummy, relationship between mental health and custody staff
- Cursory mental health screening and monitoring
- Disciplining of inmates with mental illness for disruptive behavior regardless of etiology
- Poor lighting, poor ventilation, and inadequate observation of cells
- Interview of segregation inmates occurring without privacy or confidentiality
- Vacant mental health staff positions and large clinician caseloads
- Unavailability of psychotherapy and group programs
- Regular labeling of self-injurious and suicidal inmates as malingerers
- Psychiatric medication as the sole therapeutic modality for most inmates
- Unavailability of maximum-security residential care
- Severely limited or unattainable psychiatric hospitalization

psychiatric hospitalization. In the face of such physical resource inadequacies, only abbreviated and often substandard mental health care may be rendered—even if a clinician works in a segregation facility where collegiality and compassion are evident. If a mixture of indifference and resource limitations is present, a culture of neglect nearly invariably arises. Table 10–2 lists characteristics common to segregation facilities that provide substandard mental health care.

MENTAL HEALTH TREATMENT IN SEGREGATION

Screening and Diversion

Although formal policies may differ, intervention for mentally ill inmates potentially slated for administrative segregation should be initiated at the time of sanction consideration by an institutional rules infraction board or similar administrative body. Following a disruptive or aggressive action by a mentally ill offender, it is recommended that mental health clinicians assist custody staff in determining if symptoms of mental illness influenced the inmate's behavior and if the offender has adequate understanding of the disciplinary proceedings

(Metzner 2003; National Commission on Correctional Health Care 2001). Such an evaluation is crucial if the prisoner is known to be seriously and chronically mentally ill.

Inquiry by correctional mental health staff into an inmate's behavioral instability should include the offender's diagnosis, medication compliance, recently observed symptoms, and possible precipitating or mitigating factors. If the inmate's conduct is related to symptoms of mental illness, treatment rather than discipline is needed, and diversion into a secure correctional mental health unit may avert further psychiatric deterioration in an administrative segregation facility (Kupers 1999). Consider an agitated inmate with paranoid schizophrenia who attacks another inmate without provocation. Further inquiry may uncover poor antipsychotic medication compliance, the development of persecutory delusions, and recent discharge from a residential treatment unit into an outpatient setting. Despite the serious nature of the infraction, correctional mental health clinicians who advocate for diversion to a secure intermediate care facility equipped for the treatment of aggressive, seriously mentally ill inmates make a wise judgment beneficial to everyone—addressing both institutional security concerns and the prisoner's treatment needs.

Unfortunately, the majority of disciplinary circumstances are not as clear as this example. In most cases, disruptive or violent acts are in response to common emotions, including anger, hatred, lust, greed, and fear, that occur even in inmates with mental illness. In these cases, involvement of mental health services in adjudication and punitive sanction determination is less helpful. An offender with well-controlled bipolar disorder who sexually assaults another inmate provides an example. If subsequent investigation indicates the brutality was unrelated to active symptoms of his or her mental illness, placement into administrative segregation is likely unavoidable. Nevertheless, the necessary monitoring and ongoing treatment requirements of the segregated offender should become the primary focus of correctional mental health staff.

Supermaximum-Security Transfers

Transgressions of a very serious nature, such as rape or attempted escape, may trigger a recommendation that the offender be transferred to a supermaximum-security facility. At present, it is considered a best practice that inmates with serious mental illness, or those with a psychological disposition prone to behavioral decay under severe stress, be precluded from transfer to such facilities unless adequate mental health resources are available (Metzner 2002). Inmates vulnerable to deterioration in supermaximum-security facilities include those with any serious mental illness; mental retardation; cognitive disorders such as dementia; a history of self-injury or mutilation; or severe personality disorders (e.g., borderline personality disorder) and a related record of functional impairment due to depression, suicidality, or brief psychosis (Metzner 2003). Prudent record review, a clinical interview, and documentation of any exclusionary factors should occur prior to approval of an inmate for transfer to a supermaximum-security institution and also upon reception at the secure facility. Prisoners who pass through conscientious screening methods yet later behaviorally deteriorate because of the stress of supermaximum-security confinement should be transferred to a segregation facility with fewer restrictions or greater access to mental health treatment.

Scope of Mental Health Services in Administrative Segregation

Mentally ill inmates housed in administrative segregation require a full breadth of multidisciplinary care to treat active symptoms, maintain psychiatric stability, and prevent deterioration (American Psychiatric Association 2000). Professional treatment guidelines for major mental illness such as schizophrenia, bipolar disorder, and major depressive disorder are not absolved by incarceration (American Psychiatric Association 2004). Irrespective of a prisoner's security needs or prior egregious behavior, the community standard of care for the treatment of mental illness should be followed. While this is admittedly a difficult task in any segregation setting, if mentally ill inmates are consigned to long-term segregation, comprehensive mental health care must be offered. This care should include evaluation, monitoring, psychotherapy, psychiatric medication, crisis care, intermediate level care (including group programs), and acute psychiatric hospitalization. Table 10–3 lists characteristics of segregation facilities that provide effective mental health care.

Monitoring of Inmates in Segregation

Correctional mental health staff should monitor all inmates in long-term segregation confinement, but particular attention should be given to mentally ill offenders (American Psychiatric Association 2000). Weekly visits to the cell-front of mentally ill inmates for informal inquiry, and observation for signs of decline, should occur (Metzner 1997). During these "house calls," cell cleanliness, attire, attitude, attention, energy level, interaction with peers, and a general sense of well being can be judged—preferably within the context of a consultative relationship with corrections officers assigned to the unit. The findings gleaned from these cell-front parlays can be communicated to other members of the treatment team, including the treating psychiatrist. If inmates not previously identified as being mentally ill reveal indications of distress, referral for more comprehensive evaluation can be made.

TABLE 10–7. Characteristics of segregation facilities that provide effective mental health care

- Acutely mentally ill inmates with active psychosis are rarely in administrative segregation.
- Inmates with mental illness are not transferred to supermax facilities.
- Segregated inmates are frequently monitored by mental health staff.
- Collaborative professional relationship exists between mental health and custody staff.
- Disruptive inmates with mental illness are addressed by mental health staff and not routinely disciplined.
- Mental health interviews and counseling occur in private settings.
- Individual psychotherapy and group programs are available therapeutic options.
- Crisis intervention occurs promptly and without the routine assumption of malingering.
- Multidisciplinary team provides care and actively engages the inmate to meet behavioral goals.
- Psychiatric care reflects a comprehensive knowledge of the segregated offender's unique needs.
- Psychiatric hospitalization is readily available for inmates when needed.
- Inmates with serious mental illness are diverted from segregation into a secure treatment setting.
- Inmates stabilized via hospitalization are not transferred directly back in segregation.
- Maximum-security residential treatment is available.

Although cell-front interviews are meaningful and necessary, such contact is insufficient for initial comprehensive evaluation or individual psychotherapy. All therapeutic contact beyond monitoring should occur in private where confidentiality can be maintained, and preferably in a segregation mental health office or interview area designated for such a purpose. Security concerns are undeniably important but can be appropriately addressed if the inmate is shackled and a corrections officer is nearby. Clinical Case 10–1 highlights some of these important points.

Clinical Case 10–1: Monitoring of the Segregated Inmate

Mr. Doe, a young man without any known history of mental illness, was placed into administrative segregation after he had stabbed another inmate. The assault was the result of a dispute between rival prison gangs. Mr. Doe had been chosen by his gang leader to commit the offense and bear the subsequent disciplinary consequences, which he did with apparent stoicism.

Mr. Doe was seen weekly at cell-front by the mental health clinician assigned the task of monitoring inmates in segregation. Initially rather brash, Mr. Doe consistently denied any problems and often sarcastically told the mental health clinician to "leave me alone…I'm no nut case." The conversation between the two usually consisted of informal, relatively friendly banter.

After 6 months of segregation, Mr. Doe's hygiene noticeably worsened, and he began to look deconditioned, having gained 15 pounds. Ordinarily well-groomed and quite lean, he now rarely showered and had stopped exercising. Mr. Doe's cell became dirty, and his demeanor changed as well, turning sullen and unfriendly. As the weeks passed, he began pacing restlessly in his cell and started to ignore the mental health clinician entirely. Segregation unit corrections officers reported that Mr. Doe was "no problem," although they too noticed him becoming increasingly withdrawn.

Growing concerned, the mental health clinician arranged for a private interview in a nearby office, with a corrections officer nearby. Initially hesitant to speak, the young inmate admitted to feeling depressed and anxious, as well as sleeping only 3–4 hours each night. He found it very difficult to concentrate and felt that "I might be going crazy." Referral for psychiatric evaluation was made.

Mental Health Treatment Team in the Segregation Unit

The combination of cell-front visitation, psychotherapy, and consultation with security staff should occur in collaboration with a psychiatrist and other correctional mental health providers working as a team, especially in the case of segregated inmates with serious mental illness (Metzner 1997). Other treatment team members may include social workers, psychology staff, activity therapists, and representatives from custody and administration. This multidisciplinary model of care requires treatment team meetings between the segregated inmate, correctional mental health clinicians, and other correctional staff involved in their care at 30- to 90-day intervals. During these encounters, active participation by the offender should be solicited and management of the inmate's mental illness addressed. Behavioral improvement may be augmented if the prisoner is advised the treatment team will recommend eventual administrative segregation release if the inmate's disordered behavior ceases.

In high-profile cases involving behavioral instability and extreme violence, it is often beneficial for senior administrative staff, such as a deputy warden, to attend a treatment team meeting to affirm behavioral expectations leading to segregation release and also to be made aware of the mental health department's role. Such involvement should preferably occur in a venue that preserves confidentiality by principally focusing on important custodial concerns without discussion of personal information or psychiatric treatment. Involvement of administrative and custody staff is an important issue, because if mental health clinicians assigned to work in administrative segregation take an overly rigid approach to their duties, focusing exclusively on textbook symptoms of mental illness while disregarding the correctional context, treatment failure is common. A balanced effort, achieved through multidisciplinary teamwork, provides for the greatest chance of treatment success and often mends philosophical rifts between mental health and custody personnel.

Psychiatric Care in Segregation

In effective systems, a psychiatrist should play an active role in segregation facilities. Isolation may exacerbate or produce distress that requires a treatment response using psychotropic medication (Burns 2003). To be successful, the correctional psychiatrist must have a comprehensive awareness of both the patient care risks and the custodial intricacies of the environment in which care is provided. In response, prescribing practices and treatment recommendations should be adjusted accordingly. This guideline also applies to psychiatrists who use telemedicine equipment to furnish care in distant prisons and therefore do not have the opportunity to witness the correctional environment directly.

Characteristics of segregation facilities may include the inability of the medication-administering nurse to see clearly into an inmate's cell or properly determine if an inmate is "cheeking" (i.e., not ingesting) medication. Inmates in such circumstances may hoard medication and then either overdose on it or sell it to other inmates for commissary items and then acutely decompensate. Some mentally ill offenders with poor insight may refuse all medication, rendering treatment efforts useless. During summer months, segregation cells may be stifling, leading to an increased risk of hyperthermia.

A psychiatrist's treatment response to the idiosyncrasies of segregation will be distinct for each prison but may entail prescribing medication in liquid form, using drugs with a lower potential for lethality in overdose, educating nursing and corrections staff on the risk of hyperthermia, relying on medication serum levels to assist with determination of compliance, and resolutely focusing on patient education and medication compliance issues. Correctional psychiatrists who treat segregated inmates should also be vigilant for the gradual development of polypharmacy, especially when several psychiatrists provide care based on a coverage rotation, making continuity of care difficult to achieve. If several classes of psychiatric medications at increasing or maximal doses are being prescribed, one must consider the possibility of environmentally caused deterioration or treatment resistance and the need for transfer to a secure intermediate care unit. The illicit diversion of medication to other segregated inmates, or medication-seeking behavior in an offender with a history of drug addiction, should also be considered.

Psychiatrists who treat inmates in administrative segregation also require considerable patience. Strict security requirements slow the pace of work considerably, and segregated offenders often require longer interviews because of the adverse environmental circumstances and a greater need of therapeutic contact. In this setting, a psychiatrist who normally examines 15–20 inmates per day in a general population venue may see only half as many patients in administrative segregation. This should be seen not as a reflection of professional inadequacy but as a reflection of the genuine need for clinical deliberateness within the constraints of a maximum security context.

Security staff in segregation may subtly influence correctional psychiatrists to view inmates in a negative light, leading to compromised professionalism. As a result, the correctional psychiatrist may, for example, ignore signs of an inmate's emotional distress or fail to implement available modes of treatment, including hospitalization, when clinically indicated. Such a scenario may occur when the segregated offender is incarcerated for a heinous crime or if the prisoner has seriously injured a fellow staff member. Psychiatrists who choose to work in this setting should remain mindful of their role as physicians and be willing to make unpopular decisions in order to ensure patient safety and provide effective care despite their own negative personal feelings or the pointed opinion of others.

Crisis Intervention and Malingering

Effective crisis intervention services are sorely needed in administrative segregation, as inmates periodically engage in destructive or bizarre behavior related to mental illness or extreme loneliness and antipathy (Bonner 2001). Such behavior includes fecal smearing, head banging, self-inflicted lacerations, destruction of personal property, fire setting, or suicidal statements. While this behavior may at times be the product of an effort to feign mental illness, it is strongly recommended that correctional mental health clinicians consciously avoid making a reflexive diagnosis of manipulation or malingering. The stress of prolonged segregation can cause mentally ill offenders to engage in unusual acts of self-harm, such as swallowing foreign objects or consuming excrement. Inmates without a history of mental illness may become seriously depressed and consider suicide as a means to escape continued isolation. Additionally, a desperate inmate who strives to maintain some control over his or her austere environment may destroy what few personal belongings he has, making a bad situation even worse.

Offenders who engage in acts of self-injury or irrational aggression deserve prompt crisis intervention regardless of the underlying motives (National Commission on Correctional Health Care 2001). The clinical response may include suicide-watch procedures, seclusion, therapeutic restraint, emergency medication, and careful multidisciplinary evaluation. Seriously mentally ill inmates may ultimately require a more intensive level of care elsewhere. Inmates with personality disorders may benefit from more frequent and intensive therapeutic contact. Prisoners who clearly do not suffer from mental illness but who orchestrate labor-intensive mental health crises should be evaluated, counseled, and referred to proper staff for complaint resolution. Irrespective of the final conclusion, correctional mental health clinicians must act with deliberateness and caution. The risk of error can be very high, with suicide one potential result if signs of genuine distress are discounted, and explosive violence another possible outcome if release to a less secure facility occurs prematurely or without adequate forethought.

Psychiatric Hospitalization

Despite the mental health treatment team's best efforts, segregated inmates may precipitously deteriorate or harm themselves so severely that transfer to a secure psychiatric hospital facility becomes necessary. The venue of hospital-level care varies between correctional systems but commonly involves transfer to a designated prison hospital facility or, less commonly, a forensic unit of a state hospital. Psychiatric hospitalization, or any other clinically necessary medical intervention, must not be disallowed solely because of security concerns or an inmate's administrative segregation status (American Psychiatric Association 2000; National Commission on Correctional Health Care 1997). If a clinical indication of hospitalization, such as a near-lethal suicide attempt or the development of florid psychosis, arises, transfer should be expedited. It is incumbent on the hospital facility to ensure adequate security while also providing patient care.

The diversion of administrative segregation inmates into a secure residential treatment unit setting following psychiatric hospital discharge should also occur. Immediate return to segregation risks negating the clinical gains achieved during hospitalization. This is especially true if ongoing treatment requirements cannot be met or if the effects of isolation trigger exacerbation of the newly stabilized illness. This scenario often initiates an expensive and futile cycle of deterioration, hospitalization, stabilization, segregation, deterioration and rehospitalization (National Commission on Correctional Health Care 2001). Once again, intensive mental health treatment rendered in a secure setting does not pardon a mentally ill offender's malicious conduct, nor does it invite ongoing misbehavior. Indeed, such care very often leads to significant behavioral improvement and a diminishing risk of further misconduct (Haddad 1999; Lovell et al. 2001).

Maximum-Security Residential Treatment

Many factors that give rise to psychiatric instability in administrative segregation and prevent an adequate therapeutic response are negated if maximum-security residential care is made available (Eshem et al. 2001). The development of a secure intermediate-care facility, designed exclusively for the provision of mental health treatment to violent and disruptive mentally ill offenders, can pay great dividends, including a decrease in inmate aggression and subsequent disciplinary response (Condelli et al. 1993; Rayford and Trestman 2002).

Chronically mentally ill inmates who would otherwise be transferred to administrative segregation and disrupt customary unit activities can be diverted to a secure mental health unit following serious misconduct. In this manner, both institutional security needs and individual psychiatric treatment requirements may be addressed without perception that the transgression of prison rules has provoked no disciplinary response. Segregated offenders suspected of malingered psychosis may undergo psychiatric evaluation in a secure setting without risk of potentially ignoring genuine symptoms. Inmates in administrative segregation or supermaximum security facilities who develop active suicidal ideation, or otherwise behaviorally decline, can be properly evaluated and afforded care without sparing security measures. Segregated mentally ill inmates may be discharged from an acute-care facility to a secure residential program for ongoing treatment so that progress attained during hospitalization is not imperiled. Finally, prisoners thought to be entirely beyond hope, including those who engage in continual acts of irrational aggression, rebellion, and self-injury, may receive intensive evaluation and care in a setting that provides a chance of psychosocial rehabilitation and behavioral improvement when all previous correctional interventions have failed. It is with this group of offenders that a maximum-security intermediate-care unit often engenders the greatest results, and the behavioral reformation of an intractably disturbed and unmanageable inmate previously "buried" in administrative segregation may appear miraculous. These points are illustrated in Clinical Case 10–2 below.

Clinical Case 10–2: The Hopelessly Disruptive Inmate in Segregation

Following his assault of a corrections officer, Mr. Jones had been in administrative segregation for over 3 years. Having borderline intellectual intelligence, a seizure disorder, serious impulse control problems, and illiteracy, he was thought to be hopelessly disruptive. Over the course of his segregation, Mr. Jones developed a repertoire of increasingly maladaptive behaviors, including smearing and throwing feces, spitting on corrections officers, exposing himself to female staff, threatening others and himself, destroying prison property, flooding his cell, head banging, swallowing foreign objects, and self-mutilation. Increasingly restrictive privileges, isolation from other inmates, and frequent custody staff intervention failed to improve Jones's conduct. The intermittent use of restraint and suicide watch precautions, with subsequent release back into segregation, appeared to reinforce his self-injurious behavior.

Mr. Jones was admitted to a maximum-security residential treatment unit (RTU), and a multidisciplinary treatment plan was developed with input from mental health, unit management, and custody staff. Participation in a therapeutic group program for 15 hours per week was initiated. Psychiatric evaluation prompted use of a mood-stabilizing anticonvulsant for enhanced impulse control. A recreation program was begun under the supervision of an activity therapist who implemented a structured exercise regimen, and a reading tutor was assigned. Psychotherapy was initiated with the principal goals being improved impulse control and frustration tolerance. All therapeutic modalities occurred in a secure setting under the direct observation of corrections officers with specialized mental health training.

Over the course of 6 months, Mr. Jones's behavior substantially improved. A mental health professional, present at all security level review hearings, reported the progress to custody and administrative staff. Following a 6-month period entirely free of prison rule infractions or conduct reports, Mr. Jones was released to the prison general population after nearly 4 years of segregation confinement, a feat considered by many to be a "miracle."

The successful implementation of a maximum-security residential treatment unit depends on adequate human and physical resources (Haddad 1999; Metzner 1998). These include corrections officers as security escorts who have undergone additional mental health training; activity therapy staff for therapeutic group and recreational programs; psychiatric nurses; psychology staff; social workers; psychiatrists; and unit management staff sensitive to the needs of mentally ill offenders.

Supplementary mental health training for corrections officers assigned to work in a maximum-security residential treatment unit is of critical importance. Such officers should preferably be volunteers genuinely interested in correctional mental health issues and who have demonstrated both compassion and professionalism. Custody staff without additional training, randomly assigned to the mental health unit and not accustomed to working with mentally ill inmates, may inadvertently undermine the mental health treatment team's best therapeutic efforts.

The secure mental health unit should also provide adequate private office space for clerical work and treatment records; cells that afford adequate observation, communication, and ventilation; indoor and outdoor recreation facilities; and secure group program space, such as adjacent holding cells linked in a semicircle. Start-up expenses for a maximum-security residential treatment unit, although costly, may be balanced over time by decreases in the risk of litigation, psychiatric hospital care, and emergency medical care following self-inflicted injury. Morale also improves, as most corrections officers are freed to work with non–mentally ill offenders, and correctional mental health staff can focus on the mission of providing treatment in a setting that greatly enhances the prospect of therapeutic success.

CONCLUSION

Despite the many disadvantages associated with providing mental health services to segregated offenders, such efforts are indispensable and have the potential to be professionally gratifying. Prior to reaching the basement of the correctional system, mentally ill inmates in administrative segregation have repeatedly been declared failures and written off by family, the educational system, the public mental health system, the private health care sector, the juvenile justice system, and, finally, the adult criminal justice system.

Mental health providers who work in segregation units should take solace in the knowledge that their work is vitally important because they are often the last hope for inmates caught in a downward spiral of psychiatric illness and criminality. To attain any level of treatment success in this challenging setting can be very rewarding. All correctional mental health clinicians who dedicate time and effort to this underserved population should be rightfully proud of their accomplishments.

SUMMARY POINTS

- Administrative segregation is a form of prolonged solitary confinement with severe privilege restrictions.
- Supermaximum-security prisons are administrative segregation facilities designed to provide the highest level of security precautions and restricted isolation.
- Prolonged segregation confinement is potentially psychologically harmful and has significant potential for exacerbating mental illness.
- Offenders with mental illness are often placed in segregation because of behavior caused by mental illness.
- There are significant barriers to providing adequate mental health treatment to segregated offenders.
- Inmates whose unruly conduct is caused by mental illness should receive psychiatric treatment and should not be placed into segregation or be transferred to supermaximum-security facilities.
- All inmates in segregation should be monitored for signs of mental deterioration.
- Offenders with mental illness in segregation should be afforded multidisciplinary treatment via a team approach.
- Segregated inmates who engage in self-injurious behavior require comprehensive evaluation without the presumption of malingering.

- Offenders with serious mental illness in segregation should be afforded psychiatric hospitalization based on clinical need alone, irrespective of security concerns.
- Segregated offenders with mental illness who require psychiatric hospitalization should not be placed back in segregation unless adequate mental health treatment is available.
- Maximum-security residential treatment is a valuable resource in the care and management of inmates with mental illness presenting a security risk.

REFERENCES

American Psychiatric Association: Psychiatric Services in Jails and Prisons, 2nd Edition. Washington, DC, American Psychiatric Association, 2000

American Psychiatric Association: Practice Guidelines for the Treatment of Psychiatric Disorders Compendium 2004. Arlington, VA, American Psychiatric Association, 2004

Arehart-Treichel J: NASA addresses mental health of Mars-mission members. Psychiatric News 37 (February):5, 2002

Bonner R: Rethinking suicide prevention and manipulative behavior in corrections. Jail Suicide/Mental Health Update 10:7–8, 2001

Burns KA: Jail diversion and correctional psychotropic medication formularies, in Management and Administration of Correctional Health Care. Edited by Moore J. Kingston, NJ, Civic Research Institute, 2003, pp 13-1–13-13

Camp C, Camp G: Corrections Yearbook 2001: Adult Systems. Middletown, CT, Criminal Justice Institute, 2002

Cohen F: Legal Issues and the Mentally Disordered Prisoner. Washington, DC, National Institute of Corrections, 1988

Cohen F: The Mentally Disordered Inmate and the Law. Kingston, NJ, Civic Research Institute, 1998

Condelli WS, Dvoskin JA, Holanchock H: Intermediate care programs for inmates with psychiatric disorders. Bull Am Acad Psychiatry Law 21:427–433, 1993

Eshem S, Hasan A, Beven G: New treatment modality in a maximum security prison: administrative control unit for the seriously mentally ill. Correctional Mental Health Report 2:90–92, 2001

Grassian S: Psychopathological effects of solitary confinement. Am J Psychiatry 140: 1450–1454, 1983

Grassian S, Friedman N: Effects of sensory deprivation in psychiatric seclusion and solitary confinement. Int J Law Psychiatry 8:49–65, 1986

Haddad J: Treatment for inmates with serious mental illness who require specialized placement but not psychiatric hospitalization. Correctional Mental Health Report 1:49–62, 1999

Haney C, Lynch M: Regulating prisons of the future: a psychological analysis of supermax and solitary confinement. New York Review of Law and Social Change 23:477–570, 1997

Harrington SPM: Caging the crazy: "supermax" confinement under attack. Humanist 57:14–20, 1997

Holton SMB: Managing and treating mentally disordered offenders in jails and prisons, in Correctional Mental Health Handbook. Edited by Fagan TJ, Ax RK. Thousand Oaks, CA, Sage, 2003, pp 101–122

Human Rights Watch: Out of Sight: Supermaximum Security Confinement in the United States. New York, Human Rights Watch, 2000. Available at: http://www.hrw.org/reports/2000/supermax/. Accessed December 7, 2004.

Human Rights Watch: Ill Equipped: US Prisons and Offenders With Mental Illness. New York, Human Rights Watch, 2003. Available at: http://www.hrw.org/ reports/2003/usa1003/. Accessed December 7, 2004.

Kanas N: Asthenia: does it exist? (abstract). Aviat Space Environ Med 71:271, 2000

Kozerenko OP, Kozlovskaya IB, Grigoriev AI: Psychological support in long-term space flights (abstract). Avia Space Environ Med 71:349, 2000

Kupers T: Prison Madness: The Mental Health Crisis Behind Bars and What We Must Do About It. San Francisco, CA, Jossey-Bass, 1999

Lovell D, Allen D, Johnson C, et. al: Evaluating the effectiveness of residential treatment for prisoners with mental illness. Criminal Justice and Behavior 28:83–104, 2001

Metzner JL: An introduction to correctional psychiatry, Part II. J Am Acad Psychiatry Law 25:571–579, 1997

Metzner JL: An introduction to correctional psychiatry, Part III. J Am Acad Psychiatry Law 26:107–114, 1998

Metzner JL: Class action litigation in correctional psychiatry. J Am Acad Psychiatry Law 30:19–29, 2002

Metzner JL: Trends in correctional mental health care, in Management and Administration of Correctional Health Care. Edited by Moore J. Kingston, NJ, Civic Research Institute, 2003, pp 12–2 to 12–18

National Commission on Correctional Health Care: Standards for Health Services in Prisons. Chicago, IL, National Commission on Correctional Health Care, 1997

National Commission on Correctional Health Care: Correctional Health Care: Guidelines for the Management of an Adequate Delivery System. Chicago, IL, National Commission on Correctional Health Care, 2001

National Commission on Correctional Health Care: Correctional Mental Health Care: Standards and Guidelines for Delivering Services. Chicago, IL, National Commission on Correctional Health Care, 2003

Palinkas LA, Gunderson EKE, Holland AW, et al: Predictors of behavior and performance in extreme environments: the Antarctic space analogue program. Aviat Space Environ Med 71:619–625, 2000

Rayford BS, Trestman RL: The intensive mental health unit in Connecticut's Department of Correction: a model treatment program. Psychiatric Times Supplement 19:2–3, 2002

Riveland C: Supermax Prisons: Overview and General Considerations. Washington, DC, National Institute of Corrections, 1999

Toch H: The future of supermax confinement. The Prison Journal 81:376–388, 2001

CHAPTER 11

Management of Offenders With Mental Illnesses in Outpatient Settings

Erik Roskes, M.D.

The Honorable Charlotte Cooksey, Judge

Richard Feldman, LCSW-C

Sharon Lipford, LCSW-C

Jane Tambree, LCSW-C

The challenges that offenders with mental illness pose to the penal system are obvious (Human Rights Watch 2003). The penal system, designed to provide safety and security, is not well equipped to manage the needs of

The authors gratefully acknowledge the assistance of Jeffrey Metzner, M.D., Fred Osher, M.D., and Melissa Reuland, who reviewed drafts of this chapter and provided useful feedback and recommendations. The authors also acknowledge Sarah Chernish, Trisha Monroe, and Mary Geer for assistance in preparation of portions of the manuscript.

the severely mentally ill. Correctional employees often are not trained to identify or assist detainees or inmates who are experiencing psychiatric symptoms. Correctional staffs vary in their response but frequently lack the knowledge, experience, and patience to provide a therapeutic intervention. In addition, the physical plant and layout of most jails and prisons are not conducive to the provision of quality mental health care. As a result, mechanisms to encourage the release of individuals with mental illness from incarceration may practically promote more effective mental health care in the community.

Previous chapters in this book have focused on the delivery of mental health care within correctional settings. In this chapter, we focus on the management of offenders with mental illness in the community. By any accounting, there are far more offenders in community settings (parole, probation, or other forms of supervised release) than there are in jails or prisons. For example, on December 31, 2002, there were 2,166,260 inmates in federal or state prisons or in local jails (Harrison and Beck 2003). During this same time period, there were 4,748,306 individuals in the United States on probation (court-ordered terms of community supervision, with conditions, in lieu of a sentence of incarceration) or parole (proactive early release from incarceration with conditions and supervision) (Glaze 2003).

The incidence and prevalence of mental illness among offenders who reside in community settings are vastly understudied when compared with incarcerated individuals. According to the Bureau of Justice Statistics, in 1998 an estimated 16% of individuals on probation, or a total of 547,800 individuals, were mentally ill. In this study, mental illness was defined by the inmate's self-report of having a "mental or emotional condition" or as having stayed overnight in a mental hospital (Ditton 1999). A previous study (Fulton 1996) found that many states did not track parolees and probationers with mental health problems and as a result were unable to determine the prevalence rate of mental illness in this population. Of the 15 states that collected this type of epidemiological information, the prevalence rates for mental illness ranged from 1% to 11% (mean=5%) for parolees and from 3% to 23% (mean=6%) for probationers. Fulton recognized the difficulty of comparing information between jurisdictions that may use differing definitions of "mental illness." She recommended the use of the following definition for mental illness, promulgated by the National Coalition for Mental Health and Substance Abuse Care in the Justice System: "adults having a disabling mental illness, which includes schizophrenia and/or an affective disorder."

In addition to mental illness, most offenders have a comorbid substance use disorder. According to the Epidemiologic Catchment Area study (Regier et al. 1990), 90% of incarcerated inmates with mental illness also met the criteria for a substance use disorder at some point during their lifetime. Therefore, substance use treatment is a critical intervention for the vast majority of offenders when they are released into the community.

There are a variety of barriers to the community-based coordinated management of offenders with mental illnesses. One of the most important barriers is the mutual distrust that exists between mental health providers and community corrections officials (Roskes et al. 1999). Mental health professionals often view criminal justice and community corrections personnel as harsh and punitive, while criminal justice officials tend to view mental health counselors as "soft" or "bleeding hearts." At times, confidentiality issues are raised by the health care and criminal justice agencies involved in the care and supervision of such individuals as reasons for noncooperation. In addition, mental health agencies have understandable concerns regarding the cost of mental health care for court-ordered clients. Finally, mental health providers may hesitate to serve individuals with legal problems because of liability concerns.

One suggested intervention for such difficulties is *cross-training*, whereby professionals from each side of the equation are trained together and train each other. These efforts serve to open communication and break down barriers. Another potential solution is the development of specialized or intensive caseloads, through which closer monitoring and more intensive services can be provided to offenders with mental illnesses. Small, specialized caseloads offer community corrections officers an improved opportunity to establish more effective relationships with providers of mental health care (Council of State Governments 2002). While there is controversy regarding an appropriate caseload size, the U.S. Probation Office notes that, given the intensity of the needs of probationers and parolees with mental illness, "a strong case can be made for a reduced caseload size," in the range of 25 to 35 cases for a mental health specialist officer (Migdalia Baerga, Administrative Office, U.S. Probation Office, personal communication, June 7, 2004).

There are many points in the criminal justice process at which individuals with mental illness may be moved from institutional into community settings, with or without imposed conditions. In this chapter, we focus on several specific mechanisms by which defendants may avoid the criminal justice system altogether or may be court-mandated to participate in community-based treatment programs such as the following:

- Prebooking diversion opportunities
- Postbooking, pretrial diversion opportunities
- Trial strategies (e.g., mental health courts)
- Sentencing strategies: probation
- Parole and supervised release

POINTS OF CONTACT BETWEEN
THE CRIMINAL JUSTICE SYSTEM AND
COMMUNITY MENTAL HEALTH PROVIDERS

Individuals with mental illness may be diverted from the criminal justice system at a variety of points. Broadly defined, these opportunities can be divided into pre- and postbooking diversion. All diversions occur because some participant in the criminal justice system (not a mental health provider) recognizes a mental health issue in a defendant or detainee. In functioning diversion programs, this recognition leads to a referral to a mental health professional for a definitive evaluation and potential diversion from the criminal justice system into the mental health treatment system. Thus, all diversion programs require some degree of partnering between agents of the criminal justice and mental health systems. The role of the criminal justice system in deciding whether to apply legal sanctions or to divert individuals away from the system is based primarily in a balancing of the principles of *police power* (the power and responsibility to protect the safety and welfare of the public) and *parens patriae* (the responsibility to protect persons who are disabled or otherwise unable to care for themselves). An ideal diversion program should include interventions for offenders with mental illnesses at all stages of the criminal justice process (Buchan 2003). The foundation for diverting individuals from the criminal justice system begins with a partnership and genuine collaboration between law enforcement, mental health, and judicial systems.

In response to the increasing cycle of recidivism, the mental health, judicial, and law enforcement systems are beginning to work together to find solutions to the growing crisis. Buchan (2003) described several counties in which a variety of agencies have begun collaborations to develop and respond more effectively to individuals with mental illness. Formal and informal mechanisms can be established to create a positive relationship between the professions. Strategic planning and partnering occur through formal agreements with memorandums of understanding, contracts, stakeholder meetings, and sharing of a staff person by two agencies. Informal agreements can include holding joint staff/team meetings with criminal justice and mental health representatives, seeking opportunities to find commonalities between criminal justice and mental health systems, or simply having the name of a contact person from a different system to consult.

In 1998, the National Institute of Justice conducted a study examining the interactions between the mental health and law enforcement systems. This study found that less than half of the 176 big-city police departments had specific protocols for handling calls with persons exhibiting emotional disturbances (PsychJob 2000).

Many judges are not familiar with the issues raised by defendants with mental illness. This lack of awareness, coupled with a legitimate concern for public safety, may lead to a decision that incarceration is the safest course of action. Additionally, many judges may incorrectly believe that while incarcerated, detainees and inmates *as a rule* receive medication and other forms of mental health treatment. Because of these basic misunderstandings, courts are likely to treat mentally ill defendants similarly to the way they treat defendants who are not mentally ill, both at trial and at sentencing. Defendants with mental illness frequently do not receive the treatment and support that might prevent recidivism, improve their mental health, and safeguard the community (Denckla and Berman 2001).

Conventional probation supervision and services are often insufficient for the seriously mentally ill or mentally retarded offender. Many mentally ill people who commit criminal offenses are reluctant to participate in psychiatric treatment. They often miss appointments, refuse medication, and do not fully adhere to probation conditions. Moreover, because many mental health agencies are reluctant to accept individuals with criminal histories into their programs, it can be difficult to arrange treatment in the community after those individuals are released (Jemelka et al. 1989).

The lack of discharge planning, combined with the ineffectiveness of traditional probation, may play a role in the quick return of persons with mental illness to the criminal justice system. Recidivism rates are much higher than average for offenders with mental illness than for those without mental illness. In one study, researchers found that 49% of federal inmates who were mentally ill had three or more prior probations, incarcerations, or arrests as compared with 28% of those without mental illness (Ditton 1999). Of the mentally ill who are incarcerated, only 17% of prison inmates and 11% of jail inmates reported receiving any treatment while incarcerated (Ditton 1999). Furthermore, correctional facilities are often not equipped to handle people who, because of mental disabilities, cannot conform their behavior to the rules. As a result, these inmates are more likely to incur disciplinary infractions than inmates who do not have a serious mental illness. Additionally, offenders with mental illnesses, because of their symptoms, are ineligible for programs that would permit them to earn time off their sentence through programming or educational credits. These individuals tend to stay longer in jail than other people charged with similar offenses, and the confinement often leads to further decompensation (Judge David L. Bazelon Center for Mental Health Law 2003).

Because of the challenges posed by offenders with mental illness to the criminal justice system and correctional agencies, several innovative approaches are being used to divert such individuals. These approaches include prebooking diversion, postarrest and postbooking diversion, mental health services in jails, specialized mental health courts, and probation/parole/mental health services collaboration. These programs seek to address criminal behaviors of mentally ill persons and attempt to link the individuals to treatment and services. Interventions are developed to address the underlying causes of the offender's behavior in an effort to prevent recidivism.

PREBOOKING DIVERSION

Police Involvement With Individuals With Mental Illness

Law enforcement officers are routinely dispatched to respond to persons with a mental illness as a peacekeeping function, and in some jurisdictions these interactions occur on a daily basis. By default, police officers are often the first responders to persons experiencing a psychiatric crisis. Ron Honberg, Director of Legal Services for the National Alliance for the Mentally Ill, reported, "In effect, police have become the front-line crisis respondents in many jurisdictions. It is really a reflection of the lack of appropriate treatment options for people" (Psych Job 2000).

During these police encounters, as in others, there is a societal expectation that if a crime has been committed, an arrest of the alleged perpetrator of that crime is warranted. However, since the late 1980s, the law enforcement profession has been challenged to develop alternatives to arresting and detaining individuals whose illegal behavior apparently stems from mental illness. This is especially true when the crime committed is a misdemeanor or nuisance crime. In the absence of *formalized* agreements or partnerships, mental health and law enforcement systems are not likely to find mutually acceptable alternatives to arrest (Psych Job 2000).

Both mental health and law enforcement professionals have speculated that individuals with mental disorders have increasingly been shifted from the mental health system into the criminal justice system. This phenomenon has been termed the "criminalization of mentally disordered behavior" (Teplin 2000) and is sometimes referred to as *transinstitutionalization*. According to Teplin (2000), the probability of being arrested was 67% greater for people who exhibited signs of a mental disorder than for those without an apparent disorder. Both police and mental health professionals emphasize the role of prebooking diversion as an ideal alternative to the "criminalization" of people with mental illness.

According to the Criminal Justice/Mental Health Consensus Project (Council of State Governments 2002), written protocols should be developed to include approaches to assist officers in effectively managing situations involving individuals with mental illness. These policies should include guidelines for law enforcement to assess the situation effectively, assurance of on-scene safety, development of partnerships with the mental health and judicial systems, implementation of appropriate responses, and comprehensive training.

Types of Police–Mental Health Collaborations

The first opportunity for prebooking diversion occurs at the scene of the disturbance. On-scene expertise in mental illness issues is crucial to the effective management of a mentally ill person suspected of committing a crime. This type of expertise can be provided by specially trained police officers or by mental health professionals (Council of State Governments 2002). Three major models of police–mental health services collaboration have been developed in various jurisdictions around the United States: specialized police response teams, specialized mental health response teams, and blended police and mental health response teams. While there are pros and cons for the various models, each jurisdiction should determine what components best suit its needs. Factors involved in deciding what type of collaboration is most appropriate include geographic size, location, and funding. Regardless of the approach accepted, law enforcement officers are responsible for ensuring safety at the scene, recognizing the presence of mental illness, determining whether a serious crime has been committed, and formulating an appropriate disposition (Council of State Governments 2002).

Specialized Police Response Teams

Following the tragic shooting of a mentally ill person by a police officer in Memphis, Tennessee, an innovative program for jail diversion and improvement of police response for mentally ill persons in crisis was developed (Cochran et al. 2000). Patrol officers in Memphis volunteer and are selected to participate in a 40-hour specialized training program led by mental health providers, family advocates, and mental health consumer groups. Having completed the training, these patrol officers become part of an elite specialized response team. Rather than having only a few officers available to respond to a crisis (as with other models), the Memphis model has multiple officers trained who are accessible for a quick response. These officers are on-duty during all shifts and perform routine patrol duties when not involved in the specialized crisis intervention tasks for which they are trained.

Through emergency communication dispatchers, one of the crisis intervention team (CIT) officers is deployed to all crisis calls. The officer responds to the scene immediately, assesses the situation to determine the nature of the complaint and the degree of risk, ensures safety, and determines the most appropriate intervention (Cochran et al. 2000). A National Institute of Justice study examined the effectiveness of various crisis response models (Steadman et al. 2000). While the results indicate that all three models divert mentally ill persons from jail, the Memphis program resulted in the lowest arrest rate among calls involving a subject with mental illness. Similar models exist in other jurisdictions, including Los Angeles, California (Lamb et al. 1995, 2002).

One of the aspects of systems change in Memphis has been the development of the "no wrong door" or "single point of entry" approach. In researching the problems of access to mental health care for individuals in police custody, the collaborating law enforcement and mental health systems found that a major barrier faced by police officers was that the treatment systems could easily refuse to accept individuals because of clinical and fiscal "silos." Thus, an individual with a psychotic illness who is also high on cocaine stopped by police for a nuisance crime such as loitering or trespassing could be refused by mental health providers because of the substance use disorder, and, conversely, by substance abuse providers for having untreated mental illness. This issue was resolved in Memphis by the development of a "single point of entry" to the treatment system at the University of Tennessee Hospital Psychiatric Emergency Department, by which the police officer is permitted to rapidly divert the individual, without arrest, into the treatment system.

Specialized Mental Health Response Teams

In this model, mental health clinicians, who are typically part of the local mental health services system, respond in pairs to persons in crisis. The mobile response teams work to develop a relationship with the police department (Cochran et al. 2000). The mobile crisis team (MCT) can be dispatched through a hotline, by a local mental health authority, or by police officers. If a crime has not been committed, the MCT can provide transportation to a community crisis bed program, hospital, or other mental health facility (Council of State Governments 2002).

Blended Police and Mental Health Response Teams

A blended response model includes pairing a police officer with a civilian mental health professional. The civilian clinician rides along with officers as a specialized team or meets the officer on the scene once it has been deemed safe (Council of State Governments 2002). The crisis team can be dispatched through the emergency communication dispatchers, a crisis hotline, or the mental health authority.

Baltimore County (Maryland) Model

Baltimore County Crisis Response was developed through the partnership of the local mental health authority, the police department, and a community mental health provider. Much as in the Memphis model, clinical and police members of the Baltimore County mobile crisis team participate together in a specialized 40-hour training program. In addition, team members receive joint training in police officer survival tactics. This joint training in mental health and law enforcement results in an innovative, hybrid mobile crisis team model. A first-responder team, consisting of police officers and mental health professionals (both dressed in similar street attire), responds in an unmarked police car. If the situation can be stabilized following an initial response by the police–mental health services team, a separate mental health team (consisting of clinicians) provides follow-up services for a period of 10 days to ensure that the person in crisis is connected to mental health services.

Jurisdictions interested in improving the overall police response and increased likelihood of diversion from the criminal justice system can begin by establishing cross-training programs between law enforcement and mental health professionals (Council of State Governments 2002). Police training should be provided in three forums: at the academy level (upon admission to the police department), through annual in-service (mandatory), and through specialized programs (elective participation in a 40-hour intensive training on mental illness). Training in the academy should contain, at a minimum, an overview of mental illness, substance abuse, and psychotropic medications; communication/crisis deescalation techniques; role-playing of actual responses; and treatment resources (Cochran et al. 2000). The purpose of training officers is not for officers to become diagnosticians, but rather to educate them about the presence of mental illness and to have them consider how the mental illness may have contributed to the person's criminal activity (Council of State Governments 2002). Cross-training enhances police officers' knowledge of mental illness, improves mutual understanding with the mental health system, and provides officers with an understanding of the rationale behind and the importance of implementing the least restrictive alternative possible to prevent the unnecessary incarceration of a mentally ill person in crisis. Psychiatrists and other mental health providers can participate in this training and contribute to improved communication between clinicians and officers. This improved communication ultimately will lead to an increase in diversion and a reduction in the criminalization of behaviors related to mental illness. Additionally, administrators of mental health and law enforcement agencies can work together to improve the systemic response, as demonstrated by the Memphis "no wrong door" approach (Cochran et al. 2000).

Outcomes

Police–mental health services collaborations have demonstrated improved outcomes on a variety of measures. For example, these joint efforts have reduced the arrest rates for incidents of police intervention in situations involving citizens with mental illness. Nonspecialized police interventions result in a 21% arrest rate (Sheridan and Teplin 1981) compared with a 2%–13% arrest rate when the police response involves a specialized, collaborative model (Lamb et al. 1995; Steadman et al. 2000). Similarly, in Los Angeles in 2001, less than 2% of police–mental health evaluations (114 arrests in 6,575 interventions) resulted in an arrest (Pacific Clinics 2002).

Police time is also reduced in such models. For example, in Los Angeles, the initial responding nonspecialized officers are able to transfer control of the situation to the specialized team within 40 minutes, as compared with a total time of 3.2 hours that the average involuntary civil commitment takes (Pacific Clinics 2002).

POSTARREST AND POSTBOOKING DIVERSION

Diversion can be accomplished at a variety of points once a person has been arrested and processed into the criminal justice system (postbooking). The first possibility for diversion is upon completion of the booking process when the commissioner or magistrate is setting bail or permitting release on recognizance. During this hearing, the commissioner can refer a defendant to a mental health professional or team for consideration for diversion. On the basis of the findings of the evaluation, a commissioner has the authority to release a defendant pending trial under special conditions that may include a mental health treatment plan. The defendant must comply with these conditions until trial in order to remain at liberty. Monitoring of the treatment plan can be assigned to a monitoring agency to ensure that the defendant is in fact following the order for release. A consequence of noncompliance can be revocation of the recognizance order and incarceration pending trial. Oversight of the plan and support of the individual are often critical in helping the defendant to remain motivated and engaged in treatment.

A second opportunity for postbooking diversion can occur at the formal bail review in which a judge is reconsidering the bail amount or a release with or without conditions. This process is consistent with the pretrial process described in the previous section. Often the diversion team is consulted by the court, defense counsel, prosecutors, or correctional staff.

A different mechanism for postbooking diversion requires the cooperation of the prosecutor's office. Under this model, an accelerated hearing date is sought for the mentally ill defendant. Bringing the defendant before the court earlier than the scheduled court date allows for expedited release if the court is in agreement with the plan. This accelerated processing may help such defendants remain engaged in prearrest community services and benefits that would be lost if they were forced to spend more time incarcerated pending trial.

Monitoring is a key component of any successful diversion program in that it allows the court to feel confident that the diverted defendant or probationer is complying with conditions of release. Monitoring agencies can include a general or trained probation agent/officer and/or a clinical team employed by the court and tasked with monitoring compliance and ensuring adequate and appropriate clinical care.

In his testimony before the U.S. Congress in September 2000, Dr. Bernard Arons (2000) stated that there were only about 50–55 "true jail diversion programs" nationwide. Several key elements were associated with successful programs:

- Involvement by all relevant mental health, substance abuse, and criminal justice agencies from the start
- Regular meetings between key personnel
- Encouragement of integration of services through the efforts of a designated liaison person working with corrections, mental health, and judicial staff
- Strong leadership
- Nontraditional and creative case management approaches

Forensic Alternative Services Team (FAST) in Baltimore, Maryland

FAST is a program run under the auspices of the Medical Service of the Circuit Court of Maryland for Baltimore. The program is grant funded through Baltimore Mental Health Systems (the mental health authority for the city) and has been in operation for approximately 12 years. Staffing includes six master's-level clinicians and one administrative assistant. The program diverts defendants at the booking/bail review phase, at accelerated trial dates, and at existing trial dates. Occasionally, the team is asked to consider a sentence modification to divert defendants already sentenced to the Division of Corrections (which could be considered postsentence diversion). Staff personnel are located in the Baltimore jails and in each district court (the lower-level trial court) in the city. FAST can also access the circuit court (the higher-level trial court, and the venue for all jury trials in Maryland) to divert the offender as needed.

To gain entry into FAST, the defendant is required to

- Be an adult.
- Be diagnosed with a major mental illness and/or illnesses associated with trauma.
- Be charged (most often at the district court level) with a relatively minor offense.
- Be amenable to community-based treatment.
- Be willing to participate in community supervision by FAST.

Like most diversion programs, FAST prefers that the defendant's participation in the diversion agreement is voluntary. A level of coercion on the part of the court to "convince" the defendant to accept the conditions of release may occur under certain circumstances. To determine program eligibility, the clinician conducts psychosocial evaluations, during which he or she balances individual defendant characteristics and history, program criteria, and community safety risks. If the defendant is eligible, an individualized treatment plan is created and offered to the court at the designated hearing. With the court's approval, the defendant is released under court order to comply with the terms of the release agreement.

The clinician who presents the original treatment plan to the court becomes the monitor of this defendant's compliance with release conditions. The clinician typically meets with the defendant and receives written and telephone documentation from the community mental health provider. The clinician also provides support to the community providers by making home visits, encouraging compliance, and helping to modify plans when needed.

If the defendant does not adhere to the terms of his or her agreement, FAST personnel respond quickly and the presiding judge is notified. Depending on the stage at which the defendant was diverted to community treatment, the responses by FAST can include an upgrade in the level of mental health or substance abuse treatment, a request for bail revocation, or a recommendation for probation revocation. FAST presents information to the court regarding compliance, and the court may modify the original disposition. Clinical Case 11–1 provides an example of how the FAST clinician can provide a parole intervention.

Clinical Case 11–1: Parole Intervention

Mr. J is a 46-year-old man who was observed in the hallway of the courthouse by a FAST clinician demonstrating clear signs of mental illness. When approached, Mr. J stated that he thought he was supposed to be in court but was not sure where. The FAST clinician determined that Mr. J was 2 days late for a court hearing on a trespassing charge, for which the judge had issued a bench warrant. With the assistance of the public defender, the judge agreed to recall the bench warrant. A new court date was assigned.

In the interim, Mr. J was evaluated as suffering from bipolar disorder and AIDS dementia. Given his continued behavioral disorder, he required the assistance of the FAST clinician to appear for and sit through his hearing several weeks later. At that time, the case was postponed for 90 days to give the FAST clinician time to obtain appropriate treatment. The treatment plan ultimately developed included psychiatric care, mobile treatment, and a day program (with transportation). Mr. J responded well to these treatments, and the case was dismissed at the time of the postponed hearing.

FAST continues to face challenges, primarily regarding the inability of the program to meet the demands and the difficulties of serving individuals with comorbid mental illness and substance use disorders. Finally, supervised housing with an appropriate level of program structure is extremely limited. These shortcomings present the court, and FAST by extension, with the dilemma of needing to achieve rapid case disposition but being unable to do so because of inadequate community resources.

Outcomes and Caveats

Data regarding the effectiveness of jail diversion programs are beginning to emerge. The Substance Abuse and Mental Health Services Administration (SAMHSA) of the U.S. Department of Health and Human Services has undertaken a multisite study of jail diversion programs across the country (Steadman et al. 1999b). While the evaluation of the effectiveness of jail diversion is a complex task (Draine and Solomon 1999), initial results indicate that jail diversion leads to decreased jail time and no increase in arrest rates or recidivism. There was, however, no evidence of clinical or social improvements (F. Osher, personal communication, December 1, 2003; see also Steadman et al. 1999a).

The most parsimonious explanation of these findings is that, absent improvements in the mental health and social service system to which people are diverted, jail diversion programs have only limited impact on the lives of people with mental illness. This situation is often termed the "Diversion to what?" question. However, the importance of these data should not be minimized, as jail time alone is traumatizing for many, and reducing it alone has some value. That this reduction in incarceration occurs without an apparent decrease in public safety, even in the absence of positive clinical outcomes, is cause for optimism.

SPECIALIZED MENTAL HEALTH COURTS

Origin and Rationale

Over the previous few decades, a few jurisdictions have made attempts to manage mentally ill defendants in a less punitive and more therapeutic way. In the 1960s, courts in Chicago and New York practiced what was known as "therapeutic disposition" of such cases. Chicago courts could order psychiatric screening, allow psychiatrists and social workers to make sentencing suggestions, and give nonpenal sentences such as outpatient treatment or civil commitment to offenders with mental illnesses. Often when the referrals resulted in these therapeutic dispositions, the criminal charges were dismissed (Mathews 1970; cited in Goldkamp and Irons-Guynn 2000).

In New York, offenders with mental illnesses were diverted to health care treatment at the time of arrest and avoided the courts entirely. Police officers had the option of taking arrestees to Bellevue or Elmhurst Hospital's prison wards, both of which were administered by the Department of Corrections and linked the mental health and criminal justice systems' efforts on behalf of these individuals. The court could also refer defendants for competency-to-stand-trial and criminal-responsibility evaluations. Under these orders, the hospital treatment team prepared a report that answered the court-ordered legal question and made recommendations regarding appropriate treatment (Mathews 1970; cited in Goldkamp and Irons-Guynn 2000).

These early initiatives were the precursors to the modern mental health court. Like other diversion programs, mental health courts seek not only to address the criminal behaviors of the mentally ill defendant but also to link the defendant to treatment and services. These specialty courts attempt to address the underlying problems of each defendant in an effort to prevent recidivism and to promote ongoing connection to community mental health services.

Development of Mental Health Courts

Mental health courts are modeled after the drug courts created in southern Florida in the early 1990s (Denckla and Berman 2001). As in the approaches adopted by the drug court model, the mental health court judge takes a hands-on role in managing the defendant's case and uses treatment as a public safety tool rather than relying solely on incarceration, fines, or other forms of punishment (Goldkamp and Irons-Guynn 2000). Under this new model, the courts attempt to attack the root of the problem by focusing on reasons that underlie why the defendant became involved in the criminal justice system (Goldkamp and Irons-Guynn 2000).

The first mental health court began operation in Broward County, Florida, in 1997. Since that time, there has been a proliferation of these courts around the country in recognition of the need for this type of initiative. In 2000, the U.S. Congress passed the America's Law Enforcement and Mental Health Project Act, allowing local jurisdictions to receive federal funds to create or expand existing mental health courts (Judge David L. Bazelon Center for Mental Health Law 2003).

The mental health court model is based on the premise that the criminal and juvenile justice systems are ineffective providers of mental health services. The rationale behind the development of this specialized court system is twofold: 1) a mental health court can properly address the mental illness underlying a criminal defendant's actions, and 2) the specialty court can assign an appropriate treatment for that criminal defendant (Judge David L. Bazelon Center for Mental Health Law 2003). Rather than imprisoning or fining the mentally ill defendant, the mental health court can provide that individual with psychiatric treatment and other necessary services. With such assistance, the system aspires to address each defendant's mental illness and thereby hopes to reduce the recidivism of mentally ill defendants. Unlike the regular criminal court, the mental health court seeks to help the mentally ill defendant on a long-term basis. Once the defendant is in the program, the court retains jurisdiction over him or her, enabling the judge to monitor the defendant's progress until the completion of the program by the offender (Goldkamp and Irons-Guynn 2000).

Screening and Evaluation for Mental Health Court Admission

All mental health courts share common features. The identification of potential candidates for the mental health court requires screening and referrals of defendants soon after their arrest. This initial stage is vital if the offender is to be offered a timely opportunity to participate in the program. Newly incarcerated detainees must be screened for mental illness within 24–48 hours of their entry into the criminal justice system (Goldkamp and Irons-Guynn 2000). Jail staff, family members, and defense attorneys are generally responsible for identification of appropriate candidates (Denckla and Berman 2001).

After being identified as potentially eligible, these offenders must be evaluated to determine if their illness is severe enough to qualify for services and whether they have a history of violence. Criteria for "serious mental illness" vary from state to state. In some jurisdictions, participants must have organic brain impairment, developmental disability, or an Axis I diagnosis as assessed by DSM-IV-TR (American Psychiatric Association 2000a). In other jurisdictions (e.g., King County, Washington), the defendant need only have a diagnosis of mental illness or obvious signs of serious mental illness (Goldkamp and Irons-Guynn 2000).

The second factor considered in determining eligibility for mental health court admission is the nature of the crime with which the defendant is charged. Most jurisdictions limit eligibility to those persons with mental illnesses with a nonviolent misdemeanor charge, although a few jurisdictions do allow participation with a nonviolent felony charge. The target populations of these courts include perpetrators of minor crimes, generally misdemeanors or "quality of life" ordinance violations such as disorderly conduct. Either the mental health court judge or the treatment team has the final decision about eligibility (Goldkamp and Irons-Guynn 2000).

Finally, all mental health courts require the defendant's voluntary assent or consent to participation. As noted earlier and discussed in detail below, this consent may be "coerced" or negotiated rather than truly voluntary.

Mental Health Court Program

Entry into the program varies by jurisdiction and generally occurs either prior to or after conviction. Some jurisdictions use a nonconviction approach, and the mentally ill person is sentenced before the case is adjudicated; if the defendant completes the program, the charges may be dismissed. Other jurisdictions require the defendant to plead guilty before entering the program; however, the plea may be withdrawn or expunged upon successful completion of the program. Another approach is to allow a deferred adjudication or deferred sentence to be entered pending completion of the program (Goldkamp and Irons-Guynn 2000).

Once the defendant is admitted into the mental health court program, a treatment team oversees his or her case. This treatment team may include the judge, probation officers, clinical supervisors or coordinators, case managers, defense attorneys and prosecutors, and jail liaisons, each of whom is accountable to the court. This team works together to link the participants with appropriate treatment services, often including residential or other supportive housing placements. The participation of the court ensures the presence of a central figure to coordinate these services, monitor the defendant's progress, and provide accountability for the treatment process. The judge presides formally over any legal matters at the entry and completion stages of the process. The judge also routinely meets with the participant and provides rewards or sanctions as appropriate. Sanctions may be of a punitive nature (e.g., time in jail) or therapeutically oriented (e.g., increased intensity of treatment). Treatment providers in such settings can assist judges in making decisions regarding determining if therapeutic approaches or criminal justice sanctions are indicated. Most mental health court programs last from 12 to 18 months and have a subsequent probation period (Goldkamp and Irons-Guynn 2000).

Outcomes and Caveats

It is too early to determine whether mental health courts are truly succeeding in preventing recidivism or whether the treatment programs are successful in helping mentally ill offenders stabilize in the community. However, the development of mental health courts reflects a change in attitude in the criminal justice system toward offenders with mental illnesses. These mental health courts represent a fundamental philosophical shift away from the traditional adversarial process and punish orientation of the judiciary to a more hands-on therapeutic jurisprudence approach. Such alternative methods should continue to be considered, explored, and modified. Additionally, clinical outcome research and program evaluation are required to determine if mental health courts are having the desired effect or if, as has been found in some studies of intensive supervision probation (Draine and Solomon 1994; Solomon et al. 1994)–the increased focus on these defendants may result in their being more likely to remain involved in the criminal justice system.

SENTENCED INDIVIDUALS

The Presentence Investigation

The sentencing of defendants varies by jurisdiction. Historically, in the 1920s and 1930s, a medical model of corrections developed in which sentencing became based on a defendant's individual characteristics rather than simply on the crime committed. During this time, the use of a presentence investigation, or PSI, report came into common use. Over time, two major types of PSI reports have been developed: offender based and offense based. The former is prepared for the sentencing court in order to describe the offender and offer background information to be used by the judge in making sentencing decisions. Inherent in this format is the possibility of rehabilitation and community integration. As sentencing approaches became more punitive during the 1950s and 1960s, determinate sentences with less judicial discretion were emphasized. Guideline sentencing, legislated in a more conservative social environment, encouraged punishment that was more uniform among offenders (offense based). In addition, the individuality of offenders was felt to be less important in sentencing than the nature of the offense and the role of the convicted offender in that offense (Sullivan 2002).

In jurisdictions that continue to allow for a substantial judicial discretion in sentencing or in cases in which diminished capacity may be at issue, mental health evaluations are beneficial supplements to PSIs. Mental health evaluations are usually requested by defendants seeking to establish mental illness as a mitigating factor in the commission of an offense, to rebut expert testimony by the state, or to assist in determining postsentence treatment requirements in the community (U.S. Sentencing Commission 2002). Such evaluations may be used by judges to determine appropriateness for probation with mandated community treatment, as opposed to (or in addition to) a term of incarceration. As an example, federal probation officers, in the preparation of a PSI in which mental health is to be raised as a possible mitigating factor arguing for release, base a recommendation for release on answers to the following questions (Federal Judicial Center 2003):

- Does the severity of a mental illness impact management of risk or compliance with standard conditions of release?
- Does a disorder create a risk issue?
- Is the offender willing to voluntarily submit to treatment?

These reports often play a major role in the development of specialized conditions of probation or, eventually, parole.

Court-mandated supervision of an offender in a community setting has been described as "a means to engage the offender [in] improving compliance with general societal norms, including conditions of release" (Taxman 2002, p. 20). Interventions and supervision strategies must address each individual's specific needs in order to achieve positive outcomes. Ideally, these individuals should be provided with a plan that integrates or coordinates a variety of services and approaches, including psychiatric treatment, psychotherapy, substance use treatment, case management, and rehabilitative (including psychosocial, vocational, and residential) services.

Types of Postconviction Release

Judges can impose a term of *probation* as an alternative to incarceration for defendants or convicted of minor crimes. Probation can also be imposed before judgment in cases where sentencing is offered before a trial to give a defendant a chance to reform. In each of these cases, conditions are imposed on the defendant. The defendant must comply with these conditions on pain of return to court for a violation of probation hearing. *Parole,* by contrast, is a form of early release from jail or prison, with conditions similar to those of probation imposed on the offender. Parole is affirmatively granted by an official body (often called a parole commission), and an offender must demonstrate a level of compliance with conditions of incarceration and a degree of readiness to return to the community.

Finally, in many jurisdictions, incarcerated individuals can be released early on the basis of behavioral requirements during their time in jail or prison. This form of release, often called *mandatory* or *supervised release,* is distinguished from parole in that it is a passive process. In other words, no decision is made about an individual defendant. Instead, "good time" can be earned, and additional time can be earned by participation in programs, based on statutorily defined calculations. Noncompliance with conditions of parole or supervised release can result in a return to incarceration and imposition of the remainder of the sentence.

In all of these forms of release, *standard* and *special conditions* may be imposed. Standard conditions include requirements regarding living situation, work obligations, reporting to a supervising officer, payment of fees, avoidance of firearms and drugs, and obedience to the law. Special conditions are individualized and can include such requirements as participation in psychiatric or addiction assessments or attendance at a treatment program. These conditions are analogous to those imposed in postbooking diversion programs and in mental health courts.

Collaborative Programs

Programs that have demonstrated success in the management of court-ordered individuals have a high degree of collaboration and cross-training (Roskes and Feldman 1999; Roskes et al. 1999). These programs include personnel from a variety of treatment disciplines, including psychiatrists, nurses, social workers, case managers, addictions counselors, and rehabilitation staff, as well as community corrections officials. In addition, these programs have a highly developed "treatment first" orientation. A treatment-first philosophy forces providers from both mental health and criminal justice to seek a treatment intervention when things are going poorly rather than jumping quickly to a punitive or correctional intervention. Often, the latter takes the form of a good cop/bad cop conversation with a client in which the client is placed in a forced-choice situation. Roskes and colleagues (1999) have described a number of successful interventions under this paradigm. Clinical Case 11–2 provides an example of how various treatment approaches function in a multidisciplinary fashion in a collaborative program.

Clinical Case 11–2

Mr. A is a 45-year-old man with bipolar disorder and cocaine dependence who was convicted of bank robbery a number of years before. He had spent about 8 years in prison prior to his first parole. He was re-incarcerated after only 8 months in the community, having relapsed on cocaine and discontinuing his psychiatric treatment. He had two more cycles of release and re-incarceration. The latest parole was by far the most successful, lasting over 2 years.

He presented one day with racing thoughts, disorganized thinking, and denial of his illness. He repeatedly denied cocaine use and insisted that he was taking his medications, lithium and olanzapine, as prescribed. He readily agreed to provide urine and blood samples to confirm his abstinence and compliance with the medication regimen. Because his psychiatrist was concerned, he contacted Mr. A's parole officer, who came to the clinic. The psychiatrist offered Mr. A a voluntary hospitalization in an attempt to intervene in an apparent manic decompensation. Mr. A refused. The parole officer indicated that, given what he was seeing, he had serious concerns about Mr. A's adherence to treatment and compliance with other conditions of his release. The parole officer continued, saying "If you don't go into the hospital, I will have to give some serious thought to seeking a revocation of your parole. I don't want you to go back to prison, but.." After some discussion, it became apparent that Mr. A was concerned about not being home the following week when his disability check was due to come in the mail. "Where I live, if you aren't home, your mail isn't delivered."

Given Mr. A's reality-based concerns, the psychiatrist offered Mr. A a course of partial hospitalization. Mr. A agreed and was accepted into a local partial program, where his medications were readjusted. The decompensation resolved in about 4 weeks and Mr. A continued in outpatient treatment. He remained in the community, fully compliant with the conditions of his parole, for three more years until he died of a sudden heart attack.

At times, relationships between mental health providers and community corrections can be formalized through contractual agreements. In 1978, the Administrative Office of the U.S. Courts was authorized by federal legislation to contract for drug treatment services. This contractual capacity was expanded to include mental health treatment. Later, the authority to enter into such contracts was delegated by federal district courts to each local or regional U.S. probation office in order to permit flexibility in meeting the needs of each office (Hughes and Henkel 1997). The federal probation system has been at the forefront of the development of the specialized probation officer. Specialties include both mental health and substance abuse specialists, among others (Freitas 1997). In other instances, informal relationships develop between parole and probation officers and mental health providers or agencies. These agencies work with clients and come to view the officer as another referral source.

SPECIAL TOPICS

Medication Management of Court-Ordered Outpatients

Many, if not most, individuals who are in community treatment by court order will be required by that court order to take medication as prescribed. Some court orders may specify, for example, the type or name of the medication and even the dosage or a dose range. These court orders are less preferable than court orders that consist of a more general statement, as the specific court order precludes the clinician from reacting to changes in the individual patient's clinical condition. In addition, a specific court order eliminates the negotiation that must take place in community care between the doctor and the patient around medication issues.

In the community care of court-ordered patients, a common strategy to ensure medication compliance is the use of long-acting intramuscular antipsychotics. In addition, for appropriate patients, medications that require serum monitoring of therapeutic concentration can be useful in that the blood level serves as a proxy for medication compliance.

Newer antipsychotics (e.g., risperidone, olanzapine, quetiapine, ziprasidone, aripiprazole) are often preferred by patients because of their improved tolerability. While not without disadvantages, these medications, when used in appropriate cases, can lead to more successful community tenure of court-ordered patients. Clozapine, in addition to being used to successfully treat many patients with previously treatment-resistant psychosis, may have a specific neurochemical role in the treatment of aggression (Hector 1998; Spivak et al. 1997). One study has found a reduction in arrest rates in patients with psychotic disorders taking clozapine compared with those taking other anti-psychotics. If nothing else, the requirement for regular blood testing necessi-tates frequent contact with mental health care providers, which may result in an improved therapeutic alliance. Similarly, other medications that require frequent blood testing and monitoring of serum levels (e.g., lithium, valproic acid) can be used as proxies for medication compliance.

Working With Insanity Acquittees in the Community

While not technically a part of the correctional system, in many ways, the in-sanity defense system mirrors the criminal justice system. There are, how-ever, several key differences that may be relevant to the community provider working with such patients. The similarities begin at the onset of the legal process. An individual is charged with a crime, but rather than plead not guilty or engage in a plea bargaining process, the individual, his attorney, other legal actors (including the judge or even the prosecuting attorney), or correctional staff raise concerns regarding mental health issues. This may happen at any point prior to trial and may result in a competency to stand trial assessment. Some individuals, though remarkably few, will plead insan-ity in those states permitting such a defense. For example, Janofsky and col-leagues (1996) found that only 190 defendants, out of more than 60,000 (0.3%) indicted defendants, in Baltimore during 1991 entered a plea of insan-ity. Nearly all withdrew the plea prior to trial. Many fewer will be adjudicated as "not guilty by reason of insanity" (NGRI) or "not criminally responsible." Janofsky et al. (1996) reported that only 8 defendants (0.01%) were ultimately adjudicated not criminally responsible by reason of mental disease or defect.

Upon this adjudication, the defendant is transferred out of the criminal justice system and into the mental health system, though often to a forensic high-security hospital that has many of the same security issues that apply to jails and prisons. Maryland's statute governing length of confinement of NGRI acquittees is characteristic of these confinement laws. According to this statute, the NGRI acquittee is hospitalized until such time as he or she is no longer "a danger, as a result of mental disorder or mental retardation, to self or to the person or property of others if discharged" (Maryland Anno-tated Code 2004). It is important to note that, unlike a sentence to prison, in which the term of confinement is defined, confinement to a psychiatric hos-pital subsequent to a successful insanity defense may be indeterminate and does not depend on the nature of the crime committed (Jones v. U.S. 1983). However, some states, such as Oregon, have restricted the maximum length of criminal commitment to the maximum sentence a defendant could have received for the instant offense (Oregon Counseling, undated).

States vary in their approach to conditional release of NGRI acquittees. In some states (e.g., Maryland), a judicial process places the burden on the detained patient to demonstrate by a preponderance of the evidence that if released, he or she would not pose "a danger, as a result of mental disorder or mental retardation, to self or to the person or property of others" (Maryland Annotated Code 2004). Other states, such as Oregon, commit the individual determined insane under state law to the supervision of an administrative board. This board, which in Oregon is termed the Psychiatric Security Review Board, bears responsibility for all decisions as to release and rehospitalization (Oregon Counseling, undated).

Upon release, the individual is subject to a variety of conditions that generally include a specified housing arrangement and required participation in mental health and substance abuse treatment. Clinicians working with such individuals in community settings have a dual role as clinical providers and as agents of public safety. This role is functionally identical to working with individuals who, by court order, are mandated to treatment by judges as a condition of probation or by parole boards as a condition of parole or supervised release.

Management of Individuals With Complex Comorbidities

One of the issues facing all community mental health providers is the difficulty in working with people with mental illness who have comorbid conditions. In forensic populations, as noted earlier, a significant majority of individuals with mental illness also have substance use disorders. For example, in a study of 16 individuals under federal supervision requiring psychiatric treatment, 94% of the individuals had comorbid mental illness and addiction (Roskes and Feldman 1999). These disorders must be managed in an integrated fashion in community settings in order to maximize the chances for the individual to succeed in his or her community placement (Minkoff 2001; Pita and Spaniol 2002). Ideally, a single program should manage both the mental illness and the substance use disorders in court-ordered patients. Random urine screens can be extremely helpful in ensuring that the patient is remaining abstinent and can also serve as a tool for maintaining a connection between the patient and the clinical program.

Medical comorbidity is also very common in this population. Roskes and Feldman (1999) found that nearly 60% of the individuals in their study suffered from a variety of medical problems, ranging from quiescent hepatitis C infection to recurrent metastatic lung cancer. The role of the psychiatrist and other members of the mental health team, both in assisting in the diagnosis and in ensuring adequate medical care, is significant and often undervalued in community mental health settings.

Coercive Treatment in a Community Setting

As in correctional institutions, clinicians working with patients under a court order may find themselves in a dual-agency role in which they are hired by the agency but provide treatment to the inmate. Treatment under any kind of court order presents moral and ethical dilemmas unique to the coerced treatment paradigm (Monahan et al. 2003). When working in a court-mandated treatment setting, clinicians must recognize that the therapeutic relationship is itself contaminated by the coercive nature of the court order that brings the patient into treatment. This coercion can be used to assist the patient in achieving his or her goals, such as obtaining stable housing (which is often initially court-mandated) or avoiding a return to jail, prison, or the hospital (see Clinical Case 11–2 earlier in this chapter).

Clinicians serving court-ordered clients serve two masters: the patient and the public safety monitoring agency (Packard 1989). Such dual-agency dilemmas can arise in several ways, as in the following examples:

- A provider may find that his patient has encountered legal problems, and the court may order compliance with ongoing treatment. This provider now serves as a public safety agent in addition to the preexisting pure clinical role.
- A forensic evaluator may recommend treatment to the court and have the court order the defendant to undergo that treatment with the evaluator.
- A clinician providing court mandated treatment may be asked to answer ongoing public safety questions or to testify regarding public safety issues.

The last item above is probably the most common situation and is the only one that a clinician working with court-ordered patients should expect as a matter of course. In these treatment situations, the clinician must be responsive to questions from public safety agents regarding attendance, adherence to treatment requirements, and maintenance of sobriety. Many public safety agencies send regular questionnaires to providers treating court-ordered patients and expect feedback on these questionnaires. It is imperative for these providers to provide patients with ongoing information regarding communication between the provider and the public safety agency and to obtain ongoing consent for that communication. Refusal to give such consent should be clarified with the patient, and the patient should be made aware that the clinician will be required to report the patient's refusal to consent to information transfer.

It is clear that treatment under these paradigms may be coercive. Many individuals come to treatment under these court orders as less than fully willing participants, and it is a challenge to the therapeutic skills of the provider to engage such clients. The degree of coercion even among court-ordered patients is rather variable, however. For example, individuals found NGRI and then conditionally released generally will not be released until they assent to ongoing care in the community. In contrast, people released on probation may not have undergone nearly as much institutionally based treatment. In the authors' experience, such individuals are much more likely to test the clinician's ability to provide structure and safety, as they have not received the intensive treatment and psychoeducation in the jail or while released on bail awaiting trial.

Indirect support for this concept comes from the very low rate of rearrest (3.4%–7.8% rearrests per year) among conditionally released NGRI acquittees (Wiederanders et al. 1997). In comparison, by the end of 2002, 50% of all parolees in general had a rearrest or other unsatisfactory end to their parole (Bureau of Justice Statistics, undated). Of note, however, is that there is some research demonstrating lower recidivism among offenders with mental illnesses when compared with offenders without mental illness, and that the risk factors for recidivism are no different for individuals with mental illness than they are for those without mental illness (Bonta et al. 1997).

The Testifying Clinician

At times, clinicians caring for individuals under court order may be called to testify regarding a patient. Most of the time, the clinician is being asked to testify as a fact witness—that is, to advise the court as to details of compliance with treatment as defined by the court order requiring that treatment. On less frequent occasions, the clinician may be asked to provide opinion testimony as an expert witness. In general, clinicians working with court-ordered patients should only testify under court order and should strenuously avoid being drawn into other, nonmandatory witness roles.

Testifying as a fact witness generally raises no issues for the treating clinician, provided that the clinician has advised the patient of the need to share information with the court or the supervising agency from the outset of the court-ordered treatment and on a frequent basis during that treatment. Requests for such testimony may be built into the court order, which may require periodic reports to the court. (This may happen, for example, in a mental health court model or in a supervised-release model that requires monthly or quarterly reports.) Alternatively, a clinician may be called only when things are going badly. Most patients treated under this rubric are aware of the need for such information sharing. When done well, this open sharing of information, with the consent of the patient, serves to improve the care delivered to the patient and results in an increased chance for successful community treatment (Heilbrun and Griffin 1998).

Assuming the role of an expert witness raises more difficult ethical issues, as the expert role calls for more than simple reporting of facts. The expert witness can be asked to provide opinions on a variety of questions, such as dangerousness risk and competency to proceed with trial in new cases. As in many areas of correctional psychiatric practice, this form of dual agency is ethically difficult. The clinician asked to testify as an expert witness has two potentially conflicting obligations: his or her fiduciary responsibility toward his patient and his or her legal mandate to testify truthfully. Most forensic academicians strongly discourage blending the clinician and expert roles, and the American Psychiatric Association's *Guidelines for Psychiatric Services in Jails and Prisons,* 2nd Edition (American Psychiatric Association 2000b) explicitly endorses this separation of roles. However, there are times when a clinician cannot escape such requests from a court. It is important to recognize that such expert testimony, regardless of the content, may irrevocably alter the quality of the therapeutic relationship. Such risks should be explained to the court prior to testifying in order to attempt to preserve the therapeutic alliance for future treatment efforts.

A clinician who chooses to work with court-ordered patients can do several things to avoid the need to be called to court to testify. First and foremost, clear communication with the patient that the clinician will be sharing information, with the patient's consent, with a supervising agency or court must occur from the outset and throughout the course of treatment. This serves both to keep the court-ordered nature of the treatment at the forefront of the patient's and clinician's minds and to avoid subsequent misunderstandings. Should a patient refuse consent, efforts to treat the patient should be terminated and the refusal to grant consent alone should be communicated to the court or supervising agency.

Second, adherence to reporting schedules should be maintained. These reports should be made completely and in a timely fashion. If this approach is adopted when things are going well, the supervising agency is able to respond quickly if and when things begin to turn sour (e.g., as evidenced by missed appointments or noncompliance with medications).

Finally, reporting of problems as soon as they happen is imperative. Such reporting permits the clinician and the supervising agency or court to work together to craft a clinical intervention under a treatment-first philosophy before legal action becomes necessary. For example, if a patient develops early signs of mania and substance use and is suspected of noncompliance with medication, a conference can be held with the patient, the clinician, and the supervising agent. Various clinical options (e.g., increased frequency of visits to the clinician, partial or inpatient hospitalization, emergency testing of medication levels, urine toxicology screens) can be presented to the patient. Only when all clinical interventions fail should legal consequences be considered. Provided that there is good communication between the clinician and the supervising agency, such interventions result in improved community tenure and minimal use of legal sanctions (Roskes et al. 1999).

CONCLUSION

In this chapter, we have described a variety of collaborative models used by criminal justice and mental health professionals in the community, along the entire spectrum of community criminal justice opportunities, from arrest through the postsentence conditional release process. While there are a number of difficulties involved in taking on this work, paramount among them the conflicts encountered in taking on a dual role, these difficulties can be overcome with adequate motivation, interest, and training. Some of the common denominators in successful collaborative programs include a willingness to develop an understanding of the "other" system, the motivation to learn each other's language, and an ability to set aside stereotypes and take each case as it comes. Providers must develop an ability to see the human being behind the rap sheet and to develop a relationship with that person. In the end, working with such individuals has obvious public safety implications: people with mental illness and legal involvement are all around us in our communities. Clearly, these individuals are better cared for and our society is a better and safer place if we participate as providers in their return to and retention in our communities.

SUMMARY POINTS

- Diversion represents opportunity for persons with mental illness to be diverted from the criminal justice system.
- Mental health courts examine underlying mental illness that contributes to a defendant's action and assign treatment.
- Probation is an alternative to incarceration.
- Parole is a form of early release from jail or prison.
- Mental health evaluations are often helpful supplements to presentence investigations.
- Clinicians working with court-ordered clients may have a challenging dual-agency role.

REFERENCES

American Psychiatric Association: Diagnostic and Statistical Manual of Mental Disorders, 4th Edition, Text Revision. Washington, DC, American Psychiatric Association, 2000a

American Psychiatric Association: Guidelines for Psychiatric Services in Jails and Prisons, 2nd Edition, Washington, DC, American Psychiatric Association, 2000b

Arons BS: Testimony before US Congress, September 21, 2000. Available at: http://www.house.gov/judiciary/aron0921.htm. Accessed June 10, 2004.

Bonta J, Law M, Hanson K: The prediction of criminal and violent recidivism among mentally disordered offenders: a meta-analysis. Psychol Bull 123:123–142, 1997

Buchan L: Ending the cycle of recidivism: best practices for diverting mentally ill individuals from county jails. National Association of Counties, June 2003. Available at: http://www.naco.org. Accessed October 24, 2003.

Bureau of Justice Statistics, Office of Justice Programs: Probation and parole statistics. Washington, DC, U.S. Department of Justice. Available at: http://www.ojp.usdoj.gov/bjs/pandp.htm. Accessed October 27, 2003.

Cochran S, Deane MW, Borum R: Improving police response to mentally ill people. Psychiatr Serv 51:1315–1316, 2000

Council of State Governments. Criminal Justice/Mental Health Consensus Project, 2002. Available at: http://consensusproject.org. Accessed October 24, 2003.

Denckla D, Berman G: Rethinking the revolving door; a look at mental illness in the courts. New York, Center for Court Innovation, 2001. Available at: http://www.courtinnovation.org/pdf/mental_health.pdf. Accessed June 10, 2004.

Ditton PM: Mental health and treatment of inmates and probationers (NCJ 174463). Washington, DC, Office of Justice Programs, Bureau of Justice Statistics, U.S. Department of Justice, July 1999. Available at: http://www.ojp.usdoj.gov/bjs/pub/pdf/mhtip.pdf. Accessed August 4, 2003.

Draine J, Solomon P: Jail recidivism and the intensity of case management services among homeless persons with mental illness leaving jail. J Psychiatry Law 22:245–261, 1994

Draine J, Solomon P: Describing and evaluating jail diversion services for persons with serious mental illness. Psychiatr Serv 50:56–61, 1999

Federal Judicial Center: Supervising defendants and offenders with mental disorders–participant guide. VHS (#AVA21221VNB5CFP) distributed by the Federal Judicial Center. Available at: http://www.fjc.gov. Accessed June 10, 2004.

Freitas SI: Mentally disordered offenders: Who are they? What are their needs? Federal Probation, March 1997, pp 33–35

Fulton B: Persons with mental illness on parole and probation: the importance of information, in Community Corrections in America: New Directions and Sounder Investments for Persons With Mental Illness and Codisorders. Edited by Lurigio A. Seattle, WA, The National Coalition for Mental and Substance Abuse Health Care in the Justice System, 1996. Available at: www.nicic.org/pubs/1996/014000.pdf. Accessed August 13, 2003.

Glaze L: Probation and parole in the United States, 2002 (NCJ 201135). Washington, DC, Office of Justice Programs, Bureau of Justice Statistics, U.S. Department of Justice, August 2003. Available at: http://www.ojp.usdoj.gov/bjs/pub/pdf/ppus02.pdf. Accessed June 10, 2004.

Goldkamp JS, Irons-Guynn C: Emerging judicial strategies for the mentally ill in the criminal caseload: mental health courts in Fort Lauderdale, Seattle, San Bernardino, and Anchorage (NCJ 182504). Washington, DC, Office of Justice Programs, Bureau of Justice Assistance, U.S. Department of Justice, April 2000. Available at: http://www.ncjrs.org/pdffiles1/bja/182504.pdf. Accessed June 10, 2004.

Harrison P, Beck A: Prisoners in 2002 (NCJ 200248). Washington, DC, Office of Justice Programs, Bureau of Justice Statistics, U.S. Department of Justice, July 2003. Available at: http://www.ojp.usdoj.gov/bjs/pub/pdf/p02.pdf. Accessed June 10, 2004.

Hector RI. The use of clozapine in the treatment of aggressive schizophrenia. Can J Psychiatry 43:466–472, 1998

Heilbrun K, Griffin PA: Community based forensic treatment, in Treatment of Offenders With Mental Disorders. Edited by Wettstein RM. New York, Guilford, 1998, pp 168–210

Hughes J, Henkel K: The federal probation and retrial services system since 1975: an era of growth and change. Federal Probation, March 1997, pp 103–111

Human Rights Watch: Ill-equipped U.S. prisons and offenders with mental illness. New York, Human Rights Watch, 2003. Available at: http://www.hrw.org. Accessed October 24, 2003.

Janofsky JS, Dunn MH, Roskes EJ, et al: Insanity defense pleas in Baltimore City: an analysis of outcome. Am J Psychiatry 153:1464–1468, 1996

Jemelka R, Trupin E, Chiles J: The mentally ill in prison: a review. Hosp Community Psychiatry 40:481–491, 1989

Jones v U.S., 463 U.S. 354, 103 S.Ct. 3043 (1983)

Judge David L. Bazelon Center for Mental Health Law: Criminalization of people with mental illnesses: the role of mental health courts in system reform. Available at: http://www.bazelon.org/issues/criminalization/publications/mentalhealth-courts/mentalhealthcourts.pdf. Accessed October 21, 2003.

Lamb HR, Shaner R, Elliott DM, et al: Outcome for psychiatric emergency patients seen by an outreach police-mental health team. Psychiatr Serv 46:1267–1271, 1995

Lamb HR, Weinberger LE, DeCuir WJ: The police and mental health. Psychiatr Serv 53:1266–1271, 2002

Maryland Annotated Code, Criminal Procedure Article, §3-114, 2004. Available at: http://www.lib.umd.edu/RARE/MarylandCollection/MDResourceGuide/MD AnnCodes.html. Accessed June 10, 2004.

Mathews AR: Mental Disability and the Criminal Justice System. Chicago, IL, American Bar Foundation, 1970

Minkoff K: Developing standards of care for individuals with co-occurring psychiatric and substance use disorders. Psychiatr Serv 52:597–599, 2001

Monahan J, Swartz M, Bonnie RJ: Mandated treatment in the community for people with mental disorders. Health Aff 22:28–38, 2003. Available at: http://www.medscape.com/viewarticle/462070_print. Accessed October 8, 2003.

Oregon Counseling. Guilty except for insanity (GEI) and psychiatric security review board (PSRB) jurisdiction. Available at: http://www.oregoncounseling.org/Laws Rights/GuiltyExceptInsanity.htm. Accessed June 10, 2004.

Pacific Clinics. Mental Health Law Enforcement Programs, 2002. Available at: http://www.pacificclinics.org/mental_health_law_enforcement_pr.htm. Accessed June 10, 2004.

Packard WS: Forensic evaluation and treatment in the same institution: a moral dilemma, in Correctional Psychiatry. Edited by Rosner R, Harmon RB. New York, Plenum, 1989, pp 187–195

Pita DD, Spaniol L: A Comprehensive Guide for Integrated Treatment of People With Co-occurring Disorders. Boston, MA, Boston University Center for Psychiatric Rehabilitation, 2002

Psych Job: The Memphis PD's crisis intervention team reinvents police response to EDPs. Law Enforcement News (John Jay College of Criminal Justice/CUNY), December 15/31, 2000. Available at: http://www.lib.jjay.cuny.edu/len/2000/12.31/. Accessed June 10, 2004.

Regier DA, Farmer ME, Rae D, et al: Comorbidity of mental disorders with alcohol and other drug abuse. JAMA 246:2511–2518, 1990

Roskes E, Feldman R: A collaborative community based treatment program for offenders with mental illness. Psychiatr Serv 50:1614–1619, 1999

Roskes E, Feldman R, Arrington S, et al: A model program for the treatment of mentally ill offenders in the community. Community Ment Health J 35:461–472, 1999

Sheridan EP, Teplin L: Police-referred psychiatric emergencies: advantages of community treatment. J Community Psychol 9:140–147, 1981

Solomon P, Draine J, Meyerson A: Jail recidivism and receipt of community mental health services. Hosp Community Psychiatry 45:793–797, 1994

Spivak B, Mester R, Wittenberg N, et al: Reduction of aggressiveness and impulsiveness during clozapine treatment in chronic neuroleptic-resistant schizophrenic patients. Clin Neuropharmacol 20:442–446, 1997

Steadman HJ, Cocozza JJ, Veysey BM: Comparing outcomes for diverted and non-diverted jail detainees with mental illnesses. Law Hum Behav 23:615–627, 1999a

Steadman HJ, Deane MW, Morrissey JP, et al: A SAMHSA research initiative assessing the effectiveness of jail diversion programs for mentally ill persons. Psychiatr Serv 50:1620–1623, 1999b

Steadman HJ, Deane MW, Borum R, et al: Comparing outcomes of major models of police responses to mental health emergencies. Psychiatr Serv 51:645–649, 2000

Sullivan J: The history of the presentence investigation report. San Francisco, CA, San Francisco Center on Juvenile and Criminal Justice, 2002. Available at: http://www.cjcj.org/pubs/psi/psireport.html. Accessed November 11, 2003.

Taxman F: Supervision: exploring the dimensions of effectiveness. Federal Probation, September 2002, pp 14–27

Teplin L: Keeping the peace: police discretion and mentally ill persons. National Institute of Justice Journal, July 2000. Available at: http://www.ncjrs.org/pdffiles1/jr000244c.pdf. Accessed October 24, 2003.

U.S. Sentencing Commission: Determining the sentence (Chapter 5), in U.S. Sentencing Commission 2002 Federal Sentencing Guideline Manual. Available at: http://www.ussc.gov/2002guid/CHAP5.htm. Accessed November 11, 2003.

Wiederanders MR, Bromley DL, Choate PA: Forensic conditional release programs and outcomes in three states. Int J Law Psychiatry 20:249–257, 1997

Legal Issues Regarding the Provision of Mental Health Care in Correctional Settings

Fred Cohen, LL.B., LL.M.

Joan B. Gerbasi, J.D., M.D.

Inmates in jails and prisons, before or after conviction, have a constitutionally based claim to adequate treatment for their serious mental illness. Custodians and clinicians alike may not be deliberately indifferent to an inmate's need for treatment of a serious mental or physical illness (Estelle v. Gamble 1976). These two sentences seem reasonably straightforward, yet they contain some basic legal concepts that are arcane, others that are not clearly defined, and some that are not always agreed on.

How is mental illness defined for correctional treatment purposes? What is a *serious* mental illness? What is deliberate indifference? What constitutes adequate treatment, and what are the consequences of failure to provide it? These questions and their answers rest on the more basic platform of why inmates are constitutionally entitled to care when nonoffending and seriously ill free persons are not so entitled.

In this chapter, we discuss the legal issues relevant to correctional mental health care. In the first section, we outline the constitutional basis of the right to treatment in jails and prisons and the scope of that right. In the second section, we outline the type and extent of care that is legally required and, in the third section, address a variety of procedural issues that arise in caring for mentally ill inmates. For a more comprehensive discussion of legal issues relevant to correctional psychiatry, the reader is directed to Fred Cohen's text *The Mentally Disordered Inmate and the Law* and its 2003 cumulative supplement (Cohen 1998, 2003).

THE BASIC PREMISE: THE LEGAL RIGHT TO TREATMENT

It is a general principle basic to our scheme of government that absent a "special relationship," of which physical custody is one, our government does not owe any affirmative obligations to its citizens. The government has no general obligation to provide housing, employment, safety, or medical care to the general population. However, when an individual is in the state's custody, this lack of obligations changes. In *DeShaney v. Winnebago Department of Social Services* (1989), the U.S. Supreme Court explained the constitutional basis of the government's basic obligation to protect and care for its citizens. In the Court's opinion, Chief Justice Rehnquist wrote,

> [W]hen the State takes a person into its custody and holds him there against his will, the Constitution imposes upon it a corresponding duty to assume some responsibility for his safety and general well-being. The rationale for this principle is simple enough: when the State by the affirmative exercise of its power so restrains an individual's liberty that it renders him unable to care for himself, and at the same time fails to provide for his basic human needs—e.g., food, clothing, shelter, medical care, and reasonable safety—it transgresses the substantive limits on state action set by the Eighth Amendment and the Due Process Clause. (489 U.S. 189, 200)

DeShaney accomplishes at least two significant things. It makes clear that without actual physical custody, government has no obligation to provide services. However, with official custody there arises an obligation to protect and preserve life, including the treatment of serious medical and mental illnesses.

Duty and the Mental Element

In law, where one party has a duty, someone else possesses a right. The duty at hand is the provision of treatment for seriously ill inmates, who, in turn, have a right to at least minimally adequate care. Under what conditions does that duty to provide care arise? The answer is not so simple. Part of the difficulty stems from the fact that mental illness is not necessarily obvious. It can often be discovered only by mental health evaluation. Under what circumstances, then, must psychiatric care be given? Does an inmate need to request care in order for the duty to arise, or are there certain situations that require evaluation and treatment, regardless of whether the inmate has requested treatment?

The U.S. Supreme Court has twice addressed this issue. First, in *Estelle v. Gamble* (1976), the Court elucidated the general duty. In that case, Mr. Gamble, a prisoner in a Texas state prison, injured his back while performing a prison work assignment. He complained of pain and received multiple evaluations and treatments but reported that his pain persisted. After being disciplined for failure to work and placed in solitary confinement, Gamble instituted a civil rights action for damages under 42 U.S.C. § 1983 against certain prison officials, including the chief medical officer of the prison. He claimed that his Eighth Amendment rights had been violated. The Eighth Amendment to the U.S. Constitution, as made applicable to the states through the Fourteenth Amendment, prohibits cruel and unusual punishment. Gamble argued that the officials' alleged failure to deliver appropriate medical care constituted such punishment.

The Court reviewed the history of the Eighth Amendment and noted that the primary concern of the drafters of the Constitution was "'torture[s]' and other 'barbar[ous]' methods of punishment," but that, over time, the Eighth Amendment has been interpreted to prescribe punishments that "are incompatible with the evolving standards of decency that mark the progress of a maturing society" (429 U.S. 97, at 102; internal citations omitted). The Court stated that denying inmates needed medical care rises to this level:

> An inmate must rely on prison authorities to treat his medical needs; if the authorities fail to do so, those needs will not be met. In the worst cases, such a failure may actually produce physical 'torture or a lingering death,' the evils of most immediate concern to the drafters of the Constitution. (429 U.S. 97, at 103)

The Court further stated, however, that in order to successfully allege a violation of Eighth Amendment rights, an inmate must show that prison officials showed *deliberate indifference* to the inmate's serious medical needs:

> [D]eliberate indifference to serious medical needs of prisoners constitutes the "unnecessary and wanton infliction of pain," proscribed by the Eighth Amendment. This is true whether the indifference is manifested by prison doctors in their response to the prisoner's needs or by prison guards in intentionally denying or delaying access to medical care or intentionally interfering

with the treatment once prescribed. (429 U.S. 97, 104–105; internal citations and footnotes omitted)

The *Gamble* Court did not, however, define deliberate indifference. It did state that mere negligence in diagnosing or treating a medical complaint would not be sufficient to state a valid claim under the Eighth Amendment. According to the *Gamble* Court, "Medical malpractice does not become a constitutional violation merely because the victim is a prisoner. In order to state a cognizable claim, a prisoner must allege acts or omissions sufficiently harmful to evidence deliberate indifference to serious medical needs. It is only such indifference that can offend 'evolving standards of decency' in violation of the Eighth Amendment" (429 U.S. 97, 106; footnotes omitted). In Mr. Gamble's case, the Court observed that he had been seen by medical personnel 17 times over a 3-month period and had been provided treatments for his complaints, albeit not the ones Mr. Gamble thought he should have. They concluded that this care did not constitute deliberate indifference.

It was not until 18 years later that the Supreme Court finally defined the seemingly oxymoronic term *deliberate indifference*. The case of *Farmer v. Brennan* (1974) involved Dee Farmer, a preoperative male-to-female transsexual who was beaten and raped in the general population of a federal prison. She alleged a violation of her Eighth Amendment rights and claimed that the failure to house her in segregation constituted deliberate indifference to her psychiatric disorder. In ruling that her rights had not been violated, the Court stated that deliberate indifference is more than negligence (the failure to use such care as a reasonably prudent person would use under similar circumstances), but less than acts or omissions for the purpose of causing harm or with knowledge of a likely harmful result. It specifically defined deliberate indifference as subjective recklessness: the responsible party must know of and disregard the inmate's condition and needs. It is the knowing disregard of an excessive risk to an inmate's health or safety; the official must know the facts creating the risk and must actually draw the inference as to risk. The Court did state that proof of actual knowledge can include the obviousness of a risk and its disregard, despite a defendant's impassioned, "I didn't know." The Court emphasized that liability in civil actions such as medical malpractice brought in state courts may exist when acts or omissions are not accompanied by the knowledge requirement of the deliberate indifference standard. However, without the actual knowledge of the risk, the act or omission cannot be condemned as the infliction of punishment prohibited by the Eighth Amendment.

Deliberate indifference, then, is the culpable mental state required to support either an Eighth Amendment claim for damages or injunctive-type relief in an individual or class action. However, it is important to remember that individual health care professionals may still be found personally liable in medical malpractice. Physicians and other professionals have an additional duty to practice within the relevant standard of care in their profession. This is as true in jails and prisons as it is in the community. Therefore, although malpractice, or negligence, alone will not support a constitutional claim, it will support a state law–based claim.

An Ohio court recently defined medical malpractice as follows:

> [I]n order to establish medical malpractice, it must be shown by a preponderance of the evidence that the injury complained of was caused by the doing of some particular thing or things that a physician or surgeon [in this case a psychiatrist] of ordinary skill, care and diligence would not have done under like or similar conditions or circumstances, or by the failure or omission to do some particular thing or things that such a physician or surgeon would have done under like or similar conditions and circumstances, and that the injury complained of was the direct result of such doing or failing to do some one or more of such particular things. (Pratt v. SOCF 2003)

Although exact standards vary from state to state, a claim of medical malpractice requires that the plaintiff prove four elements: 1) the defendant owed a duty to the plaintiff, 2) this duty was breached by care that was below the relevant standard of care, 3) the breach was the legal cause of the plaintiff's injury, and 4) the plaintiff suffered actual damages.

Consider the above case of *Pratt v. SOCF,* a case in Ohio in 2003. The plaintiff inmate Pratt received an initial intake screening by a nurse and was evaluated soon thereafter by a psychiatrist and a multidisciplinary treatment team. Pratt was continued on the mental health caseload, but medication was deemed not clinically indicated. Pratt subsequently sued and based his claim for damages on a delay in receiving psychiatric medication. This claim was rejected as neither malpractice nor deliberate indifference. Viewed in the light most favorable to plaintiff Pratt, this is at most a disagreement as to a course of treatment. Liability will not be found when, as here, there is a reasonable exercise of professional judgment. If Pratt, for example, had been receiving psychotropic medicine at the prison from which he transferred and that medication was summarily discontinued without a study of the records or individual diagnosis, then a good case for deliberate indifference—to say nothing of the easier-to-prove malpractice—could exist.

"Serious Medical Needs"

Although the Supreme Court has provided a definition of deliberate indifference, it has not similarly defined or described what constitutes a "serious medical need." *Estelle v. Gamble* (1976) dealt with medical treatment and not psychiatric care. *Bowring v. Godwin* (1976) was the first federal decision to clearly extend the *Estelle v. Gamble* requirements to psychiatric care. In its decision, the court noted:

> We see no underlying distinction between the right to medical care for physical ills and its psychological or psychiatric counterpart. Modern science has rejected the notion that mental or emotional disturbances are the products of afflicted souls, hence beyond the purview of counseling, medication and therapy. (551 F.2d 44, 47)

It is now well settled that psychiatric care is included within the Supreme Court's definition of "serious medical needs."

The requisite seriousness of an illness is not as clearly defined. Since an inmate's basic right to treatment flows from the Eighth Amendment's proscription of cruel and unusual punishment, the Supreme Court would likely look to the extent of present suffering and future consequences of a failure to medically intervene to determine whether an illness is "serious." The various federal courts of appeal have grappled with the meaning of *serious* and have developed two competing tests, with several variations of each. One is the "obvious to a layman" test described in *Ramos v. Lamm* (1981), a 1980 Tenth Circuit decision in which the court stated, "A medical need is serious if it is one that has been diagnosed by a physician as mandating treatment or one that is so obvious that even a lay person would easily recognize the necessity for a doctor's attention." (639 F.2d 559, 575; citation omitted). The second test is the "doctor's judgment" test, coupled with the extent of pain and consequences of failure to intervene. Under this test, a medical condition is sufficiently serious if a doctor "would find [it] important and worthy of comment or treatment" and if failure to treat the condition could result in further significant injury or the "unnecessary and wanton infliction of pain" (McGuckin v. Smith 1992).

In Ohio, influenced by the consent decree in *Dunn v. Voinovich* (1993), the Ohio Department of Rehabilitation and Correction uses the following definition:

> A substantial disorder of thought or mood that (1) significantly impairs judgment, behavior, or the capacity to recognize reality or cope with the ordinary demands of life within the prison environment and (2) is manifested by substantial pain or disability. Serious mental illness requires a mental health diagnosis, prognosis, and treatment, as appropriate, by mental health staff. It is expressly understood that this definition does not include inmates who are substance abusers or substance dependent (including alcoholics and narcotic addicts), or inmates convicted of a sex offense who are not otherwise diagnosed as seriously mentally ill.

While not suggesting that this definition is judicially required, we are confident that it would be judicially approved. We recognize also that ultimately professional judgment will hold sway and that reasonable disagreements will occur. Correction officials, however, who rely on expert clinical judgment utilizing this definition certainly will not be deliberately indifferent on the "seriousness" issue.

Often a legal battle over whether a disorder is "serious" enough is actually a battle over whether the condition at issue is a disease. Gender identity disorder (GID) is an excellent example of a disorder for which there is debate about, first, whether it fits the requisite medical model and, second, the seriousness of the disorder, the necessity for treatment, and the types of treatment indicated. *Kosilek v. Maloney* (2002) determined that GID is a serious mental disorder and that clinical judgment is required to determine the appropriateness of treatment. The treatment choices ranged from supportive counseling to hormonal treatment to surgery.

In *Kosilek,* the Massachusetts Department of Corrections had adopted a freeze-frame policy and focused on Kosilek's medical status at the time of his arrest. For Kosilek this meant he did not get hormones, since he was not legally taking them in the community. While holding that an inmate is not entitled to the best or most desired treatment, Federal District Court Judge Wolf also held that clinical judgment, and not economics or political repercussions, must dictate the treatment.

While the law clearly is lacking a precise definition of *seriousness,* some generalities in assessing seriousness may be distilled from the case law outlined in Table 12–1 (Cohen 1998, pp. 4–36).

TABLE 12–1. Important points from case law regarding assessment of serious medical needs

- To successfully allege that an illness was not appropriately assessed and treated, the diagnostic test or evaluation not completed must have been one of medical or psychiatric necessity. An inmate's reports of minor aches, pains, or distress will not establish such necessity.

- A desire to achieve rehabilitation from alcohol or drug abuse, or to lose weight to simply look or feel better, will not suffice.

- A diagnosis based on professional judgment and resting on some acceptable diagnostic tool (e.g., DSM-IV-TR) is presumptively valid.

- A decision by a mental health professional that mental illness is not present is presumptively valid.

- While "mere depression" or behavioral and emotional problems alone do not qualify as serious mental illness, acute depression, paranoid schizophrenia, "nervous collapse," and suicidal tendencies do qualify.

Pretrial Detainees

The discussion thus far has focused on the Eighth Amendment's prohibition against cruel and unusual punishment as the source of an inmate's right to medical treatment. Eighth Amendment rights do not, however, attach until a defendant has been convicted of a crime. In *Bell v. Wolfish* (1979), the U.S. Supreme Court held that in contrast to a convicted prisoner's right not to be subjected to cruel and unusual punishment, pretrial detainees could not be punished *at all*. As such, the Eighth Amendment cannot be the source of protection for inmates in jails who are awaiting trial.

Pretrial detainees, however, are entitled to at least the same degree of care as are inmates in prison (Hott v. Hennepin County 2001). The source of this right, however, is the due process clause of the Fourteenth Amendment. The clause states, "[No State] shall deprive any person of life, liberty, or property, without due process of law" (U.S. Constitutional Amendment XIV, § 2). *Due process* is a complicated legal doctrine that includes both a procedural and a substantive component. In our context, it is the substantive component—the term *liberty* itself—that contains the detainee's right to medical care. Deliberate indifference to the serious medical needs of pretrial detainees violates the due process clause because such conduct "could well result in the deprivation of life itself" (Fitzke v. Shappell 1972; quoting from McCollum v. Mayfield 1955). The *Fitzke* court stated:

> An individual incarcerated, whether for a term of life for the commission of some heinous crime, or merely for the night to "dry out" in the local drunk tank, becomes both vulnerable and dependent upon the state to provide certain simple and basic human needs....Denial of necessary medical attention may well result in disabilities beyond that contemplated by the incarceration itself....[F]undamental fairness and our most basic conception of due process mandate that medical care be provided to one who is incarcerated and may be suffering from serious illness or injury. (Fitzke v Shappell, 468 F.2d 1072, 1076; emphasis and internal citations omitted)

As described later in this chapter, inmates in jail present different problems than inmates in prisons. Long-term care is not an issue, but short-term care, acute crisis treatment, substance intoxication and detoxification, and management of suicide risk are all present. Jail programs must, therefore, be aware of these different needs and adjust their diagnostic (or screening) and treatment programs accordingly.

SYSTEM ASSESSMENT— WHAT IS ADEQUATE CARE?

The foundational litigation of the 1970s focused on prisons and jails that had virtually no system for providing mental health care. These earlier "no care" cases have morphed into hundreds of essentially quality-of-care or denial-of-access cases, since every jurisdiction now has some type of mental health care system (Human Rights Watch 2003). Despite this large and growing body of case law, a handful of important federal decisions have established some basic requirements for constitutionally adequate care. In 1980, a federal district court in Texas initially decided the case of *Ruiz v. Estelle* (1983), a class action lawsuit attacking the mental health system in the Texas Department of Corrections. In finding the conditions in Texas prisons unconstitutional, Judge Justice identified six components for a minimally adequate mental health treatment program:

1. A systematic program for screening and evaluating inmates must be in place to identify those who require mental health treatment.
2. Treatment must entail more than segregation and close supervision of the inmate patients.
3. Treatment requires the participation of trained mental health professionals, who must be employed in sufficient numbers to identify and treat in an individualized manner those treatable inmates with serious mental disorders.
4. Accurate, complete, and confidential records of the mental health treatment process must be maintained.
5. Prescription and administration of behavior-altering medications in dangerous amounts, by dangerous methods, or without appropriate supervision and periodic evaluations are unacceptable.
6. A basic program for the identification, treatment, and supervision of inmates with suicidal tendencies is a necessary component of any mental health treatment program.

Since the *Ruiz* decision, additional cases have made it clear that a constitutionally adequate system would also include adequate human and physical (bed space) resources dedicated to mental health and an effective process of inmate access to such resources. There are no legally mandated ratios for staff or beds; it is the availability of care by persons trained to provide it that matters, not whether one is top-heavy with doctors or whether hospital care is within or outside the Department of Corrections. The courts will not judge a system by measuring outcomes; *it will judge it by inmate access to trained caregivers in an environment conducive to treatment.*

In *Langley v. Coughlin* (1989), the New York prison system was found to be unconstitutional. The district court developed an extensive checklist for adequate access and care that was even more detailed than the list developed in *Ruiz*. In the *Langley* court's opinion, the following factors would be unacceptable characteristics of a mental health system (Cohen 1998, pp. 7–9):

1. Failure to take a complete medical (or psychiatric) record
2. Failure to keep adequate records
3. Failure to respond to inmates' prior psychiatric history
4. Failure to at least place under observation inmates suffering a mental health crisis
5. Failure to properly diagnose mental conditions
6. Failure to properly prescribe medications
7. Failure to provide meaningful treatment other than drugs
8. Failure to explain treatment refusals, diagnosis, and ending of treatment
9. Seemingly cavalier refusals to consider bizarre behavior as mental illness even when a prior diagnosis existed
10. Personnel doing things for which they are not trained

Distinguishing *required,* as above, from *desired* is most important. Striving only to meet minimal constitutional requirements while understanding that whatever goals are set are unlikely to be met virtually ensures failure and vulnerability to lawsuits. In Table 12–2, we outline the minimum mental health treatment requirements in a correctional setting. In the appendix to this chapter, we provide a more comprehensive listing of required and desired treatment program components that serves both as a guide to program creation and as a model for quality assurance–type assessment.

Suicide Prevention

As discussed in more detail in Chapter 4 ("Suicide Prevention in Correctional Facilities"), incarcerated individuals are far more likely to commit suicide than individuals in the general population. Individuals in jails, as opposed to prisons, are particularly at risk. The stress of arrest or conviction, along with guilt and shame, often compounds other suicide risk factors individuals may have, including substance abuse. For some, facing the prospect of conviction or serving a prison sentence is unbearable, and suicide becomes the only viable option. The task for mental health professionals working in jails and prisons is to recognize these risks and implement a system of care that provides appropriate assessment, treatment, and monitoring of suicidal inmates.

Because most jail suicides take place within 24–48 hours of arrest, the initial task falls on corrections staff at intake. They must be trained to identify risk factors, take precautionary measures, and contact mental health professionals. Mental health and corrections staff should work together to develop guidelines and an action plan.

In the civil hospital setting, inpatient suicides are much more difficult to defend than outpatient suicides because inpatients are under the hospital's control and have often been admitted to the hospital to treat suicidality. In

TABLE 12–2.   Minimum requirements for mental health
treatment programs

- Mental health screening and evaluation
- Treatment, not merely segregation or medication
- Adequate numbers of trained mental health professionals
- Confidential mental health records
- Appropriate prescription of psychotropic medications
- Suicide prevention program
- Inmate access to treatment
- Adequate physical space

some respects, jail or prison is similar to the inpatient setting in that inmates
are captive in the facility and cannot seek care or help elsewhere. Under the
DeShaney principle, when the government holds a person against his or her
will, there is a duty to assume some responsibility for the person's safety and
general well-being. It may seem a natural extension of this principle that jail-
ers would be held accountable for suicides that occur within their walls.

In reality, however, liability for custodial suicide is relatively rare. Recall
that prison officials' duty to inmates is that they not be deliberately indifferent
to the inmates' serious mental illness, with a mental requirement of subjective
recklessness. To show that deliberate indifference resulted in a suicide, the
"plaintiff must show that the jail official displayed deliberate indifference to
the prisoner's taking of his own life" (Edwards v. Gilbert 1989). The deliberate
indifference standard "requires a strong likelihood rather than a mere possibility that the self-infliction of harm will occur" (Popham v. City of Talladega
1990). The official must have been aware of the risk of suicide and have dis-
regarded it.

Even in a case in which an inmate was known to be suicidal but was
placed in an inpatient psychiatric unit where he suffocated himself with a plastic bag, the reviewing court found no deliberate indifference (Estate of Max
G. Cole v. Fromm 1996). Likewise, no liability was found in a case in which
a patient told officers during the booking process that he had attempted suicide 2 days before and the officers interpreted the statement as a joke from a
"happy drunk" and did not place him in a suicide watch cell, and he hung
himself 45 minutes later (Estate of James Boncher v. Brown County 2001).
In a case in which a pretrial detainee committed suicide while on suicide
watch but during a time when staff was unavailable to monitor the cell, the
Eleventh Circuit ruled that summary judgment in favor of all defendants was
appropriate (Cagle v. Sutherland 2003). The *Cagle* court found that allowing
1 hour and 40 minutes to elapse between checks did not show deliberate in-

difference, in part because the inmate had been stripped of his belt and shoe-laces, as well as the contents of his pockets, which would have reduced his risk (he hung himself with the elastic from his underwear).

Liability, however, is not impossible, and, of course, malpractice liability may be present when constitutional violations are not. In a review of lawsuits involving custodial suicides, the following questions emerge as relevant to outcome (Cohen 1998, pp. 2–15):

1. Did the facility have a basic program or protocol in place to respond to suicidality?
2. Was adequately trained staff in place in adequate numbers?
3. Is the structure of the facility itself a contributory factor?
4. Was staff response to the actual situation in compliance with the established suicide prevention program and adequate to the demands of the situation?
5. Was the victim being monitored for suicide?
6. Were clinical (as opposed to custodial) personnel involved? If not, why not? And if so, when and how?

Confidentiality

Delivering care within the confines of a jail or prison that is on par with the relevant standard of care in the community always will be constitutionally adequate. However, the parameters of confidentiality of the clinician–patient relationship in jails and prisons are markedly different from those in the community.

Confidentiality of the clinician–patient relationship is grounded in ethical and legal principles. It rests, in part, on the assumption that a patient will be deterred from seeking care and discussing the important matters relevant to therapy if there is not some guaranteed confidentiality in that relationship. Indeed, even the U.S. Supreme Court has recognized a broad therapist–patient privilege (Jaffe v. Redmond 1996). While there are certain well-recognized limitations on the confidentiality of the relationship, including the so-called *Tarasoff* "duty to protect" exception, these exceptions are generally limited (Tarasoff v. Regents of the University of California 1976). The *Tarasoff* exception applies when a patient tells the therapist that he or she intends to harm a readily identifiable person.

In penal confinement, however, the principles may remain the same but the situation is different. Confidentiality is limited both by the various individual interests at play and by the physical environment of jails and prisons—an environment in which privacy is extremely compromised. The problem of maintaining confidentiality arises regularly with cell-front mental health contacts, particularly in segregation; special pill calls for those in general population; housing reserved for those with mental illness; and the requirement that security staff be present or nearby during individual or group treatment sessions. This list of situations alone—and there are others—demonstrates the impossibility of visual confidentiality in a jail or prison setting. The most that can be realistically required within the confines of a jail or prison is auditory privacy and the privacy of medical records. These are the areas that require legally safeguarded protection.

In general, written records in a correctional setting enjoy the same protection they enjoy in the community. Practitioners should familiarize themselves with relevant state and federal laws with respect to medical records. Generally, those laws require the patient's written consent for the release of the actual record to those outside the treatment team. However, certain information obtained in the course of evaluation and treatment is not protected and must be shared with relevant prison officials, because a prison setting creates a set of security concerns much broader than those in the outside world. For example, a patient in the community could tell his psychiatrist that he purchased an illegal gun for protection in his home without fear that the psychiatrist would notify the police. In prison, however, if a psychiatrist became aware that one of his patients had a cache of razor blades or other weapons, this information would need to be communicated to the authorities.

Recognizing that the law on point is quite unsettled, we suggest that corrections officials, working with a clinical team, develop policies guiding the sharing of limited information when an inmate is identified as one of the following:

- Being suicidal
- Being homicidal
- Presenting a reasonably clear danger of injury to self or to others, by virtue of either conduct or oral statements
- Presenting a reasonably clear risk of escape or the creation of internal disorder or riot
- Receiving psychotropic medication or being noncompliant with medication
- Requiring movement to a special unit for observation, evaluation, or treatment of acute episodes
- Requiring transfer to a treatment facility outside the prison or jail

Only that illness-related information directly related to the need should be shared, and sharing should be limited to those within the ambit of the concern or activity. It makes sense for an officer to know that an inmate on his or her unit is taking medication, that the medication causes drowsiness, and that the inmate may act in a certain fashion if noncompliant. An officer need not be told about an inmate-patient's hatred of his father, sexual conflicts, or similar matters. When an officer is part of a treatment team—an increasingly popular measure—it is absurd to pretend there is confidentiality as regards that officer. The key, however, is to build into officer training the need to not discuss the case and to impose employment-related penalties for unauthorized disclosures.

Additionally, in the forensic setting, clinicians come in contact with patient-inmates in a variety of contexts, with differing limits on confidentiality. For example, information obtained in the course of psychiatric evaluation and treatment would generally be protected, but information obtained in the context of a court-ordered evaluation would not. These evaluations include evaluations of competency to stand trial and of criminal responsibility and parole/probation reports. It is always the evaluator's responsibility to inform the person being evaluated of the purpose of the evaluation, the limits of confidentiality, and the persons to whom the information will be reported.

Even in treatment settings, clinicians should clearly specify any limits on the usually expected confidentiality of the patient–clinician relationship. This disclosure should occur at the outset of treatment, except in emergencies. Clinicians should familiarize themselves with the rules of their particular institutions in this regard. Notwithstanding these necessary limits on confidentiality, relevant ethical guidelines, such as the APA's *The Principles of Medical Ethics, With Annotations Especially Applicable to Psychiatry* (2001), should be adhered to with the greatest degree possible.

PROCEDURAL ISSUES

It may seem peculiar to lump in one section, as we do here, the legal issues of transfer of an inmate to a mental hospital, forced medication, and prison discipline. In the previous sections of this chapter, we have discussed substantive matters, that is, the "what" of a problem. Now we shift our emphasis to "how" something is done. The "how" question is process, whereas the "what" is substance.

Transfer for Treatment

In *Vitek v. Jones* (1980), the Supreme Court determined that the stigmatizing effects of a transfer to a hospital for involuntary psychiatric treatment, coupled with subjection of the inmate to involuntary treatment, represent the type of deprivation that requires the procedural due process afforded by the Fourteenth Amendment. The case involved Mr. Jones, an inmate convicted of robbery. While in prison, he was placed in solitary confinement, where he set his mattress on fire and suffered severe burns to his body. After treatment in the burn unit, he was transferred to the security unit of a prison mental hospital. Under relevant Nebraska law, the transfer required only that a physician or psychologist find that Mr. Jones suffered from a mental disease or defect and could not be given proper treatment in prison.

In finding that the Nebraska transfer scheme violated the due process clause of the Fourteenth Amendment to the U.S. Constitution, the Supreme Court observed that even after conviction and imprisonment, Jones retained a liberty interest that would be infringed on by transfer to a mental hospital. Commitment to a mental hospital was characterized as a "massive curtailment of liberty" that not only includes involuntary confinement but also causes social stigma and requires prisoners to comply with mandatory behavioral treatment that they would not have to comply with in prison.

To safeguard this liberty interest and protect it from unjust infringement, the *Vitek* court described the following minimum procedural protections that must be in place before transfers can be made:

1. A written notice to the prisoner that a transfer to a mental hospital is being considered
2. A hearing, sufficiently after the notice to permit the prisoner to prepare, at which disclosure to the prisoner is made of the evidence being relied on for the transfer and where the prisoner receives an opportunity to be heard in person and to present documentary evidence
3. An opportunity at the hearing for the defense to present testimony of witnesses and to confront and cross-examine witnesses called by the state, except upon a finding, not arbitrarily made, of good cause for not permitting such presentation, confrontation, or cross-examination
4. An independent decision-maker (the person need not come from outside the prison or hospital administration)
5. A written statement by the decision-maker as to the evidence relied on and the reasons for transferring the inmate
6. Availability of "qualified and independent assistance" furnished by the state, if the inmate is financially unable to furnish his or her own (this does not include the right to legal counsel)
7. Effective and timely notice of all the foregoing rights

These are minimum safeguards, or a floor, and any jurisdiction is free to fashion a more protective procedural format. *Vitek* appears to be one of those judicial decisions that has worked its way into a general culture of compliance in the world of prisons. Few decisions will be found today even discussing *Vitek*-like issues.

Vitek applies to transfers to mental hospitals. Prison-to-prison transfers are not encompassed by due process, and neither are classification-treatment decisions that lead to housing in a prison's mental health unit. *Vitek* used the term *mental hospital* for the due process trigger. Short-term transfers for evaluation, crisis stabilization, or a similar psychiatric emergency also are not encompassed by *Vitek*.

Right to Refuse Treatment and Forced Medication

In *Washington v. Harper* (1990), a decade after *Vitek,* the Supreme Court recognized a substantial liberty interest on the part of inmates to resist unwanted psychotropic medication. The majority first held that the due process clause of the Fourteenth Amendment permits prison officials to treat a prisoner who is medically diagnosed as having a serious mental illness with antipsychotic drugs against his or her will if the inmate is dangerous to self or others and the treatment is in the inmate's medical interest. This, in effect, established the state's substantive rights and diminished those of the inmate, who, inter alia, contended that he must also be found to be incompetent to consent to medications before being forcibly medicated.

Walter Harper had extensive experience with the Washington State prison system and its efforts to provide him with mental health care. Harper at first consented to the administration of antipsychotic drugs. He then experienced side effects that caused him to say he would rather die than continue with the medication. The treating physician then followed Washington's procedures to medicate Harper over his objection. The Washington policy provided for both the substantive and procedural grounds for the incursion on the inmate's protected liberty interest.

The Court upheld the Washington procedural format without expressly providing a minimally acceptable procedural format. The Washington format included various procedural protections, including a hearing before an internal independent committee; the right to notice; the opportunity for the inmate to present his own evidence at the hearing and to cross-examine the hospital's witnesses; the assistance of a lay adviser who understands the relevant psychiatric issues; and the right to an appeal. Importantly, the Court held that an internal committee, and not a judicial decision-maker, would fulfill relevant due process requirements (Washington v. Harper 1990).

Harper, like *Vitek,* is not applicable to a psychiatric emergency in which medication is a part of a control arsenal that includes seclusion, restraint, or even a chemical spray. *Harper* issues, again like those pertaining to *Vitek,* now are rarely litigated.

Disciplinary Proceedings

Under certain conditions a prison inmate is entitled to a due process (or *Wolff*) hearing before disciplinary punishment may be imposed. In *Sandin v. Conner* (1995), the Court held that a due process hearing is not required unless there may be an atypical, significant deprivation, which is the liberty interest protected here by the due process clause of the Fourteenth Amendment. Prior to *Sandin,* disciplinary segregation itself would require a so-called *Wolff* hearing. Now extraordinarily long terms in segregation are found not to require such a hearing, which is even less procedurally demanding than those required in *Vitek* or *Harper.* The niceties of the hearing process and liberty interest analysis are beyond the scope of this chapter. Suffice it to say that the *Wolff* hearing format remains unchanged, although the number of occasions when such is required was reduced by *Sandin.*

If an inmate, then, is constitutionally entitled to a disciplinary hearing—and that includes the right to be present—must the inmate be competent in the sense of being triable? Does an inmate's serious mental illness afford a defense to the charge? Should an inmate's mental illness be considered as part of any dispositional process?

As for competency, no hearing should be viewed as constitutionally acceptable unless the inmate understands the charges, is able to participate in his or her own defense, and understands the consequences of such a hearing. There is virtually no case law on point, but every correctional system should be certain that there is a procedure to establish on the record the trial (or hearing) competency of an accused.

There is no formal recognition of an administrative insanity defense. That is, no matter how ill the inmate is, no matter how directly related to the illness the misconduct and harm are, prison officials legally need not excuse the misconduct on the basis of mental illness. However, many jurisdictions informally allow their hearing officials to find an inmate with mental illness guilty and then impose a "time served" sanction. Additionally, an inmate's mental illness always should play a role in fashioning a disposition. Someone involved in treatment should advise the disciplinary officials of the likely impact on treatment of a particular disposition, especially when segregation is possible.

Segregation

A flashpoint for many mentally ill prisoners is being placed in some form of segregated housing. The behavior of some inmates with serious mental illness can become a nightmare for staff. Locking up the "disturbed, disruptive inmate," to borrow Hans Toch's (1997, p. 126) term, moves the problem somewhat out of sight, but it hardly addresses the inmate's condition. Indeed, the problems are likely to be exacerbated and the disruptiveness merely transferred to a different area. Chapter 10 ("Offenders With Mental Illnesses in Maximum- and Supermaximum-Security Settings") describes in detail the challenges facing offenders with mental illness in maximum and supermaximum security settings.

Mental health services are difficult and expensive to deliver in these settings. For example, if a psychiatrist is able to see eight inmate-patients a day in a less secure setting, the doctor likely will see only four because of the search and escort delays. Too often, there simply are no services, with the possible exception of "drive-by" mental health rounds.

The number of inmates held in segregation on any given day is unknown, but a recent study estimated that number as 20,000 inmates, with the mentally ill disproportionately represented (Human Rights Watch 2000, p. 3). Fred Cohen recently testified:

> [In] all of the systems that I have studied in one fashion or another, if a prison system has gone bad or is bad…in its provision of mental health care, what you have to do is go to the segregation units and you will find the sickest people locked down, unattended to, and it is the way that a malfunctioning prison system operates to hide their mentally ill. [I have found this in]…every system that I have ever looked at and the poorer the system, the more serious the conditions, the [worse the] deterioration, [the more] terrible [the] nightmare for the inmate. (Testimony of Fred Cohen 2001)

Placing the mentally ill inmate in segregation either as discipline or for administrative purposes raises a number of legal issues. If the inmate is seriously mentally ill and adequate treatment, however defined, is somehow provided, the environment itself may be attacked as so counterproductive that the placement violates the Eighth Amendment.

In *Jones El' v. Berge* (2001), involving the Wisconsin Supermax in Boscobel, Judge Barbara Crabb granted the plaintiff-inmates' request for a preliminary injunction that encompasses supermax prisons and that also plainly implicates segregation units within other prisons having conditions of confinement as stringent as a supermax. In brief, the court ordered that inmates identified as seriously mentally ill may not be housed at Wisconsin's supermax and that supermax inmates at risk of having serious mental illness must be evaluated pursuant to the court's order. A few prisoners identified as seriously mentally ill and previously transferred were ordered not to be returned to supermax.

Ohio, as a matter of policy, excludes the seriously mentally ill, as well as a group collectively characterized as "at risk," from its supermax. Ohio does have a high-security intensive treatment unit at the Southern Ohio Correctional Facility, which is designed for short-term placements. Indeed, the 40-cell unit has done just that, processing inmates from the unit to a residential treatment unit and ultimately into the general prison population.

It is clear that seriously mentally ill persons cannot simply be locked away in supermaxes or similarly restrictive segregation settings. On the other hand, some inmates with serious mental illness may be so disruptive and self-destructive that for their own protection and the protection of staff, relatively short-term high-security settings are required and are likely permissible, if adequate treatment is required (Lovell et al. 2000).

The Human Rights Watch (2003), in its study of prisoners and offenders with mental illness, captured the issues and needs beautifully when it noted:

> Mental health experts told us progress is possible, but requires paradigm shifts in which correction officials must relinquish some of the usual rules by which prisons operate. Facilities would have to be run according to treatment protocols as determined by mental health staff. Public officials would have to support a form of incarceration that differed markedly from the traditional prison and be willing to stand up to critics who would argue that such treatment-oriented facilities "coddled" the worst prisoners. Another obstacle, of course, would be funding. No one doubts that a treatment-oriented milieu for mentally ill prisoners who are disruptive must be labor-intensive—and hence expensive. Yet until the expense is undertaken, the vicious cycle of segregation and decompensation and short-term hospitalization will continue until the prisoners are ultimately released, at least as sick as they were upon entry into the criminal justice system, from prison back into the community. (p. 163)

Discharge Planning

As noted earlier, the *DeShaney* principle requires actual official custody before any duties to protect or treat arise. Logically, then, the duty to provide care should end at the back door to the prison as it begins at the front door. In this instance law and policy may actually trump logic. There is a nascent movement to extend the right to care, and the duty to provide it, at least for a brief period after discharge. When a seriously mentally ill inmate is released on parole, and a modified type of custody exists, an argument for continuing obligation may be a bit easier.

Wakefield v. Thompson (1999) opened the door to the expansion of the *DeShaney* principle, holding that a state must provide an outgoing prisoner who continues to require psychotropic medication with a supply sufficient to ensure availability during the time reasonably necessary to consult a doctor and receive a new supply. *Wakefield* did not mandate a community treatment plan, it did not require that government provide access to a doctor and medication, and it did not require that housing be made available. Thus, *Wakefield* is a very small step from the back door into the community, but legal developments often surge after such a small step.

Brad H. v. City of New York (2000) represents such a surge, although the duty of care is based exclusively on New York State law. The settlement gives jail inmates who receive mental health treatment while they are in New York City jails improved access to medications, Medicaid, treatment and services in the community, public benefits, housing or shelter, and transportation upon their release (Barr 2003). *Brad H.* is of no precedent-setting value outside of New York, based as it is on a New York law that requires that mental health treatment providers offer discharge planning to all patients. Litigants in other jurisdictions must find a similar state law or seek to expand the constitutionally based *Wakefield* claim.

That claim may be entitled one of "continuing obligation"—that is, having injected the state into the illness and treatment of a person, there is an obligation to continue that treatment. *Lugo v. Senkowsky* (2000) builds on *Wakefield* by holding that when surgery was performed on a prison inmate who required follow-up surgery for removal of a stent, the now-paroled inmate was entitled to that follow-up procedure.

Aftercare is an idea whose time may have arrived, nudged along by a few groundbreaking decisions. The American Association of Community Psychiatrists in December 1998 issued a strong position statement supportive of discharge planning along with detailed guidelines.

CONCLUSION

Convicted prisoners and pretrial detainees have a constitutional right to treatment of their serious mental illnesses. The right is founded in the Eighth and Fourteenth Amendments to the U.S. Constitution and mandates that prisons and jails not be deliberately indifferent to the inmate's serious medical needs. Deliberate indifference, however, is a relatively minimally demanding legal standard and requires actual knowledge of and disregard of a risk of harm. While constitutional liability will not attach absent this subjective recklessness, clinicians are still held to the malpractice negligence standard with respect to state law claims.

The past several decades have seen growing litigation about the extent of care that is constitutionally required. In general, services must be offered that are adequate to detect, assess, and treat serious mental illnesses and prevent suicide. Additionally, inmates must have ready access to those services. The quality of services offered must be tailored to the special needs of the prison environment, including a recognition of risks present in that environment, such as the increased risk of suicide. Over the past several decades, we have also seen judicial attention to the rights of inmates and a recognition that, despite their criminal status, inmates continue to be entitled to many of the procedural and substantive protections available to free individuals.

SUMMARY POINTS

- A "special relationship" arises in corrections when an individual is placed in official custody thereby creating an obligation to protect and preserve life.
- The Eighth Amendment prohibits cruel and unusual punishment of persons convicted.
- Deliberate indifference to needed medical care for convicted inmates with serious medical needs violates the Eighth Amendment.
- An inmate cannot be automatically transferred from a prison to a hospital for involuntary psychiatric treatment without procedural protections.
- Under certain conditions a prison inmate is entitled to a due-process hearing before disciplinary punishment may be imposed.

REFERENCES

American Psychiatric Association: The Principles of Medical Ethics, With Annotations Especially Applicable to Psychiatry. Washington, DC, American Psychiatric Association, 2001

Barr H: New York City agrees to provide services for jail releasees with mental illness. Correctional Mental Health Report 5:1, 2003

Bell v Wolfish, 441 U.S. 520 (1979)

Bowring v Godwin, 551 F.2d 44 (4th Cir. 1976)

Brad H. v City of New York, 712 NYS.2d 336 (Sup. Ct. 2000); 716 NYS.2d 852 (N.Y. App. Div. 2000)

Cagle v Sutherland, 334 F.3d 980 (11th Cir. 2003), rehearing, en banc, denied, 2003 U.S. App. LEXIS 25460 (11th Cir. 2003)

Cohen F: The Mentally Disordered Inmate and the Law. Kingston, NJ, Civic Research Institute, 1998

Cohen F: The Mentally Disordered Inmate and the Law, 2003 Cumulative Supplement. Kingston, NJ, Civic Research Institute, 2003

DeShaney v Winnebago Department of Social Services, 489 U.S. 189 (1989)

Dunn v Voinovich, Case No. C1-93–0166 (S.D. Ohio 1993)

Edwards v Gilbert, 867 F.2d 1271 (11th Cir. 1989)

Estate of James H. Boncher v Brown County, 272 F.3d 484 (7th Cir. 2001)

Estate of Max G. Cole v Fromm, 94 F.3d 254 (7th Cir. 1996), cert. denied, 117 S.Ct. 945 (1997)

Estelle v Gamble, 426 U.S. 97 (1976)

Farmer v Brennan, 511 U.S. 825 (1994)

Fitzke v Shappell, 468 F.2d 1072 (6th Cir. 1972)

Hott v Hennepin County, 260 F.3d 901 (8th Cir. 2001)

Human Rights Watch: Out of Sight: Super-Maximum Security Confinement in the United States. New York, Human Rights Watch, 2000. Available at: http://www.hrw.org/reports/2000/supermax/html. Accessed on December 30, 2004.

Human Rights Watch: Ill-Equipped: U.S. Prisons and Offenders With Mental Illness. New York, Human Rights Watch, 2003. Available at: http://www.hrw.org/reports/2003/usa1003/html. Accessed on December 30, 2004.

Jaffe v Redmond, 116 S.Ct. 1923 (1996)

Jones El' v Berge, 164 F.Supp.2d 1096 (W.D. Wis. 2001)

Kosilek v Maloney, 221 F.Supp.2d 156 (D. Mass. 2002)

Langley v Coughlin (715 F.Supp. 522, 540–541 (S.D.N.Y. 1989), aff'd, 888 F.2d 252 (2d Cir. 1989)

Lovell D, Cloyes K, Allen D, et al: Who lives in super-maximum custody? A Washington State study, Federal Probation, Vol 64, 2000

Lugo v Senkowsky, 114 F.Supp.2d 111 (N.D. N.Y. 2000)

McCollum v Mayfield, 130 F.Supp. 112 (N.D. Cal., 1955)

McGuckin v Smith, 974 F.2d 1050 (9th Cir. 1992)

Popham v City of Talladega, 908 F.2d 1561 (11th Cir. 1990)

Pratt v SOCF, WL 22285922, 2 (Ohio Ct. Cl. 2003)

Ramos v Lamm, 639 F.2d 559, cert. denied, 450 U.S. 1041 (1981)

Ruiz v Estelle, 503 F.Supp. 1265, 1339 (S.D. Tex. 1980), aff'd in part, 679 F.2d 1115 (5th Cir. 1982), cert denied, 460 U.S. 1042 (1983)

Sandin v Conner, 515 U.S. 472 (1995)

Shannon B: Diversion of offenders with mental illness: recent legislative reforms Texas style, Ment Phys Disabil Law Rep 20:431, 1996

Tarasoff v Regents of the University of California, 551 P.2d 334 (Cal. 1976)

Testimony of Fred Cohen, Preliminary Injunction Hearing, Austin v Wilkinson, No 4:01 CV 0071 (N.D. Ohio, September 24, 2001)

Toch H: Corrections: A Humanistic Approach. New York, Harrow & Heston, 1997

Vitek v Jones, 445 U.S. 480 (1980)

Wakefield v Thompson, 177 F.3d 1160 (9th Cir. 1999)

Washington v Harper, 494 U.S. 210, 215–217 (1990)

APPENDIX:
REQUIRED AND DESIRED TREATMENT PROGRAM COMPONENTS IN CORRECTIONAL SETTINGS

1. *Diversion of selected offenders with mental illness.* There is a virtual unanimity in the literature, and among experts, that too many prisoners with serious mental illness are swept into jail and prison, often for minor offenses. A progressive system would provide legal authorization for pretrial examinations and diversion to treatment where appropriate (Shannon 1996).

2. *Identification of inmates with mental illness upon entrance to the system.* Unless the system has in place mechanisms to identify those needing care, either at reception or after confinement, it simply cannot meet its treatment obli-

gations. Better systems will have a computerized classification and tracking system.

3. *Identification for appropriate care of those inmates with alcoholism, drug addiction, some form of sexual dysfunction, or problems associated with domestic violence, including "battered woman syndrome."* The conditions noted here generally fall outside of legally mandated care. Compliance with basic legal requirements, as noted, would encompass only the seriously mentally ill. However, a correctional system that is responsive to these impaired individuals is one that is a "full service" system and that in itself is deemed desirable.

4. *Training of staff on the signs and symptoms of mental disorders.* Identification of those who need care does not end at the front door, nor is it limited to mental health specialists. Security staff, especially those assigned to mental health special care units and to segregation units, must be able to identify those who need care and understand the behavior associated with the condition or any medications involved.

5. *Quantity and quality of human resources available for the various tasks associated with mental health treatment.* Mental health staff should be appropriately licensed and multidisciplinary and should function administratively in an integrated fashion. Staffing ratios for psychiatrists, psychologists, social workers, and others should be established at least as a rough guide for judging the objective quality of a system. Opportunities will exist for staff development and enrichment. "Burnout" and "dry out" seem endemic to staff members in this highly charged work area, and comprehensive programs will provide opportunities for growth and respite.

6. *Quantity and quality of physical resources available.* Obviously, a certain amount of physical space designed for various treatment or program objectives must be available. The available space should be designed to meet the needs for hospitalization: longer-term care needs not necessitating hospitalization; crisis care needs (e.g., suicide-watch placements); and perhaps needs for transitional care units and a special needs unit (e.g., housing for dually diagnosed inmates). Use of a "least restrictive environment" approach suggests enhanced concern for the inmates' needs.

7. *Access to care.* Without ready access to diagnosis and care, human and physical resources become virtually meaningless. Ensuring access calls for a study of waiting lists, response to "kites" (i.e., inmate written requests), knowledge by security staff and inmates on how to gain access, and appropriate training and orientation of inmates on gaining access. A model system would perform regular audits, question inmates and staff, assess the orientation process, and even do emergency "trial runs." In evaluating access, one necessarily also evaluates the relationship between security and mental health staff. Without a collaborative approach, no system will function very well.

8. *Content of records.* Records are crucial to the legal requirement of continuity of care. They are evidence of the care and are also instrumental in ensuring its quality. As a barometer of the quality of care, regular progress notes and a comprehensible individual treatment plan demonstrate whether appropriate care is being given and accommodate the regular personnel changes that are endemic to corrections. The legal concern here is with continuity of care, and it is the mental health record that is a necessary, although not sufficient, factor in meeting that obligation.

9. *Medication management.* There should be reasonable access to a psychiatrist and to a formulary that does not restrict access to the newer psychopharmacological agents. There must also be regular monitoring and testing. In systems that have rapid turnover or that use *locum tenens* (i.e., substitute) psychiatrists, special attention must be paid to medication practices, especially changes in medication.

10. *Restorative opportunities.* For the seriously mentally ill, medication may well be the treatment of choice, but it should not be the only treatment or programming available. For those not taking medication, it is even more important to have a full range of activities, along with individual and group therapy. These activities can include work opportunities, structured physical activities, horticultural programs, guide-dog training, vocational training, and the like. Programs dealing with anger management, social skills, and educational opportunities often enhance restorative opportunities.

11. *Management information system (MIS).* A model MIS should be computerized and used for needs assessment, CQI (Continuous Quality Improvement), and tracking. Model programs will produce concrete examples of how the MIS is used in the system.

12. *Data/research on treatment outcomes.* Comprehensive programs will not be content to simply "build, hire, and provide access." They will be concerned with the articulation of treatment objectives and be engaged in acceptable research on outcomes.

13. *Economy of scale.* Are the administrative and organizational structures designed to provide the maximum care for the funds allocated? Are services regionalized (or clustered)? Are services shared and accessible? Are the *actual* costs known?

14. *Policy procedure: contemporary, comprehensive, accessible.* In the interest of uniformity and consistency of practice, a system must have contemporary policy and procedures on point. They should be readily available and understandable. Special attention should be paid to issues such as transfer from correctional settings to mental hospitals, forced medication, restraints and isolation, disciplinary proceedings, confidentiality, consent, and suicide. These areas generate the most legal concern and have the clearest legal mandates.

15. *Discharge planning.* A comprehensive care system should not end at the institution's walls. Discharge planning begins inside, and appropriate community care, including medication and housing arrangements, will be the hallmark of a comprehensive system.

16. *Quality assurance program.* An ongoing internal survey, evaluation, and feedback system, accompanied by a statutory, evidentiary privilege to safeguard such studies from disruptive discovery demands, should be part of any sophisticated system. A national report on medical care has made a powerful case for improving patient safety through a systems approach, along with enhanced individual responsibility and professional judgment (Shannon 1996).

Index

*Page numbers printed in **boldface** type refer to tables.*

285